W9-BZK-749

Churchill Livingstone's
**Dictionary** of **Sport**
and **Exercise Science**
and **Medicine**

For Elsevier:

*Commissioning Editor*: Dinah Thom
*Development Editor*: Catherine Jackson
*Project Manager*: Kerrie-Anne Jarvis
*Designer*: Stewart Larking
*Illustrations Buyer*: Merlyn Harvey
*Illustrator*: Chartwell and Graeme Chambers

Churchill Livingstone's
# Dictionary of Sport and Exercise Science and Medicine

Editor
## Sheila Jennett

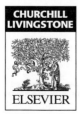

EDINBURGH LONDON NEW YORK OXFORD PHILADELPHIA ST LOUIS SYDNEY TORONTO 2008

QT
13
C53
2008

**CHURCHILL LIVINGSTONE**

© 2008, Elsevier Limited. All rights reserved.
First published 2008

ISBN: 9780443102158

**British Library Cataloguing in Publication Data**
A catalogue record for this book is available from the British Library.

**Library of Congress Cataloging in Publication Data**
A catalog record for this book is available from the Library of Congress.

**Note**
Neither the Publishers nor the Editor assume any responsibility for any loss or injury
and/or damage to persons or property arising out of or related to any use of the material
contained in this book. It is the responsibility of the treating practitioner, relying on
independent expertise and knowledge of the patient, to determine the best treatment
and method of application for the patient.

*The Publisher*

**ELSEVIER** your source for books,
journals and multimedia
in the health sciences

**www.elsevierhealth.com**

Working together to grow
libraries in developing countries

www.elsevier.com | www.bookaid.org | www.sabre.org

**ELSEVIER**   BOOK AID International   Sabre Foundation

The
Publisher's
policy is to use
**paper manufactured
from sustainable forests**

Printed in China

# Contents

List of contributors     vi
Preface     vii
Acknowledgements     viii

**A-Z**     1-408

**Appendix 1** Human Anatomy     411
1.1 Nervous system     411
1.2 Bones, joints and muscles     418
1.3 Heart, lungs, and circulation     429
1.4 Alimentary system     433

**Appendix 2** SI units and the metric system     435

**Appendix 3** Normal values     443

**Appendix 4** Nutrients     445
4.1 Macronutrients     446
4.2 Micronutrients: vitamins     447
4.3 Micronutrients: minerals     451
4.4 Ergogenic aids     455

**Appendix 5** Hormones     459

**Appendix 6** Drugs     463

**Appendix 7** Abbreviations and acronyms     471

**Appendix 8** Useful addresses and websites     479

**Appendix 9** References and further reading     481

# List of contributors

**Simon Coleman BA PhD**
Programme Leader,
Applied Sport Science,
Department of Physical Education, Sport and Leisure Studies,
University of Edinburgh, UK

**Sheila Jennett MD PhD FRCP(Glasg)**
Emeritus Professor of Physiology,
Hon Senior Research Fellow, Institute of Biomedical and Life Sciences,
University of Glasgow, UK

**John MacLean MBChB MRCGP FFSEM(UK)**
Medical Director, The National Stadium Sports Medicine Centre, Glasgow, UK;
Clinical Lecturer in Sport and Exercise Medicine,
University of Glasgow, UK

**Dalia Malkova MSc PhD**
Senior Lecturer, Human Nutrition Section,
Division of Developmental Medicine,
University of Glasgow, UK

**David Markland BA(Hons) PhD C. Psychol**
Senior Lecturer,
School of Sport, Health and Exercise Sciences,
Bangor University, UK

**Neil Spurway MA PhD**
Emeritus Professor of Exercise Physiology,
Hon Senior Research Fellow, Institute of Biomedical and Life Sciences,
University of Glasgow, UK

# Preface

Science and medicine related to sport and exercise have emerged and developed rapidly as disciplines over recent decades, with expansion of courses of study that train and qualify increasing numbers for the related activities and professions. The UK's first two university-level courses in Sports Science started in 1975; there are now about 150. Along with expansion, there has been enhanced breadth, with many modern courses placing equal or greater emphasis on non-sporting exercise: recreational and health-promoting for those relatively fit or therapeutic for those with medical problems. Sport and exercise medicine has developed more recently this side of the Atlantic at both the undergraduate level and that of professional recognition.

Relevant research, publications, societies and conferences have burgeoned in parallel with these developments, as well as internet coverage – where it may not always be easy to select the most useful and scientifically reliable sites. With this dictionary, commissioned by Churchill Livingstone, we offer a source of basic information for initial ready reference over the whole field. Broadly, this includes the subspecialties concerned with muscle function and training, control of movement, biomechanics, nutrition, sports psychology and sport and exercise medicine, as well as relevant anatomy, physiology, biochemistry and pharmacology. In the main alphabetical text we have aimed to make definitions, descriptions and recommended usage as clear and accurate as brevity allows, and with illustrations where appropriate. The appendices provide complementary detail in figures, text and tables, standard units and terminology and notes on resources for further information and study.

I and my fellow contributors hope that this will be a useful pocket companion for those involved in any capacity in the many associated fields of interest.

*Sheila Jennett*
*Glasgow 2007*

# Acknowledgements

The Editor thanks Sarena Wolfaard, Dinah Thom and Catherine Jackson of Elsevier, for initiating the project, commissioning the book and for guidance during preparation. Also Neil Spurway for the proposal of editorship, and for help and support throughout; and, indirectly, Chris Brooker, editor of the *Churchill Livingstone Pocket Medical Dictionary* which served as an example and a source for some text and appendix material, and whose notes from experience in editing that and other dictionaries were helpfully made available. Grateful thanks especially to all the contributors who made time for this task within their busy professional lives, for their patience with editorial suggestions and requests, for their assistance with decisions on coverage and with preparation of appendix material, as well as writing their share of the entries in the main text.

We all thank the following people who read, before submission, the whole of the main text, or all components related to their particular expertise, and made helpful suggestions for additions or amendments:

*Andy Cathcart*
*Peter Clarke*
*Desmond Gilmore*
*Stanley Grant*
*Ian McGrath.*

We also thank these who wrote, rewrote or advised on the content of some individual entries:

*Heather Cubie*
*Bill Ferrell*
*Margaret Gladden*
*Ian McGrath*
*David Miller*
*Tasha Miller.*

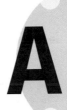

**abdomen** region of the body between the thorax (separated from it by the **diaphragm**) and the pelvis; colloquial *belly*. The *abdominal wall* consists of skin, connective tissue including a variable amount of fat, and muscles. A continuous thin membrane, the *peritoneum*, lines the wall and covers all the organs in the *abdominal cavity*. *See fig appendix 1.4.*

**abdominal breathing** *see* **diaphragm**.

**abdominal cramps** tight, constrictive, usually intermittent abdominal discomfort, usually the result of spasm of an internal organ, e.g. bowel spasm related to gastroenteritis or menstrual cramps. Not to be confused with muscular cramp from contraction of the abdominal wall musculature, possibly secondary to trauma. *See also* **stitch.**

**abdominal injury** damage to the abdomen and/or its contents. Can occur in sport, especially contact sports. Injury may be superficial, to the abdominal wall only, but significant trauma can damage the internal organs and lead to significant blood loss. Accumulation of blood in the abdominal cavity may be undetected, with potential fatality.

**abdominal muscles** layers of muscle in the abdominal wall. The *rectus abdominis* muscles, strap-like, lie vertically each side of the midline; their action can be important in breaking the force of a blow. A 'three-ply' layer of flat muscles, each with the fibres running in different directions (*external* and *internal oblique*, and *transverse*) extend from the lower ribs to the hip bone, and from the sheath of the rectus muscles to the lumbar spine, thickest in the flanks. Actions include: forward flexion and rotation of the trunk; assisting expiration during deep breathing or against airway obstruction, by contracting as the **diaphragm** relaxes, or acting together with the contracting diaphragm to raise abdominal pressure in straining (urination, defaecation, childbirth) and in vomiting. *See appendix 1.2 fig 4.*

**abdominal pain** discomfort in the abdomen which may result from a variety of medical conditions related to one or other of the abdominal organs, or from injury, particularly during contact sports. Medical advice should be sought and physical activity should cease.

**abduction** movement sideways of the arm at the shoulder, of the leg at the hip, of a finger, thumb or toe away from the middle of the hand or foot; *abductor* a muscle with this action; opposite of **adduction**. *See appendix 1.2 fig 3.*

**ability** the physical and/or cognitive capability to perform a task without further training. *perceived ability* a person's perception of their specific abilities within a given domain, such as in football versus in another sport. *See also* **capacity, skill, performance.**

**abrasion** superficial injury to skin or mucous membrane from scraping or rubbing.

**absolute threshold** in psychophysics, the smallest magnitude of a sensory input that can be detected, typically defined as the magnitude that can be detected over a proportion of presentations (e.g. 75%). Also known as *absolute limen. See also* **difference threshold**.

**absorption** *see* **intestinal absorption**.

**acceleration** change in motion of a body or object: the rate of change of velocity with respect to time. *linear acceleration:* the rate of change in linear velocity with respect to time; related to force by Newton's second law of motion (often stated as force = mass × linear acceleration). Measured in metres per second squared (m.s$^{-2}$). *angular acceleration:* the rate of change in angular velocity with respect to time. Measured in degrees per second squared ($°.s^{-2}$) or radians per second squared (rad.s$^{-2}$); related to moment by Newton's second angular law of motion (moment = moment of inertia × angular acceleration). *tangential acceleration:* the acceleration of an object or body acting at a tangent to its direction of motion, e.g. when it is moving in a circle or around a curve. *instantaneous acceleration:* acceleration measured over a very short (infinitesimal) period of time, effectively a continuous measurement of acceleration. *See also* **gravitational acceleration.**

**accessory bone** the *os trigonum* in the **ankle joint** – a bone present in only <10% of the population. In practice, rarely injured in sport but can be confused on X-ray with an avulsed fragment of bone or loose body.

**accident rates** accidents are common in sport, particularly in contact sports, and result in a significant workload for hospital A&E departments. Currently there are 20 million sports injuries in the UK each year, 50% of them football related, at an estimated cost in treatment and lost productivity of £1 billion.

**acclimation** artificial approximation to natural acclimatization, to either heat or altitude, achieved by exposure in a thermal or hypobaric chamber for several hours a day, typically for 2–3 weeks before going to the challenging new environment.

**acclimatization** adjustment of physiological processes in response to a change from the accustomed environment: to heat or cold, or to high altitude. For example, repeated exercise in the heat leads to an increase in maximal sweating rate, but with reduced sodium concentration in the sweat; low oxygen content in the blood at high altitude leads among other adjustments to increased breathing and cardiac output, assisting oxygen supply. *See also* **altitude acclimatization**, **heat acclimatization**, **sweating**.

**acetabulum** (from the Latin for a vinegar-cup) the cup-shaped cavity on each side of the pelvis into which the head of the femur fits, forming the 'ball-and-socket' of the **hip joint**. *See appendix 1.2 fig 1.*

**acetylcholine (ACh)** a substance made in certain nerve cells and released from their axon terminals at a junction or **synapse** in the process of *cholinergic* transmission of impulses (1) from motor nerves to skeletal muscle, (2) from one nerve to another in the nervous system (in the brain, and in autonomic ganglia), (3) at parasympathetic nerve endings (e.g. those that slow down the heart rate, stimulate secretion from glands or activate smooth muscle in the gut). Cholinergic receptors occur in two different pharmacological groups: *nicotinic*, e.g. at skeletal muscle motor endplates, and *muscarinic*, e.g. in cardiac and smooth muscles. *See also* **neuromuscular junction, neurotransmitter, parasympathetic nervous system.**

**acetyl coenzyme A** an important metabolic intermediate, involved in various metabolic pathways, including glucose and fatty acid oxidation, and degradation of some amino acids. It also represents a key intermediate in lipid biosynthesis. Commonly referred to as *acetyl CoA*. *See also* **Krebs cycle.**

**acetylsalicylic acid** better known as *aspirin*. Developed by the pharmaceutical group Bayer in Germany in 1899. Used at lower doses (2–3 g per day) as an analgesic and antipyretic. At higher doses (>4 g per day) it is a very powerful anti-inflammatory agent and therefore effective in soft tissue injury, but its use is limited by gastric side effects. *See also* **non-steroidal anti-inflammatory drugs.**

**achievement goal** a goal focused on demonstrating high ability to oneself or others, or to avoid demonstrating low ability.

**achievement goal orientation** a person's general tendency to act in an ego-involved or task-involved manner.

**achievement motivation** form of motivation characterized by a competitive drive to meet high standards of performance, also known as *need for achievement*.

**Achilles tendon** a large tendon (*aka **tendo calcaneus***) at the back of the ankle, joining the main **calf** muscles (gastrocnemius and soleus) to the heel bone (calcaneum). The tendon is commonly injured in sport either by direct trauma (resulting in partial or complete rupture) or by repeated micro-trauma or overuse resulting in inflammation. *Achilles tendonitis* is most commonly the result of poor technique, poor footwear, hard running surface, high-intensity or long-distance running. Treatment is with **RICE**, anti-inflammatory medication, a heel raise and correction of causes. Surgery may be required in severe cases. *Achilles bursitis* is inflammation of the **bursa** (a 'bag' of fluid) that separates the tendon from the back of the calcaneum. *See appendix 1.2 fig 6.*

**acidaemia** lower than normal **pH** of the blood. *See also* **acidosis.**

**acid–base balance** refers to the mechanisms that keep body fluids close to their normal **pH** (i.e. neither too alkaline nor too acidic), vital for normal cellular function. *See also* **acidosis, alkalosis.**

**acidosis** condition due to decrease in **pH** of body fluids, from accumulation of acid or depletion of alkali. *metabolic acidosis* can occur by accumulation of $H^+$ during high-intensity exercise, due mainly to an increased rate of anaerobic glycolysis and therefore of lactic acid production. Pathological causes include diabetic ketoacidosis and severe kidney disease. *respiratory acidosis* is caused by carbon dioxide retention due to inadequate ventilation, in lung disease, or in respiratory depression by drugs. In *compensated acidosis* pH may be normal, with a high blood bicarbonate concentration (due to increased renal retention) when the cause was respiratory, or with a low blood carbon dioxide (due to **hyperventilation**) when the cause was metabolic. *See also* **glycolysis, lactic acid.**

**acquired immune deficiency syndrome (AIDS)** denotes a particular stage of infection with the **human immunodeficiency virus (HIV).** The criteria for defining an illness as AIDS, in a person infected with HIV, are those of the US Centers for Disease Control and Prevention (CDC); they include certain infections and cancers, and/or specified low levels of immune system cells in the blood.

**acromioclavicular joint** the small synovial joint above the shoulder, between the outer end of the clavicle and the acromion process of the scapula, linking them to form the shoulder girdle. Parts of the trapezius and deltoid muscles are attached to the joint capsule. Commonly injured in contact sports especially rugby. *See appendix 1.2 fig 4A.*

**actin** globular protein molecule which readily links with others (with consumption of ATP) to form long, double-helical strands. Such *actin filaments* are found in a wide variety of animal and plant cells, as well as forming the structural core and main (but not only) component of the *thin filaments* in the **myofibrils** of all animal muscles. Actin is thus a protein of great evolutionary antiquity and vertebrate striated muscles are unusual only in having a very high content of it (80% of total protein), and in its highly ordered locations within the cells, where thin filaments alternate with thick filaments containing actin's partner protein **myosin**, to form the cross-striated pattern. *See also* **muscle, muscle fibres;** *appendix 1.2 fig 7.*

**action** in addition to its general meaning, the name for a force applied to a body or object. Often used with *reaction* in a simple expression of Newton's third law of motion.

**action potential (AP)** transient voltage change propagating along the membrane of nerve, muscle or other excitable cell; the means whereby information flows rapidly along the cell's length. Triggered by a small **depolarization,** an AP consists of further depolarization and often an over-shoot to an inside-positive **membrane potential.** The depolarization/positive swing is caused by the in-flow of sodium and/or calcium ions, according to the tissue, and the return to normal inside-negative po-tential by the subsequent outflow of potassium ions. Metabolic energy is used in maintaining the differences between the intracellular and extracellular concentrations of these ions, but not in the AP itself. *See also* **electromyography (EMG), nerve fibre, neuro-muscular junction, sarcoplasmic reticulum (SR), t-tubes.**

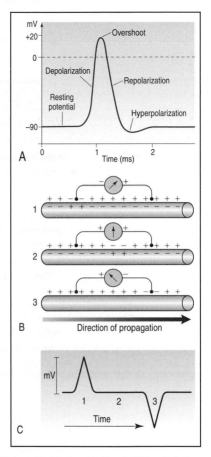

Action potential propagating along a nerve fibre. A, AP recorded between electrodes inside and outside an axon. B, Voltmeter placed to record the potential difference between external electrodes at two points along an axon. This and the voltage differences across the membrane ( + − ) are indicated for three successive stages of propagation (1, 2, 3). C, Record of voltage changes with time, corresponding to stages 1, 2, 3, in digram B.

**activation** initiation of a response in an effector (i.e. a muscle or gland).

**active movement** movement by the person's own effort, as distinct from passive movement.

**actomyosin ATPase** *see* **muscle enzymes**.

**acupuncture** the practice of inserting fine needles into specific parts of the body for therapeutic purposes, as in traditional Chinese medicine. Energy known as *qi* is believed to flow through channels ('meridians') linked to particular organs and functions; along these, needles are inserted at selected points to stimulate or depress the energy flow. Used in the treatment of a variety of diseases, for relief of pain or for production of anaesthesia.

**acute injury** refers to the first 24–48 h after an injury due to a traumatic episode, such as one sustained during a sporting activity.

**adaptive behaviour** a change in behaviour to successfully meet changes in environmental circumstances.

**adaptive thermogenesis** the thermic effect of factors such as cold, heat, fear, stress and various drugs that can increase the rate of energy expenditure above normal baseline levels.

**addiction** dependency on chemical substances such as drugs, alcohol and tobacco. Also more recently applied in exercise settings to a dependency on regular exercise. *See also* **exercise dependence**.

**adduction** movement of the arm inwards to the side of the body, of a leg inwards towards the other leg, of a thumb, finger or toe towards the middle of the hand or foot; *adductor* a muscle with this action. Opposite of **abduction.** *See appendix 1.2 fig 3.*

**adenosine** nucleotide consisting of a base, adenine, and a sugar, ribose.

**adenosine mono-, di- and triphosphates (AMP, ADP, ATP)** molecules in which one, two or three phosphate groups are combined with the ribose unit of adenosine. ATP is the key energy currency of every living cell. It is synthesized anaerobically by **glycolysis** and aerobically by **oxidative phosphorylation**, and is hydrolysed to ADP and a phosphate ion ('inorganic phosphate', $P_i$) by the *ATPases* of myosin, membrane pumps and all other energy-requiring systems. Accumulation of ADP, and even more so of AMP, signifies ATP depletion and stimulates ATP resynthesis. *See also* **creatine kinase** (*fig*), **phosphocreatine.**

**adherence** extent to which a person maintains a behavioural regimen, such as regular exercise. *See also* **compliance**.

**adipose tissue** specialized connective tissue where fat is stored (mainly subcutaneous; also around some organs, e.g. kidneys and heart); its cells, the *adipocytes,* are a major storage site for fat in the form of **triacylglycerols** (triglycerides) which can be mobilized by enzyme action **(hormone-sensitive lipase)** to provide fatty acids via the blood for energy metabolism, as in endurance exercise or in starvation. Also provides a protective and insulating layer. *See also* **body composition, body fat, glucose, growth hormone.**

**adjective checklist** in psychometrics, a list of adjectives that can be endorsed as applying or not applying to oneself or others.

**adolescent athlete** an athlete in the period between the onset of puberty and full maturity. This is the period of final bone growth and skeletal maturation, which increases the risk from contact injuries to the epiphyses (the ends of the long bones, not yet fused with the main shaft). The psychological changes that accompany the physical changes may result in problems with **self-esteem, compliance** and **motivation.**

**adrenal glands** endocrine glands sited above each kidney. The outermost region, the *adrenal cortex*, secretes **steroid hormones**: the **glucocorticoids** (principally cortisol), **mineralocorticoids** (principally **aldosterone**) and **androgens** in both male and female. The inner *adrenal medulla* secretes the catecholamines, mainly adrenaline and noradrenaline, under the control of the **sympathetic nervous system.** *See also* **adrenocorticotrophic hormone (ACTH), hormones, steroids;** *appendix 5.*

**adrenaline (***epinephrine***)** a catecholamine, one of the hormones secreted from the adrenal medulla into the blood stream, in response to stimulation by the **sympathetic nervous system**, increasing in circumstances requiring urgent and demanding action. Prepares the body for 'fight or flight' or for any other enhanced activity by increasing the heart rate and force, selectively increasing blood flow to muscle and mobilizing glucose from liver glycogen stores. Acts on **adrenoceptors** via the circulating blood, also as a neurotransmitter but, in mammals, only within the central nervous system.

**adrenergic** term used generically to describe nerves which liberate either **adrenaline (***epinephrine***)** or **noradrenaline (***norepinephrine***)** as a neurotransmitter from their endings; also in common usage in USA as an adjective for things associated with adrenaline or noradrenaline such as receptors. *noradrenergic* is sometimes used specifically to describe noradrenaline-releasing nerves. *See also* **adrenoceptors.**

**adrenoceptors** transmembrane proteins on cells that are activated by noradrenaline released at sympathetic nerve endings or by circulating catecholamines. There are three main types: *alpha-1 (*$\alpha_1$*), alpha-2 (*$\alpha_2$*)* and *beta (*$\beta$*)* which mediate responses by different cellular mechanisms and are activated preferentially by different agonists. Each type has three subtypes. All subtypes respond strongly to **noradrenaline,** $\beta$ most strongly to **adrenaline,** and certain synthetic dugs can distinguish between $\alpha_1$ and $\alpha_2$. Such differences account, for example, for smooth muscle relaxation in some tissues ($\beta$-mediated vasodilatation in skeletal muscle; bronchodilation in the lungs) and vasoconstriction in others ($\alpha$-mediated, in gut and skin) during heightened sympathetic activity. International agreement is for 'adrenoceptor' but the use of '*adrenergic receptors*' is still common in the USA.

**adrenocorticotrophic hormone (ACTH)** a hormone secreted into the bloodstream by the **anterior pituitary**; acts on the adrenal cortex, promoting the secretion of corticosteroids. ACTH secretion is itself regulated by the *ACTH-releasing hormone* from the hypothalamus. This in turn is susceptible to many influences within central nervous system, taking part in responses to many types of injury or stress.

**aerobic** dependent on oxygen.

**aerobic capacity** maximum rate at which an animal or human subject can take up oxygen from the air; also known as **maximal oxygen consumption (uptake) ($\dot{V}O_{2\,max}$)**. Aerobic capacity of individual muscles is the maximum rate at which they can utilize oxygen. *See also* **aerobic power.**

**aerobic endurance** period for which aerobic work can be maintained by an individual; may vary from a few tens of seconds in a sedentary person and a few minutes in a sprint or power athlete, to more than 24 h in an ultra-marathoner.

**aerobic exercise** exercise furnished with energy by aerobic metabolism; regular repetition enhances the capacity of the cardiorespiratory system to deliver oxygen to muscles. Compare **anaerobic exercise.**

**aerobic metabolism** *see* **glycolysis, oxidative phosphorylation**.

**aerobic power** a term that is widely, but loosely, used as interchangeable with **aerobic capacity,** or $\dot{V}O_{2\,max}$ though the units for this are those of oxygen uptake rate, not power; 'aerobic power' would more properly refer to mechanical power output at $\dot{V}O_{2\,max}$.

**aerobic threshold** *see* **metabolic and related thresholds**.

**aerobic training** training aimed at enhancement of **aerobic power** or **endurance**; consists of intensive (for power) or sustained (for endurance) exercise below $\dot{V}O_{2\,max}$. *See also* **target heart rate.**

**aetiology (etiology)** strictly, the study of the causation of a condition but more commonly used to refer to causative factors themselves. *aetiological factors* those responsible for the origin and progress of a disorder or disease and 'of unknown aetiology' meaning that the cause is obscure.

**affect** in psychology, a general term for subjectively experienced feelings encompassing emotion and mood. *adj affective. affective response* subjectively experienced feeling in response to an environmental event. *positive affect* a general dimension of affect reflecting a state of enthusiasm and alertness. *negative affect* a general dimension of affect reflecting a state of distress, subsuming various negative moodstates including fear, anger, shame and guilt. *See also* **circumplex model.**

**afferent** means 'going towards'. Describes nerves that carry impulses towards the central nervous system, or to relay stations outside it, from neural receptors (e.g. sensory nerves from the skin, those conveying proprioceptive information from muscles and joints or visceral afferents from internal organs). Also describes blood or lymph vessels in which flow is towards some point of reference, e.g. afferent arterioles to the glomeruli of the kidney. Opposite of **efferent.**

**affordance** a property of an object or a feature of the environment that offers an organism the opportunity to act in a particular way.

**ageing and exercise** certain risks, especially involving the cardiovascular system, increase with age. Ageing is associated with degenerative conditions; there is a reduction in bone density and deterioration of lung function, aerobic fitness and muscle strength. The benefits of activity in advancing years include a reduced incidence of heart disease, maintenance of bone mineral content (reducing fracture risk), muscle strength and balance (reducing falls) and an increased life expectancy. *See also* **osteoporosis.**

**aggression** behaviour with the intent of causing harm to another individual or group.

**agonist** an agent having a positive action. (1) In pharmacology, a chemical agent that causes a response by a cell when it binds selectively to a specific receptor. Usually refers to a drug which imitates the action of a hormone or neurotransmitter. (2) With reference to skeletal muscles, one, or a group, which is initiating or maintaining a positive action, e.g. the biceps when flexing the elbow. *See also* **antagonist, reciprocal inhibition.**

**agreeableness** one of the **big five** personality factors characterized by a tendency to be kind, generous, sympathetic and unselfish.

**airway(s)** the passage(s) from the mouth or nose via the pharynx, larynx, trachea and the branching **bronchial tree** to the alveoli of the lungs. Airway (singular) usually refers to the upper airway (upper respiratory tract) which may need to be cleared of inhaled or vomited material, e.g. before mouth-to-mouth (or -nose) resuscitation. Airways (plural) refers to the bronchial tree within the lungs, particularly in the context of chronic obstructive airways disease and **asthma**, when the smallest branches are narrowed. *See appendix 1.3 fig 4.*

**alanine (Ala)** an **amino acid**, one of the 20 building blocks of **proteins** in food and in the body. Not an 'essential' amino acid in the diet as it can be made in the body from other substances.

**alcohol** ethyl alcohol (ethanol) in alcoholic drinks is one of a group of organic compounds. The anxiety-reducing effects of alcohol can improve confidence and performance, particularly in sports where fine motor control is required, e.g. by snooker players or marksmen. In many sports, particularly team sports, alcohol intake is a part of the culture. Because of the well-known diuretic properties, athletes should be advised against alcohol consumption when fluid replacement is a priority, and alcohol can impair both performance and recovery after exercise. It is banned in some sports (e.g. motor racing, skiing).

**aldosterone** hormone secreted by the adrenal glands, at a rate regulated by the level of sodium in body fluids. Acts in the kidneys to enhance reabsorption of sodium, reducing its loss in the urine. Similar action on sweat glands reduces sodium loss when sweating rate is high. *See also* **hormones**; *appendix 5.*

**Alexander Technique** a form of psychophysical re-education. Based on the observation that unconscious habits, which disturb our postural reflexes, are associated with problems of health and performance, it promotes better co-ordination and control, aiming either to remove the cause of, or simply prevent, many forms of ill health, chronic pain, poor posture and inadequate performance. Developed in the late 1890s by an Australian actor who studied and improved his own vocal problems, the Technique is now widely recognized as a fundamental tool for establishing good co-ordination, balance and poise. It is valued by athletes as a way to improve performance and prevent or resolve injuries. It is taught on a one-to-one basis and teachers will usually have attended a three-year training course or its equivalent.

**alexithymia** a personality trait characterized by difficulty in recognizing or describing one's emotions.

**alimentary** pertaining to the gut and its functions. *alimentary tract* the whole passage from mouth to anus, via the *oesophagus*, *stomach*, and **intestines**. *alimentary system* the tract and all that happens within it, including eating, **digestion**, absorption and excretion, and the movement of the contents by the intestinal smooth muscle. *See fig appendix 1.4.*

**alkalosis** condition following increase in **pH** of body fluids, from accumulation of base or depletion of acid. *metabolic alkalosis* is associated with loss of gastric acid with excessive vomiting, and *respiratory alkalosis* with excessive loss of carbon dioxide due to **hyperventilation** from any cause, including the physiological response to hypoxia at high altitude. In *compensated alkalosis* pH may be normal, with a low blood bicarbonate concentration (due to increased renal excretion) when the cause is respiratory, or with a raised blood carbon dioxide (due to hypoventilation) when the cause is metabolic. *See also* **acid–base balance.**

**allergy** an **immune response** induced by exposure to an *allergen* causing a harmful hypersensitivity reaction (*allergic response*) on subsequent exposure. *See also* **immunity**.

**alpha-agonist** in full *alpha (α) adrenoceptor (or adrenergic) agonist* a naturally occurring substance or a drug that acts specifically on cellular alpha-adrenoceptors. *See also* **adrenaline, adrenoceptor, sympathetic nervous system.**

**alpha (α)-blocker** a substance that interferes with the action at the adrenoceptor of an α-adrenergic agonist. In full *alpha (α) adrenoceptor (or adrenergic) antagonist.* Can be selective for alpha-1 ($\alpha_1$), alpha-2 ($\alpha_2$) or their further subtypes. *See also* **adrenoceptor.**

**alpha (α)-ketoglutarate** an intermediate in the Krebs cycle; may be depleted in the late stages of endurance exercise, suggesting potential utility as an anticatabolic agent.

**alpha (α) motor neurons** the final pathway for activation of skeletal muscles; neurons with cell bodies in the central nervous system (brain stem or spinal cord), and myelinated nerve fibres that terminate in motor endplates at **neuromuscular junctions**. *See also* **gamma (motor) system, motor unit.**

**alpha (α) receptor** *see* **adrenoceptor**.

**alpha (α)-tocopherol** the most biologically active form of *vitamin E*, which is the most important antioxidant in cell membranes. Its principal function is to stabilize the structural integrity of membranes by breaking the chain reaction of lipid peroxidation. Vitamin E is also essential

for normal function of the immune system. *See also*
**reactive oxygen species, vitamins;** *appendix 4.2.*

**altitude** the height above sea level. As atmospheric (barometric) pressure decreases progressively with increasing altitude, from the standard 1 atmosphere at sea
level, the partial pressure of oxygen ($PO_2$) decreases
proportionately; the air still contains the same ~21% of
oxygen but there are fewer molecules of oxygen per unit
volume. There is also a drop in temperature and humidity, but the essential problem for human life and activity
is shortage of oxygen (**hypoxia**).

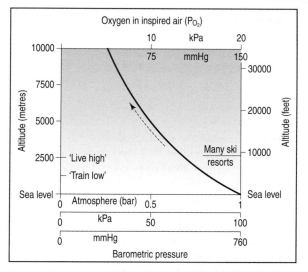

Altitude: relation between decreasing barometric pressure and $PO_2$ and levels for
athletic training. *Broken arrow*: altitude sickness possible in the unacclimatized.

**altitude acclimatization** physiological adjustments that help to compensate mainly for the shortage of oxygen. When blood is inadequately oxygenated in the lungs, the hypoxic condition (low $PO_2$) of blood and tissues stimulates changes in: (1) **ventilation:** increase in rate and depth of breathing brings the partial pressure of oxygen in the lungs (and therefore in the arterial blood) closer to that in the air, whilst decreasing the partial pressure of carbon dioxide ($PCO_2$); the resulting **alkalosis** is gradually corrected and the hyperventilation later diminishes; (2) **cardiac output (CO):** initial increase at rest, and at any level of activity, provides greater blood flow to the tissues in compensation for the lowered oxygen content of the blood. Over a few days CO decreases again for any given $\dot{V}O_2$ until it has returned to sea-level values, with tissues extracting more oxygen per litre of blood (i.e. the **arteriovenous difference** increases); (3) *oxygen transport and delivery*: after an initial increase in haematocrit due to reduction in plasma volume, stimulation of erthropoietin secretion enhances red blood cell production in the bone marrow, raising the red cell count and **haemoglobin** (Hb) concentration in the blood; this increases the amount of oxygen that can be carried per litre of blood at the lowered saturation (but the polycythaemia increases blood viscosity). The affinity of Hb for oxygen is modified by an increase in the enzyme 2–3 DPG, causing a rightward shift in the **oxyhaemoglobin dissociation curve**; this assists offloading in the tissues at a any given local $PO_2$, but can be offset by a leftward shift of the curve due to low arterial $PCO_2$. There are also changes in cellular metabolism. The timing and effectiveness of these adjustments vary among individuals, as does tolerance of the negative effects. *See also* **acclimation, altitude sickness, altitude training, chemoreceptors, erythropoiesis, hypoxia, partial pressure.**

**altitude sickness** (*altitude illness*) may occur at altitudes higher than about 8000 ft (~2500 metres) above sea level, although it has been reported between 1500 and 2500 metres. Incidence is related to the height attained and the rapidity of ascent, as well as to individual susceptibility. Problems range from mild nausea, headache and disordered sleep (*acute mountain sickness*) to pulmonary oedema (with cough and frothy sputum) and cerebral oedema (with neurological symptoms and mental confusion) which can be fatal. All are direct or indirect results of low partial pressure of oxygen ($PO_2$) in the atmosphere. Prevention may include premedication and staging the ascent; those who develop symptoms should go no higher whilst they persist, and descent as a medical emergency may be necessary if symptoms are severe.

**altitude training** training at real or simulated altitude sufficient to reduce oxygen partial pressure ($PO_2$) significantly below that at sea level, undertaken with a view to increasing haematocrit and so oxygen-carrying capacity of the blood, and thus enhancing sea-level aerobic performance. Individual responses vary widely and other effects can be deleterious (e.g. muscle mass is reduced and blood viscosity is increased). A 'live high (e.g. 2500 m), train lower (e.g. 1250 m)' strategy is currently more favoured, as the training itself can then be close to sea-level intensity, while haematocrit increase is still achieved during the less active periods. Some research has suggested that altitude training may also improve sea-level endurance performance by enhancing the **running economy** (oxygen consumption at a given speed) of the athletes. *See also* **altitude acclimatization.**

**ambient temperature and pressure** the temperature and pressure (atmospheric, barometric) of the body's surroundings. Used when correcting a volume of saturated gas (at ATPS) to standard temperature and pressure dry (STPD), e.g. when measuring the volume of expired gas for assessment of oxygen uptake.

**amenorrhoea** absence of menstruation. *primary amenorrhoea* when the menstrual periods have not started by the appropriate age. *secondary amenorrhoea* when periods stop after they have been established. *See also* **female athletic triad.**

**amino acids** organic acids in which one or more of the hydrogen atoms is replaced by the amino group, $NH_2$. They are the end-products of digestion of dietary protein and from them the body synthesizes its own proteins. Within the body amino acids also act as precursors of many other molecules essential for life. Amino acids may be categorized as essential or non-essential. *essential amino acids:* those that must be provided in the diet since the human body does not have the enzymes for their synthesis; of the 20 amino acids that are present in proteins or as free amino acids in the body, nine are 'essential' (histidine, isoleucine, leucine, lysine, methionine, phenylalanine, threonine, tryptophan, valine). Of these, three are known as *branched-chain amino* *acids (BCAA)*: *leucine* is oxidized to a significant extent during exercise, and tracer studies that follow leucine kinetics are often used as an estimation of protein turnover; *isoleucine* and *valine* can also serve as fuel sources. It has been claimed that ingestion of BCAA before and during exercise may improve the physiological and psychological responses, and that BCAA with **arginine** and/or other amino acids may promote **growth hormone** release, but other studies do not support this. There are no known toxic effects. *See also* **ergogenic aids, gluconeogenesis;** *appendix 4.4.*

**amnesia** partial or complete loss of memory, due either to brain damage (traumatic, vascular or degenerative) or psychological disorder (e.g. in dissociative states when the memory 'rejects' unpleasant events). Associated not uncommonly in sport with **head injury.** *anterograde amnesia* refers to impaired recall for events following brain damage; *retrograde amnesia* refers to failure of recall for events prior to the insult; the duration of *post-traumatic amnesia* is related to the severity of brain damage in head injury.

**amotivation** a state of lacking any motivation to engage in an activity, characterized by a lack of perceived competence and/or a failure to value the activity or its outcomes. *See also* **learned helplessness.**

**amphetamines** potentially harmful group of stimulant drugs currently banned in sport. Scientific evidence as to their beneficial effect is lacking. These drugs primarily affect the central nervous system resulting in euphoria, increased alertness and aggression. Side effects are common and include drug dependence, depression, impaired co-ordination and judgement, reduced perception of fatigue, cardiovascular effects (increased blood pressure and cardiac output) and an increase in metabolic rate. Also known as 'speed,' 'uppers' and 'pep pills', they were previously prescribed (and are still used illegally) to assist weight loss.

**anabolic agents** substances which have an anabolic effect (tissue building and energy storing). *See also* **anabolic steroids.**

**anabolic steroids** usually refers to a group of synthetic drugs based on the male sex hormone *testosterone* secreted by the testes, and having similar anabolic and other androgenic actions to this and other **androgens** from the adrenal cortex in both sexes. These drugs are misused in sports, especially where enhanced power and strength are beneficial such as weight lifting and cycling. Used in conjunction with a training programme, they lead to an increase in muscle size and power. They may also lessen fatigue and improve tissue repair. Use in children can lead to premature fusion of the epiphyses, stunting skeletal growth. Side effects are common and potentially serious. They include psychological changes (notably aggression), liver damage, cardiovascular (raised blood pressure) and endocrine effects (masculinization in females, testicular atrophy and reduced sperm count in males.) *See also* **adrenal glands, hormones;** *appendix 5.*

**anabolism** *see* **metabolism.**

**anaemia** lower than normal concentration of **haemoglobin** in the blood, due to a low red blood cell (RBC) count and/or less than normal haemoglobin content in each RBC. Has a variety of causes, most commonly deficiency of iron (required for haemoglobin synthesis) or chronic blood loss. Symptoms include general weakness, shortness of breath and pallor. *iron deficiency anaemia* is seen not uncommonly in sport and is usually a combination of poor dietary intake and menstrual blood loss. As a result the use of iron supplementation is recommended at a higher than usual **ferritin** level. *See also* **iron, minerals**; *appendix 4.3.*

**anaerobic** independent of oxygen.

**anaerobic capacity** the total amount of energy that can be obtained from anaerobic sources (**creatine phosphate** breakdown and anaerobic **glycolysis**) in a single bout of continuous exercise. Strictly a theoretical concept, since some contribution from aerobic metabolism cannot be prevented in any real-time measurement. Estimated by total work output in 30 s (**Wingate test**) or 90 s cycle ergometer tests, or by treadmill running up a steep gradient; the longer test periods more closely extract all possible energy from the anaerobic systems, but cannot avoid a small yet significant aerobic contribution.

**anaerobic exercise** exercise at an intensity exceeding aerobic capacity, which therefore draws a significant fraction of its energy from anaerobic sources. Sprints of any form, jumps and forceful throws are examples. In sustained anaerobic exercise, metabolic products accumulate rapidly; this is indicated by the continual increase of blood **lactate** concentration throughout the period of effort, but other products such as phosphate ions,

ADP, AMP and adenosine contribute much more to the fatigue which forces termination of the effort after some 10–120 s, depending on its intensity. Also known as *supramaximal exercise.* Compare **aerobic exercise.**

**anaerobic metabolism** *see* **glycolysis, lactate**.

**anaerobic power** maximum rate of power production, typically measured by **Margaria stair test** or first 5 s of a **Wingate test.**

**anaerobic threshold (AT)** *see* **metabolic and related thresholds**.

**anaerobic training** training at exercise intensities which cannot be maintained by oxygen intake, and are therefore sustainable for not more than a few tens of seconds without a rest interval.

**anaesthetic** literally, without sensation. A substance administered in order to allow surgical procedures that would normally cause pain. A *general anaesthetic*, given by inhalation or injection, acts in the brain and causes loss of consciousness; a *local anaesthetic*, injected into the relevant tissue, prevents transmission along sensory nerves. *vb anaesthetize* to administer an anaesthetic; *anaesthetized* or *under anaesthesia* the state of the patient so treated.

**analgesic** a drug used to relieve pain. *See also* **acetylsalicylic acid, non-steroidal anti-inflammatory drugs (NSAID), opiates**; *appendix 6.*

**anaphylaxis** a dramatic and dangerous reaction by the immune system, caused by release of inflammatory mediators (such as histamine) from mast cells on exposure to an allergen. Characterized by urticaria ('hives'), pruritus (itching), angio-oedema ('welts'), respiratory distress, vascular collapse and shock.

**anatomical position** standard position of the body used when describing body parts and their relation to each other: standing erect, facing forward, feet together and arms at the side with the palms facing forward. In this

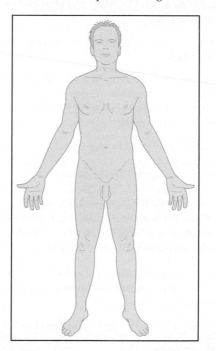

The anatomical position.

position: *superior*/*inferior* = nearer head/feet; *anterior*/ *posterior* = nearer front/back; *medial*/*lateral* = nearer to/further from the midline; *proximal*/*distal*: in the limbs nearer to/further from the trunk; in other structures (e.g. blood vessels, digestive tract) nearer to/further from point of origin.

**androgens** steroid hormones secreted by the adrenal cortex in both sexes and by the testis, responsible for male characteristics and male reproductive function; involved also in the synthesis of oestrogens in the ovary. (Applies also to synthetic hormones with similar action). *See also* **anabolic steroids, hormones**; *appendix 5.*

**angina (pectoris)** severe but temporary attack of cardiac pain that may radiate from the chest to the arms, throat, lower jaw or the back. Caused by *myocardial ischaemia* (inadequate blood flow to the heart muscle). Often the attack is induced by exercise (*angina of effort*).

**angiotensin** substance derived from *angiotensinogen* in the blood, by the action of the enzyme *renin* secreted by the kidneys. *angiotensin-converting enzyme (ACE)*: an enzyme, principally in kidney and lung endothelia, which catalyses conversion of the inactive form angiotensin I in the blood to angiotensin II; this in turn stimulates release of **aldosterone** from the adrenal glands and hence sodium reabsorption in kidneys. This *renin-angiotensin-aldosterone system* is important in the normal regulation of blood volume and arterial blood pressure. There are recent indications that either ACE itself, or perhaps some other molecule(s) whose biosynthesis is enhanced in parallel by the ACE gene, favour(s) various aspects of physical performance.

**angle of incidence** the angle at which a body, object or vector is moving relative to another (e.g. a stationary surface or environmental factor such as wind), often prior to a collision. Example: when playing a snooker ball at a cushion, the angle between the ball's direction of travel and the cushion.

**angle of pull** the angle at which a muscle pulls relative to the long axis of the bone on which it pulls. Example: the angle between the biceps brachii tendon and the radius in the forearm.

**angle of reflection** after a collision, the angle at which one object is moving relative to another (usually a stationary surface or environmental factor such as wind). Example: after a snooker ball has hit a cushion, the angle between the ball's direction of travel and the cushion. It is not necessarily the same size as the angle of incidence. Also known as *angle of rebound*.

**angle of release** the angle made between the velocity vector of a body or object (usually the **centre of mass**) and the ground or other fixed reference frame. Also known as *angle of projection* or *angle of take-off*.

**angular momentum** *see* **momentum**.

**ankle injury** *see* **anterior talofibular ligament, eversion, footballer's ankle, inversion**.

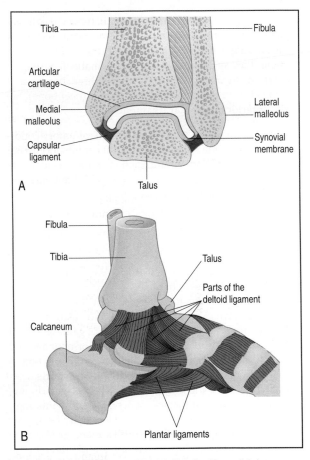

(A) Vertical section through the ankle joint. (B) Left ankle, medial view.

**ankle joint** the synovial hinge joint between the lower ends of the tibia and fibula, and the talus, where its saddle-shaped upper surface lies in the socket flanked at the sides by the medial and lateral malleoli. Strengthened by ligaments between these three bones, and also between them and the calcaneum (heel bone). *See also* **anterior talofibular ligament**.

**ankylosing spondylitis** a progressive inflammatory condition affecting the spine and sacroiliac joints, occurring most commonly in young men. Characterized in its later stages by ossification of the spinal ligaments and ankylosis (fixation) of the sacroiliac joints. *aka bamboo spine*.

**annulus fibrosus** the fibrous ring which encircles each **intervertebral disc**.

**anorexia** lack of appetite for food; *anorexia nervosa* a psychological illness characterized by an avoidance of food intake leading to severe weight loss, associated with excessive exercising, purging and disturbance of body image; may involve intense fear of gaining weight even when it is already well below the norm for age and height. May disturb reproductive hormone function in young women, causing **amenorrhoea**. The sports most often associated include 'aesthetic sports' (e.g. diving, figure skating, gymnastics, synchronized swimming), those in which low body mass and low body fat appear to be a physical and biomechanical advantage (distance running, road cycling, triathlon) and those with weight categories for competition, (lightweight rowing, weight lifting, wrestling). *anorexia athletica* similarly disordered eating plus compulsive exercising.

**antacid** a substance that neutralizes acidity. Used in alkaline indigestion remedies.

**antagonist** an agent having a counteractive effect on the action of another agent. (1) In pharmacology, a chemical agent (naturally occurring substance or drug) which prevents cells from responding to a particular **agonist** by competing at binding sites on or in the cell. (2) With reference to skeletal muscles: one, or a group, which opposes the action of another, e.g. the triceps may 'antagonize' flexion of the elbow by the biceps. Antagonistic pairs of muscles allow coordinated control. *See also* **reciprocal inhibition.**

**anterior compartment syndrome** *see* **compartment syndrome**.

**anterior cruciate ligament** *see* **cruciate ligaments**.

**anterior pituitary** endocrine gland, part of the pituitary gland at the base of the brain. Secretes **growth hormone** (with widespread actions on growth and metabolism), *prolactin* (promoting lactation) and *'trophic' hormones* that regulate in turn the endocrine secretions of the adrenal cortex, of the thyroid gland, and those from the gonads involved in reproductive function. All these secretory functions are themselves controlled by 'releasing' and in some instances also 'inhibitory' hormones from the **hypothalamus** via local blood vessels. *See also* **hormones, posterior pituitary;** *appendix 5.*

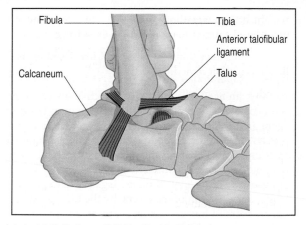

Anterior talofibular ligament. Right ankle, lateral view.

**anterior talofibular ligament** the ligament on the outside of the **ankle joint**, which is commonly injured in exercise. Runs from the fibula to the talus, preventing excessive forward movement of the foot relative to the tibia.

**anthropometry** physical measurements of human size, shape, proportion and **body composition** for the purposes of comparison and establishing population norms, e.g. for gender, age, weight, ethnicity/race.

**antibiotics** antibacterial substances, originally those derived from fungi and bacteria, exemplified by penicillin, but the term is now commonly used for all antibacterial drugs. Some have a narrow spectrum of activity whereas others, the broad-spectrum antibiotics, act against a wide range of bacteria.

**anticoagulant** an agent that reduces the propensity of blood to clot. Used to prevent or treat thromboembolic conditions (e.g. stroke, deep vein thrombosis). Also used to prevent clotting in blood removed for some types of laboratory examination, and in donor blood withdrawn for transfusion.

**antidepressants** drugs used to manage depression. There are three main groups: monoamine oxidase inhibitors (MAOI), selective serotonin reuptake inhibitors (SSRI) and tricyclic antidepressants (TCA). Research has shown that a structured exercise programme can have a mood-enhancing effect similar (and complementary) to that seen with the use of antidepressant medication.

**antidiuretic hormone (ADH)** *syn vasopressin*, neuroendocrine secretion from the **posterior pituitary**; acts in the kidneys to increase the retention of water when body fluid osmolality increases, e.g. with excessive sweat loss when fluid is not adequately replaced. *See also* **hydration status, hypothalamus, osmoreceptors, thirst, water balance**; *appendix 5*.

**anti-inflammatory drug** a drug which reduces the body's natural inflammatory response to tissue damage. Includes **steroids** and **non-steroidal anti-inflammatory drugs (NSAIDs)** which are the most commonly used in exercise-related injury. They reduce pain and swelling, allowing a quicker, safe return to activity. All were developed from aspirin. *See also* **acetylsalicylic acid**.

**antioxidants** defend body cells against **oxidative stress**. Increased cellular concentrations of antioxidants have been claimed to diminish exercise-induced muscle damage, thus reducing the risk of cellular injury. The endogenous *antioxidant enzymes* are superoxide dismutase, catalase, glutathione peroxidase, glutathione S-transferase and glutathione reductase; ageing is known to reduce, and exercise training to elevate, their activities. The hormone *melatonin,* secreted by the pineal gland, has antioxidant properties and there is evidence that it promotes the action of antioxidant enzymes. *antioxidant nutrients* are vitamins A, C and E, and lipoic acid; supplementation with these has been demonstrated to protect against exercise-induced oxidative stress and sometimes from delayed onset of muscle damage, but most studies show no effect on physical performance. Some antioxidants (e.g. vitamins E and A, coenzyme Q10, carotenoids) are fat soluble and located within cell membranes; others such as vitamin C are water soluble, located in the cytosol, mitochondrial matrix or extracellular fluids. *See also* **reactive oxygen species**, **vitamins**.

**antiseptics** chemical substances that destroy or inhibit the growth of micro-organisms. Some can be applied to living tissues, e.g. chlorhexidine used for skin preparation before invasive procedures and for hand decontamination.

**anxiety** a subjective experience of fear, apprehension or dread; *cognitive anxiety* the cognitive elements of anxiety including worrying thoughts, fear of failure and negative expectations about performance, also known as *cognitive stress; competitive sport anxiety* the anxiety response to competitive sporting situations or to sport competition in general; *somatic anxiety* the physiological and affective elements of anxiety including unpleasant perceptions of arousal, nervousness and tension; *state anxiety* the anxiety response to a threatening situation; *trait anxiety* a general disposition to respond to situations with a high level of state anxiety.

**aortic valve stenosis** narrowing of the aortic valve due to disease of the valve cusps. One of the causes of **sudden death** in sport. *See also* **heart**; *appendix 1.3 fig 1.*

**apnoea** absence of breathing *apnoeic adj.* Depletion of oxygen in the blood threatens survival after about 3 minutes.

**aponeurosis** ribbon or sheet of collagenous connective tissue, either as a separate structure (e.g. plantar aponeurosis in the sole of the foot) or providing a wide area of attachment for one or both ends of flat muscles (e.g. sartorius).

**appendicular skeleton** the parts of the skeleton other than the skull, vertebral column and the thoracic cage (ribs and sternum), i.e. the bones of the shoulder girdle, the pelvic girdle and the limbs. *See also* **axial skeleton**; *appendix 1.2 fig 1.*

**appetite** the drive to eat. Influenced by the status of energy balance, psychological and behavioural factors and by health status. It may be increased or decreased pharmacologically. The drive to eat can be evaluated by using visual analogue scales (VAS) for self-report ratings of hunger, desire to eat, prospective food consumption (how much food one could eat), satiety and fullness. *See also* **anorexia, bulimia, hypothalamus**.

**appraisal** in stress theories, the individual's conscious or subconscious interpretation of the significance of an event; *primary appraisal* the evaluation of the relevance of an event to the person's well-being; *secondary appraisal* the person's evaluation of whether or not they have the resources to cope with an event appraised as a threat to their well-being.

**approach-avoidance conflict** a state of behavioural ambivalence with respect to a goal.

**approach behaviour** behaviour directed toward the attainment of a desired outcome.

**aptitude** (1) natural ability to perform a task; (2) potential capacity to learn a task, given the necessary training.

**arches of the foot** the three arches (two longitudinal and one transverse) are responsible for maintaining the optimum load-bearing position of the foot and thus walking motion. In the erect position, the arches are maintained primarily by the bones and ligaments, allowing even distribution of body weight. Abnormal foot biomechanics may result in alteration of this balance of load, causing discomfort.

**arginine** an **amino acid**, one of the 20 building blocks of **proteins** in food and in the body. Not normally one of the 'essential' amino acids in the adult diet as it can be made in the body from other substances, but usually considered essential for children, as deficiency impairs growth; also in adult males deficiency has been linked to

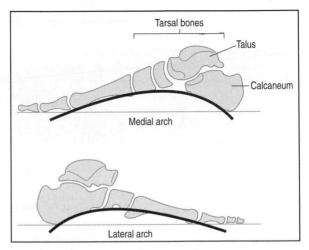

The longitudinal arches of the foot.

a low sperm count which dietary supplements can improve. One of the substances used by some athletes with the intention of stimulating **growth hormone** release, and so promoting gain in muscle mass and strength, but this action, at least by arginine taken alone, is disputed; there is better evidence for its effectiveness when combined with other amino acids. *See also* **ergogenic aids;** *appendix 4.4.*

**arousal** cognitive and physiological activation in response to a situation leading to alertness and readiness to respond. The physiological aspect is also known as *physiological arousal.*

**arrhythmia** with reference to the heart beat, any deviation from a normal rhythm. *See also* **extrasystole, fibrillation**.

**arteriosclerosis** the 'hardening of the arteries' that occurs to a variable extent with ageing. The main cause is *atherosclerosis,* when deposits known as *atheromatous plaques* are formed, mainly of **cholesterol**, in the walls of arteries and cause narrowing of the lumen, e.g. in the coronary arteries (leading to angina or thrombosis), in the cerebral arteries (leading to stroke or senile dementia) or in arteries in the legs (causing ischaemic pain when walking). *See also* **claudication**.

**arteriovenous (A-V) difference** the difference between the arterial and the venous concentration of a substance in the blood, for the whole body (when 'venous' refers to mixed venous blood in the pulmonary artery) or for an organ or region (e.g. for the tissues of the leg if 'venous' refers to blood in the femoral vein). Together with the blood flow, allows calculation of the amount removed in a given time during circulation around the whole body or region. The arteriovenous difference for oxygen is often of interest in exercise physiology. For the whole body, cardiac output ($L.min^{-1}$) $\times$ arteriovenous difference for oxygen ($L.L^{-1}$) = oxygen uptake ($L.min^{-1}$) or regional blood flow $\times$ arteriovenous difference for oxygen = regional oxygen uptake. *See also* **oxyhaemoglobin dissociation curve**.

**arthralgia** pain in a joint, especially if the absence of inflammation makes the term arthritis inappropriate. *intermittent* or *periodic arthralgia* joint pain at intervals, usually accompanied by swelling (e.g. of the knee).

**arthritis** inflammation of one or more joints which are swollen, warm to touch, tender and painful on movement. There are many causes and the treatment varies according to the cause. *arthritic adj.*

**arthrography** radiographic examination to show the internal structure of a joint, after injection of air and/or a liquid contrast medium (radio-opaque dye) into the joint cavity, to reveal more detail than an ordinary X-ray.

**arthroplasty** surgical remodelling of a joint.

**arthroscopy** procedure for visualizing the interior of a joint, using an intra-articular camera to assess, repair or reconstruct various tissues within and around it.

**articular** pertaining to a joint (an articulation). Applied to components of joints (cartilage, capsule, cavity, ligament, surfaces) and also to nerves and blood vessels supplying joints.

**articular cartilage** the layer of cartilage covering the end of a bone that forms a joint surface, providing, among its many functions, shock absorption, even distribution of load across the joint and nutrition of the underlying bone. Damage is common in sport, especially to cartilages in the **knee joint**. Permanent damage or surgical removal accelerates the development of arthritis. *See also* **meniscus.**

**artificial ventilation (artificial respiration)** restoration or maintenance of ventilation of the lungs by various means, when spontaneous breathing stops (**apnoea**) or is inadequate for any reason, including drowning, drug overdose, paralysis or weakness of breathing muscles; also when a patient's breathing is deliberately paralysed with relaxant drugs for artificial control under anaesthesia. First aid methods include mouth-to-mouth or mouth-to-nose breathing; mechanical devices include those delivering intermittent inflation from gas cylinders or continuous positive airway pressure (CPAP) for *assisted ventilation*. *See also* **cardiopulmonary resuscitation (CPR).**

**ascorbic acid** vitamin C. *See also* **vitamins**; *appendix 4.2.*

**asphyxia** total deprivation of oxygen from any cause, leading to unconsciousness and death if unrelieved; originally from the Greek, meaning absence of a pulse, which rapidly follows total lack of oxygen. Includes obstruction to breathing (e.g. *suffocation*, *strangulation*) or depletion of oxygen in the inspired gas. *See also* **apnoea, hypoxia**.

**aspiration** (1) intervention to suck out fluid from somewhere in the body, e.g. excess synovial fluid from a swollen joint or blood from a haematoma; (2) inhalation of liquid into the lungs, as when vomit is sucked into the airway from the pharynx in an unconscious accident victim. *See also* **recovery position**.

**aspirin** *see* **acetylsalicyclic acid**.

**assertiveness training** a method of developing individuals' self-confidence in interpersonal relationships.

**associative strategy** in sport psychology, a strategy used by athletes in which they focus attention on internal sensations in order to identify and reduce muscular tension by relaxation. Also known as *association*. *See also* **dissociative strategy**.

**asthma** paroxysmal **dyspnoea** characterized by wheezing and difficulty in expiration because of constriction of the airways due to spasm of the bronchial muscle (*bronchospasm*). Caused by the response of the **immune system** to a variety of stimuli. Inhaled or oral corticosteroids damp down the acute immune reaction, while inhaled $\beta_2$-receptor agonists relieve the bronchial spasm. *exercise-induced asthma*: a number of triggers are now known to produce bronchospasm and reduce performance in sport and exercise. These include intense exercise (especially combined with low fitness), respiratory tract infection, cold environmental temperature, allergens (such as pollen in hay fever), air pollution (especially cigarette smoke), certain drugs (including $\beta$-blockers) and simply exercise *per se*. Different sporting activities vary in likelihood of causing bronchospasm, e.g. it is least likely in the warm humid air of a swimming pool. *See also* **pulmonary function tests, salbutamol**.

**ataxia** lack of proper control of movements, e.g. when drunk or in neurological disease.

**atherosclerosis** *see* **arteriosclerosis**.

**athlete** increasingly favoured term for a person involved in any physically demanding sport (not only track and field athletics).

**athlete's foot** fungal infection of the skin of the foot (tinea pedis). Symptoms include intense itch, peeling and sometimes painful splits in the skin. Common in sport due to poor hygiene and use of communal changing and showering facilities. Treated by antifungal creams or dusting powders.

**athlete's heart** hypertrophy of the muscle of the left ventricle as a physiological response to training, especially endurance training. It is not considered to be pathological. Results in slowing of heart rate and changes characteristic of hypertrophy in the **electrocardiogram (ECG)**.

**athletic identity** the degree to which a person identifies with an athletic role as part of their **self-concept**.

**Atkins diet** *see* **low-carbohydrate ketogenic diets**.

**atrium** (from the Latin for cavity, entrance or passage). One of the two upper receiving chambers of the **heart**. The left atrium receives pulmonary venous blood (oxygenated, from the lungs) and the right atrium receives systemic venous blood (partly deoxygenated, from the rest of the body). *atria pl, atrial adj. See appendix 1.3 fig 1.*

**atrophy** reduction in the bulk of a body tissue or organ; occurs in muscles during prolonged bed-rest or following damage to their motor nerves (*disuse atrophy*) and in diseases of muscles themselves.

**atropine** substance that, by affecting local enzyme actions, leads to destruction (inactivation) of the neurotransmitter **acetylcholine** at parasympathetic nerve endings. By preventing parasympathetic action where there is dual autonomic innervation, atropine allows the sympathetic influence to predominate, e.g. it increases the heart rate, dilates the pupils, reduces salivary secretion and relaxes intestinal smooth muscle.

**attentional style** the way in which an individual tends to focus attention on the environment differentially along two dimensions: width (varying from a broad focus involving attention to a wide range of environmental cues to a narrow focus involving attention to a limited range of cues) and direction (directed internally on one's own thoughts and feelings versus directed externally towards objects and events outside one's body).

**attitude** a relatively enduring evaluative reaction to other individuals, situations or objects, which may be positive or negative. Typically defined as comprising affective cognitive and behavioural components.

**attribution** a person's inference about the cause of their behaviour or a behavioural outcome with regard to whether the behaviour or outcome is caused by internal factors (e.g. effort or ability) or external factors (e.g. chance or the influence of other people). *attribution theory* a theory designed to explain the types, antecedents and consequences of individuals' attributions.

**audience effects** *see* **social facilitation**.

**auricular haematoma** *see* **cauliflower ear**.

**autogenic training** a form of psychotherapy that employs self-hypnosis and relaxation techniques. Also known as *autogenics*.

**autoimmune response** action of the **immune system** against some component of the body itself, resulting in one of the many *autoimmune diseases (disorders)*.

**automatic processing** information processing that occurs without conscious attention, as in well-learned skills. *See also* **controlled processing**.

**autonomic nervous system (ANS)** the system of nerves that regulates body functions which have no direct voluntary control. Consists of motor (efferent) nerves that supply the heart, secretory glands and smooth muscle (e.g. in blood vessels, intestinal tract and airways). The two divisions of the ANS are the **sympathetic nervous system** and the **parasympathetic nervous system.** In some organs and tissues these have opposing effects, respectively promoting an increase or a decrease in activity, e.g. sympathetic nerves stimulate the heart but quieten the gut, parasympathetic vice versa. Other organs or tissues are supplied by only one of the divisions, e.g. most blood vessels only by sympathetic and digestive secretory glands only by parasympathetic. Preganglionic fibres originate within the central nervous system (CNS) and relay at ganglia outside the CNS; thence postganglionic fibres run to the relevant tissue or organ. *visceral afferents* carry information from the various sites which are subject to autonomic reflex control. *See appendix 1.1 figs 5, 6.*

**avascular** without a blood supply. *avascular necrosis* death of tissue due to lack of blood supply, usually referring to bone, following injury. Other causes in bone include hyperbaric exposure (diving), excessive intake of corticosteroids or alcohol, and some diseases. Commonly occurs after fracture of the femoral neck, leading to death of the femoral head. Also seen in fractures of the scaphoid bone in the wrist or of the head of the humerus. Often leads to **osteoarthritis**.

**avoidance behaviour** behaviour directed toward the avoidance of an undesirable outcome.

**avulsion** a forcible wrenching away, usually by injury, of a structure or part of the body, e.g. of nerves or of part of a bone.

**axial skeleton** the bones that lie centrally in the body, i.e. the skull, vertebral column, the ribs and sternum, to which the shoulder and pelvic girdles, and the limbs in turn, are linked. *See also* **appendicular skeleton**; *appendix 1.2 fig 1.*

**axilla** armpit. *axillary nerve* the main nerve passing into the arm. *axillary artery* and *vein* the main vessels serving the arm.

**axon** the long thin extension of a **nerve cell** (neuron), within a **nerve fibre,** which transmits nerve impulses (**action potentials**) to the nerve terminal in motor (efferent) nerves, or from a receptor to a nerve cell body in sensory (afferent) nerves.

# B

**back injury**  injury to the back may affect the bones (vertebral column including the sacrum, also the ilium or the ribs), muscles and ligaments. Sport-related back injuries include fractures and damage from overuse, especially to the soft tissues. Mechanical and postural causes are common and a significant cause of morbidity in the general population. Damage may be prevented by attention to posture, flexibility, muscle strength and fitness. *See also* **ankylosing spondylitis, intervertebral disc, spinal injury**.

**bacteria**  globally ubiquitous microscopic organisms, crucial to the ecosystem because of their metabolic turnover, for example, of nitrogen, carbon and sulphur. Bacteria were named from the Greek for rod, but only some (*bacilli*) are rod-shaped; others are spherical (*cocci*), curved or spiral (*vibrios, spirilla, spirochaetes*). Bacteria can be pathogenic to humans, other animals and plants, or non-pathogenic. Pathogens may be virulent and always cause infection whereas others, known as opportunists, usually only cause infection when the host defences are impaired. Non-pathogenic bacteria may become pathogenic if they move from their normal site, e.g. when normally beneficial ('probiotic') intestinal bacteria contaminate and infect a wound. Many bacteria have developed adaptations that allow them to exploit environments and survive unfriendly conditions – significantly, in modern times, enzymes that destroy antibiotics. Bacteria are classified and identified by features that include, as well as shape, staining characteristics (Gram positive or Gram negative) and whether or not they require oxygen (aerobic or anaerobic). *sing* **bacterium**. *See also* **antibiotics**.

**Baker's cyst** an enlargement of the normally small bursa in the popliteal fossa, behind the knee. May cause pain and discomfort if large or inflamed (bursitis). Named after the 19th century British surgeon who first described it, William Morrant Baker.

**balance** stability of the body, attained in the case of humans and other terrestrial animals by a continuously active process involving vestibular, visual and proprioceptive inputs causing reflex postural muscle adjustment, so as to maintain the centre of gravity directly above the supporting base of the body. *See also* **ear**.

**balanced diet** a diet which provides adequate intake of both **macronutrients** and **micronutrients**, proper regulation of metabolic processes, and maintenance of an optimal body mass. In general, dietary guidelines for the average population are also applicable to athletes, but there are differences for athletes in the recommended intake of macronutrients, in terms of grams per day, grams per day per kg body mass or percentage of energy intake from each of the main foodstuffs. *See also* **dietary reference values (DRV)**; *appendix 4.*

**ballistic movement** a movement, such as a long kick, in which a limb or part of a limb is initially accelerated forward by concentric muscle action, then swings pendulum-like through a passive (inertial or 'ballistic') phase of constant velocity, before being eccentrically decelerated.

**bamboo spine** *see* **ankylosing spondylitis**.

**Bankart's lesion** damage to the capsule of the shoulder joint at the rim of the glenoid cavity of the scapula, caused by traumatic anterior dislocation of the shoulder joint and leading to recurrent dislocation with relatively minor injury. Named after the British orthopaedic surgeon who described the lesion in the 1920s. *Bankart's operation* repairs the defect.

**banned substance** a substance which is on the list of banned **doping** classes and methods of the **World Anti-Doping Agency (WADA)** adopted (with some modifications) by the governing bodies of sport. *See appendix 6.*

**baroreceptors** sensors in the vascular system that respond to changes in pressure within blood vessels, generating afferent nerve impulses which elicit *baroreflexes*, causing appropriate corrections. The main *arterial baroreceptors* are in the wall of the *carotid sinus* on each side of the neck, where the common carotid artery divides into the internal and external carotids, and are responsible for regulation of arterial blood pressure, e.g. a rise in pressure elicits reflex reduction in peripheral resistance and/or cardiac output, via control centres in the brain stem.

**barotrauma** damage caused by change in pressure around the body (ambient pressure). Divers can be affected painfully by inequality between high ambient pressure at depth and that in closed internal air-containing spaces: the sinuses or the middle ear (*aural barotrauma:* inward bulging or at worst rupture of the eardrum, if the Eustachian tube is blocked). During surfacing the danger is *pulmonary barotrauma*: rupture of the lung surface by expanding air, with escape into the pleural cavity (pneumothorax) when surfacing without effective exhalation. *See also* **decompression illness, diving**.

**basal metabolic rate (BMR)** *see* **metabolic rate**.

**beclomethasone** an inhaled corticosteroid used in the treatment of **asthma** to reduce the inflammatory response, and used regularly as a 'preventer'.

**behaviour therapy** form of psychotherapy designed to change maladaptive behaviour patterns using the principles of classical and operant conditioning. Also known as *behaviour modification*.

**behavioural activation system (BAS)** a neurobehavioural system thought to regulate positive **affect** and **approach behaviour** in response to incentives or rewards. Individuals vary in the sensitivity of the system and it is associated with the personality factor of **extraversion**. *See also* **behavioural inhibition system (BIS)**.

**behavioural analysis** *applied behaviour analysis* application of the principles of operant conditioning to the treatment of behavioural problems. *experimental analysis of* *behaviour* application of the principles of operant conditioning to the study of behaviour. *See also* **conditioning**.

**behavioural coaching** application of the principles of operant conditioning and **cognitive behaviour therapy** to coaching, especially in sport or business.

**behavioural inhibition system (BIS)** a neurobehavioural system thought to regulate negative **affect** and avoidance behaviour in response to threats or punishment. Individuals vary in the sensitivity of the system and it is associated with the personality factor of **neuroticism.** *See also* **behavioural activation system (BAS)**.

**behavioural intention** a person's conscious or deliberate intention to engage in a behaviour.

**behaviourism** an approach to psychology which studies and interprets behaviour by objective observation of that behaviour without regard to any subjective mental processes such as ideas, emotions and will. Instead, all behaviour is held to be governed by conditioned responses.

**bends** an imprecise term traditionally used to describe some of the symptoms of **decompression illness**.

**Bernouille principle** the inverse relationship between pressure and velocity in a flowing fluid medium (liquid or gas).

**beta-agonist** in full *beta (β)-adrenoceptor (-adrenergic) agonist* a sympathomimetic drug that stimulates β-adrenoceptors. Subgroup $\beta_2$ *agonists* are used in

**asthma,** usually by inhalation, to dilate the airways by relaxing smooth muscle, acting as a 'reliever' of symptoms of wheeze, cough or breathlessness. In sport, some are allowed under doping regulations (salbutamol and terbutaline) while those with significant anabolic effects (clenbuterol) are prohibited. *See also* **adrenaline, adrenoceptor, sympathetic nervous system;** *appendix 6.*

**beta-blocker** in full *beta (β)-adrenoreceptor (or adrenergic) antagonist* a drug which blocks the stimulation of $\beta_1$-adrenoceptors in the myocardium and at other sites; used primarily in the treatment of cardiovascular disease (ischaemic heart disease and hypertension) but also in the treatment of anxiety. Banned in sport due to the beneficial effect where fine hand movement and avoidance of tremor is important such as in archery, shooting and snooker. *See also* **adrenaline, adrenoceptor, sympathetic nervous system;** *appendix 6.*

**beta-carotene** precursor of vitamin A, usually ample in a normal diet, which is converted in the body to retinol. This and other *carotenoids* also function as **antioxidants**, protecting cells against oxidation damage. Beta-carotene supplements do not appear to have any ergogenic effect. Thus, it is recommended that this pro-vitamin is best obtained through the diet. *See also* **vitamins;** *appendix 4.2.*

**beta-hydroxy-beta-methylbutyrate (HMB)** one of the newest dietary supplements on the market, which is found naturally in small quantities in catfish, various citrus fruits and breast milk. HMB supplementation has been reported to be associated with enhanced gains in muscle mass and strength during resistance training.

In addition to affecting protein synthesis, HMB is also claimed to stimulate fat oxidation. According to existing human data HMB is safe and well tolerated. *See also* **ergogenic aids**; *appendix 4.4.*

**beta-receptor** *see* **adrenoceptor**.

**bicarbonate** usually refers to sodium bicarbonate (as in 'bicarbonate of soda' or 'baking soda'). In the body it is one of the most important extracellular buffers, and the bicarbonate level is an indirect measure of the acidity of the blood. The normal range for serum bicarbonate is $22-30$ mmol.$L^{-1}$. In sport, bicarbonate supplementation is used to enhance performance in athletic events conducted at near-maximum intensity for 1–7 minutes (400–1500 m running, 100–400 m swimming, kayaking, rowing and canoeing) as they may otherwise be limited by excess hydrogen ion accumulation. *See also* **ergogenic aids**; *appendix 4.4.*

**biceps** meaning 'two-headed'. Usually refers to the *biceps brachii,* the muscle in the front of the upper arm; both heads have tendinous origins on the scapula, in front of and above the shoulder joint; their rounded bellies unite to form a single tendon which passes in front of the elbow to be inserted into the tuberosity of the radius. Its main actions are supination of the forearm and flexion of the elbow. The *biceps femoris* is one of the **hamstring muscles** in the back of the thigh. *See appendix 1.2 fig 5A.*

**bicycle ergometer** *see* **cycle ergometer**.

**big five** the widely accepted five fundamental personality factors comprising **agreeableness**, **conscientiousness**, **extraversion**, **neuroticism** and **openness to experience**.

**bile** secretion of the liver, variably stored in the gall bladder and discharged into the gut (duodenum). Contains the *bile acids,* important in the digestion and absorption of fats, and is the route for excretion of *bile pigments* (mainly bilirubin, from breakdown of the iron-containing pigments haemoglobin and myoglobin) and **cholesterol**.

**binge-eating disorder** an eating disorder characterized by a tendency to engage in episodes of binge eating. Similar to bulimia nervosa but without the accompanying compensatory behaviours such as self-induced vomiting and purging.

**binge-purge syndrome** *see* **bulimia**.

**bioelectrical impedance analysis** whole-body conductivity method for assessing **body composition**. A small alternating current flowing between two electrodes passes more rapidly through hydrated fat-free body tissues and extracellular water than through fat or bone because of the greater electrolyte content (lower electrical resistance) of the fat-free component. Impedance to electric current flow can be related to total body water content and in turn to fat-free mass, body density and percentage **body fat**.

**biofeedback** presentation of immediate visual or auditory feedback about normally unconscious body functions such as blood pressure, heart rate and muscle tension.

**biomechanical analysis** analysis of forces and motions of the human body. *qualitative biomechanical analysis* the analysis of forces and movements on (and by) the human body without regard to measurement or quantification. *quantitative biomechanical analysis* the analysis of forces and movements on (and by) the human body with emphasis on measurement and quantification.

**biomechanics** the understanding of forces and their effects on (and by) the human body and implements.

**biopsy** sample of tissue from a living subject. *biopsy vt* take such a sample.

**bipolar construct** a concept arranged along a single dimension with two opposite extremes, such as good–bad. Often used in self-report rating scales. For example, moodstates are often assessed by asking respondents to rate their mood on a set of bipolar scales such as composed–anxious, agreeable–hostile, elated–depressed.

**blister** a collection of fluid, usually serum, between the layers of the skin, causing an elevated lesion. Caused by friction, burns, local allergic responses, e.g. stings. Blisters are common with poor footwear or when exercise is of high intensity and long duration.

**blood** fluid circulating in the vascular system – the heart and blood vessels. The total volume is typically ∼5 litres in a man weighing 70 kg. The fluid *plasma,* carrying a great variety of substances, from simple inorganic ions to complex protein molecules, accounts for a little over half the blood volume and the *cells* ('formed elements') for the rest. *See also* **body fluids**, **electrolytes**, **erythrocytes**, **extracellular fluids**, **leucocytes**.

**blood coagulation** the process of clotting, which is one of the body's natural means of stopping bleeding (*haemostasis*), activated by damage to the vessel lining. Results from a complex cascade reaction, dependent on the presence of ionized calcium and involving many 'clotting factors', some always present in the blood and some released from damaged tissue and platelets. The endproduct is a mesh of fibrin in which blood cells are trapped to form a solid mass. *See also* **anticoagulant**.

**blood cells** the cells circulating in the blood stream, accounting for a little less than half the total volume: **erythrocytes** (red blood cells) smaller but in far greater number than **leucocytes** (white blood cells) and **platelets**. *See also* **haemopoiesis**.

**blood clotting** *see* **blood coagulation**.

**blood doping** a procedure banned by the **World Anti-Doping Agency (WADA)**: the administration of a blood transfusion to a sportsman or sportswoman in order to increase the oxygen-carrying capacity of the blood and as a result to improve performance. Most commonly, this involves removing up to a litre of the person's blood and storing this while the body's normal mechanisms replace the loss. At a later date, usually just prior to competition, the removed blood is transfused back into the circulation. Though banned, it is still used in some sports such as athletics and cycling as detection is difficult. The procedure is considered to be against the ethics of sport. Risks include renal damage, transmission of infection and circulatory overload.

**blood flow** quantity of blood flowing through a vessel, region or organ in unit time. Dependent on the arterial blood pressure and the resistance to flow in the local vascular bed, determined by the state of constriction/dilatation mainly of the arterioles, influenced in turn by chemical (local and hormonal) and neural (sympathetic) effects on the vascular smooth muscle.

**blood gases** normally refers to the oxygen and carbon dioxide that are dissolved in the arterial blood, following equilibration in the lungs between capillary blood and the gases in the alveoli. Measured as part of the assessment of lung function; expressed as **partial pressures** (or 'tensions') $PO_2$ and $PCO_2$. There is also a small amount of dissolved nitrogen, at a $PN_2$ in equilibrium with alveolar nitrogen. *See also* **hypoxia**, **hypercapnia**, **oxyhaemoglobin dissociation curve**.

**blood glucose** (often loosely called *'blood sugar'*) is obtained by digestion of carbohydrates and by release from liver glycogen, and is taken up by the cells of the organs and tissues for use as an energy substrate. In healthy people, blood glucose concentration is homeostatically controlled within a fairly narrow range; maintenance of the normal level is critical for the function in particular of those tissues with an obligatory demand for glucose (brain, red blood cells, renal cortex, mammary gland and testis). Hormones involved include **insulin**, tending to lower blood concentration, and **glucagon**, **glucocorticoids**, **adrenaline** and **growth hormone,** tending to raise it. It seldom falls below about $5 \text{ mmol.L}^{-1}$, even after prolonged fasting, and returns to this value within a couple of hours of the rise that follows a meal. When there is no uptake from the gut, about 8 g glucose per hour can be provided from the liver by breakdown of glycogen stores and by

**gluconeogenesis**. During prolonged exercise glucose output from the liver closely matches the increased requirement, so that the blood concentration falls only when the hepatic glycogen store is depleted, close to exhaustion. *See also* **hyperglycaemia, hypoglycaemia**.

**blood groups** classification of types of human blood, originally for defining compatibility for transfusion. *ABO groups* the four main types, named according to the antigens on the individual's red blood cells (RBC): A, B, AB (both) or O (none). (The donor's blood cells will be catastrophically hydrolysed if the recipient's plasma has antibodies to the donor cells' antigens.) An individual's blood plasma contains antibodies to whichever antigen(s) are not present on that person's own red blood cells; for example, group O (no antigens) can donate to a recipient of any group, because the recipient's plasma antigens can have no effect on the donor's red cells, and group AB (no antibodies) can receive from a donor of any group. *Rhesus (Rh) blood groups* the majority of people ('Rh positive') have another red blood cell antigen. There is no antibody to this in anyone's plasma, except when a person of the 'Rh-negative' minority has been exposed to the antigen. For example, a Rh-negative mother who has an Rh-positive baby raises antibodies that can harm a later Rh-positive fetus; likewise, a first transfusion with Rh-positive blood raises antibodies that react against a later one.

**blood loss** *see* **haemorrhage**.

**blood pressure** the pressure exerted on the blood vessel walls. Normally refers to the *arterial blood pressure*, usually expressed in millimetres of mercury (mmHg) because of traditional *sphygmomanometry* (which measures the height of a column of mercury sustained by the pressure in an inflated cuff around the arm that occludes the blood flow) but now more commonly measured by automated strain-gauge devices. Arterial blood pressure fluctuates with each heart beat between a maximum *systolic pressure (SBP)* during the ejection of blood from the heart and a minimum *diastolic pressure (DBP)* when the heart is relaxed with the aortic and pulmonary valves closed; the *pulse pressure* is the difference between them. When blood pressure is measured, values for both are quoted, e.g. 120/70 mmHg. May also be recorded directly from a cannula in an artery linked to a pressure transducer. *mean (arterial) blood pressure (MBP)* a mean value averaged over the cardiac cycle, derived from the arterial pulse pressure wave; typically closer to the diastolic than the systolic pressure such that $MBP = DBP + (SBP - DBP)/3$. *See also* **hypertension, hypotension.**

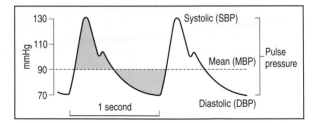

Arterial blood pressure as recorded over two cardiac cycles, at heart rate 60 beats per minute.

**blood sugar** *see* **blood glucose**.

**body building** use of exercise and diet (and often, undesirably, also drugs) to enhance size and definition of skeletal muscles. *See also* **anabolic steroids, ergogenic aids, strength training**.

**body clock** *see* **circadian rhythm**.

**body composition** whole-body composition is of interest in the contexts of control of body weight, assessment of **obesity**, and sport and exercise,. It comprises *total body fat* (essential fat plus storage fat) and *fat-free body mass (FFM)* (includes muscle, water and bone). From *body density* measurements, using established corrections and equations, the ratio of fat mass to fat-free mass can be calculated, based on the much lower density of the fat compartment. However, within the FFM, bone is more dense than muscle, so if there is either relative loss of bone density (osteoporosis) or increase in muscle mass (with training), fat percentage may be overestimated. *densitometry* techniques include underwater (hydrostatic) weighing and air displacement plethysmography. Estimates can be made of *lean body mass (LBM)*, body mass devoid of storage fat, but LBM does not exclude essential fat, so it is slightly higher than the FFM. *See also* **body fat, body fluids**.

**body discrepancy** a person's perceived discrepancy between their actual and ideal body size.

**body dysmorphia** a mental disorder characterized by a perceived defect in one's physical appearance or in a part of the body. *muscle dysmorphic disorder* a form of body dysmorphia that occurs almost exclusively in men, characterized by a perception that the body is too small and insufficiently muscular; also known as *bigorexia*.

**body fat** normal healthy values usually quoted for total body fat are 15% (12–19%) of body mass for young men and 27% (25–30%) for women, both increasing by about 5% from late teens to sixties. *essential fat* in the tissues and organs (including bone marrow, nervous system and muscle) averages 3% body mass for men and 12% for women (extra related to reproductive function); it is not a labile energy reserve, but a vital component for normal structure and function. *storage fat* represents the energy reserve that accumulates as adipose tissue beneath the skin and in visceral depots, averaging 12% body mass for men and 15% body mass for women. Methods most commonly used for estimating percentage fat are: measurement of **skinfold thickness** at prescribed sites, body density measurement, and **bioelectrical impedance analysis**. *See also* **body composition**, **body mass index**, **obesity**.

**body fluids** the total water in the body accounts for more than half of body mass (typically 45 kg in a 70 kg man). About two-thirds of the total body water (30 L) is in *intracellular fluid (ICF)* and one-third (15 L) in *extracellular fluid (ECF)* – all body fluids external to cells; of this, blood plasma accounts for ~3 L, *interstitial fluid* in the tissues and *lymph* for ~12 L. *See also* **hydration status**, **water balance**.

**body image** a person's perceptions of their own physical appearance.

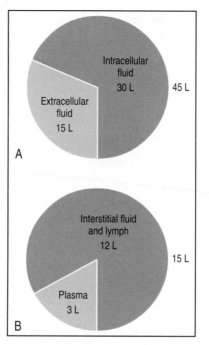

Body fluids. Typical volumes of (A) ECF and ICF. (B) The components of ECF.

**body language** non-verbal communication that expresses a person's current physical, emotional and mental state. It includes body movements, postures, gestures, facial expressions, spatial positions, attire and other bodily adornments.

**body mass index (BMI)** body mass in kg divided by height in metres squared ($kg.m^{-2}$) used to evaluate the extent of adiposity. The WHO classification for BMI is: less than 18.5, underweight; 18.5–24.9, normal weight; 25–29.9, pre-obese; 30–34.9, obese class I; 35–39.9, obese class II; greater than 40, obese class III. These predicted values cannot be used in children, pregnant women and certain other adult subjects. Also a high BMI can lead to an overestimation of fatness in relatively lean individuals with a disproportionately high muscle mass because of genetic make-up or exercise training; this applies, for example, to body builders, weightlifters or upper weight class wrestlers. *See also* **obesity**.

**body temperature** is normally regulated so as to maintain a *core temperature,* that of the blood and the internal organs, of $37°C \pm 0.5–1°C$. Determined by the balance between metabolic heat production (varying with muscular activity) and heat loss (from the skin surface, in expired air and with the excreta). Heat loss is influenced by external factors (ambient temperature, humidity, air movement and clothing) and regulated physiologically by the **hypothalamus**, via the autonomic nervous system, in response to changes in blood temperature and afferent information from skin receptors. Constriction or dilatation of skin blood vessels varies the skin temperature and hence the heat loss, effectively changing the thickness of the insulating 'shell' around the 'core'. **Sweating** is stimulated for additional evaporative heat loss and shivering for additional metabolic heat production. *See also* **heat illness, hypothermia**.

**body weight** term in common use for what is properly called *body mass* and commonly, but incorrectly, referred to in units of mass (e.g. kg). Strictly, body weight is the force due to the effect of gravity on body mass, expressed in newtons (N). *See also* **body composition**, **body mass index**.

**Bohr effect** describes a shift of the **oxyhaemoglobin dissociation curve** to the right, due to an increase in acidity, carbon dioxide tension and/or temperature of the blood; these reduce the percentage saturation of haemoglobin with oxygen, and hence the amount of oxygen carried per litre of blood, at any given oxygen tension.

**bone** a **connective tissue**, with living cells embedded in a collagen-based matrix impregnated with mineral, mostly a crystalline form of calcium phosphate. Provides skeletal framework and leverage, attachment for muscles and tendons, and stores of **calcium**, available for rapid turnover under hormonal control. Bone tissue is of two types: hard dense outer *cortical (compact) bone* and inner honeycombed *spongy (cancellous) bone* containing the red *bone marrow* where blood cells (red and white) are formed in the process of *haemopoiesis.* Yellow, fatty marrow fills a *central (medullary) cavity*.

**bone injury** broken bones are common injuries. Bruising of bone involves damage to the covering membrane, the *periosteum*, where nerves and blood vessels passing to the underlying bone can be disrupted. *See also* **fracture**.

**bone mineral density (BMD)** is measured as an indicator of *bone mass*, decreased in **osteoporosis**. Men and women who participate in strength and power activities have a bone mass as great as, or greater than, that of endurance athletes. On the other hand, the amenorrhoea that is

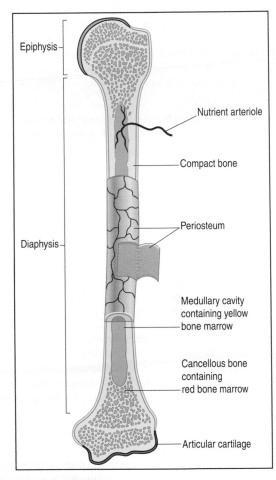

Structure of a typical long bone.

prevalent among female athletes in weight-related sports is associated with a decrease in bone mass, leaving them at increased risk of osteoporosis and stress fractures despite competitive athletic participation. *See also* **dual emission X-ray absorptiometry (DEXA), female athlete triad**.

**bone-on-bone force** the force due to contact between two bones at a joint. Includes **joint reaction force** and muscle force.

**bone scan** a radionuclear technique (using radioactive-labelled technetium-99) used in medical investigations to visualize bone and to estimate bone density. In sport, it is used in the diagnosis of bony injury, especially for suspected stress fractures which may not show up on a conventional X-ray at an early stage. *See also* **osteoporosis**.

**Borg (perceived exertion) scale** a simple method of rating perceived exertion used by coaches to gauge an athlete's level of intensity in training and competition. The commonest used is a 15-point scale, using the numbers 6–20 to describe a range of levels of exertion from very, very light (6) to exhaustion (20). Research has shown that there is a correlation between an athlete's rate of perceived exertion (RPE) and their **heart rate**, lactate threshold and $\dot{V}O_{2\,max}$. Named after Swedish scientist Gunnar Borg.

**boundary layer** microscopic layer of fluid (liquid or gas) next to the surface of a body or object moving relative to it, important in considering the **drag force** upon the object. *laminar boundary layer* layer which is next to the surface of an object, not mixing with the flow further away from the surface, and so can be considered to be a discrete layer in a plane parallel to the main flow. *turbulent boundary layer* layer which is next to the surface of an object, but in this case mixing with the flow further away from it. An example of a boundary layer change is that due to a dimpled golf ball in flight: the dimples make the boundary layer turbulent, which reduces drag caused by the pressure being lower behind the ball, so less energy is lost to the flow.

**bow legs** *see* **genu valgum**.

**boxer's fracture** a colloquial term used in sports medicine to describe a fracture of the neck of the fifth metacarpal bone due to a compressive force that causes the head of the metacarpal to bend over towards the palm, leading to a flexion deformity.

**boxing** in this popular sport each opponent attempts to score points by hitting the other on targeted areas of the body, including the head. Many of the public (and the British Medical Association) would like to see the sport banned due to the potentially serious brain damage (and occasional deaths) inflicted by intent rather than by accident. *See also* **head injury**.

**brace** a support to maintain a part of the body in its correct position.

**brachial plexus** complex system of nerves, extending from the lower neck to the axilla, derived from nerve roots of the cervical and upper thoracic segments of the spinal cord, which branch and regroup to form the nerves that supply the upper limb, including part of the shoulder region. *brachial plexus injury* is most common in sports with upper body contact such as rugby and American football (where it is called a 'stinger'), with forced lateral flexion, hyperextension or rotation of the neck. Symptoms include pain and burning sensation in the neck with paraesthesia, heaviness and weakness of the affected arm and can last from a few minutes to a few weeks. If symptoms persist, a formal neurological assessment including scanning is required, though in most cases complete resolution results.

**bradycardia** slow heart rate, defined as 60 beats per minute or less; known as *sinus bradycardia* when it arises from the normal pacemaker in the heart (the sinoatrial (SA) node), e.g. the slow resting heart rate in trained athletes, when vagal tone is increased. Pathological causes include the action of some drugs, or hormonal or electrolyte abnormalities; a fixed slow rate can arise from an abnormal focus, when the spread of excitation from the SA node is prevented by 'heart block'.

**brain** the part of the **central nervous system** (**CNS**) within the skull. Uppermost are the anatomically symmetrical left and right *cerebral hemispheres* with frontal, temporal and occipital lobes, the grey matter of the *cerebral cortex* forming the infolded outermost layer. Below the hemispheres the central *brain stem* (*midbrain, pons* and *medulla oblongata*), is in continuity with the spinal cord at the large hole (foramen magnum) in the base of the skull. The main sensory and motor nerve *tracts* to and from the cerebral hemispheres cross over in the brain stem, so brain damage on one side (e.g. stroke) disturbs function on the opposite side of the body. The *cerebellum,* also with a cortex of grey matter, lies behind and along-side the brain stem, with connections to it, and relays up and down to other parts of the CNS. *grey matter* refers to regions and clusters consisting mainly of neuron cell bodies (forming the cortical layers and more deeply the various control centres and 'nuclei'); *white matter* is composed mainly of myelinated nerve fibres in the tracts that link neurons in the different parts of the brain to each other and to the spinal cord. Interconnecting *cerebral ventricles* deep in the brain contain *cerebrospinal fluid (CSF)*, in continuity with CSF on the surface of both brain and spinal cord, where it is enclosed within mem-branous coverings, the *meninges*. *See figs appendix 1.1.*

**brain damage** in sport this is usually a result of direct trauma to the head. More common in sports such as boxing, horse riding and falls during those carried out at height. *See also* **head injury**.

**break test** isometric contraction against the examiner's manual resistance, used in clinical assessment of muscle performance.

**breath-hold** voluntary suppression of breathing move-ments. The *breath-hold time* is very variable between subjects and conditions. Starting from full lung volume, breathing air, less than one minute is usual, but longer after hyperventilation or after breathing oxygen. Although the unsuppressible stimulus to breathe at *break-point* is related to rising carbon dioxide and falling oxygen in the blood, interaction with other factors is complex, involving central respiratory rhythm, afferents from the diaphragm and decreasing lung volume. *See also* **diving**.

**breathing** the regular inflation and deflation of the lungs, serving the purpose of respiratory gas exchange *aka pulmonary ventilation.* Breathing and its pattern – the depth and frequency of breaths – are controlled by a group of neurons in the brain stem, and vary in response to changes in afferent information from several sites, notably the **chemoreceptors** (sensitive to changes in oxygen, $CO_2$ and pH in arterial blood, and to the pH in the brain) and from muscles and joints (which signal changes in activity). The output from this *'respiratory centre'* regulates, via the phrenic nerves, the frequency and strength of contraction of the **diaphragm**, which accounts alone for breathing at rest. With increasing demand, the *intercostal muscles* contribute additional lung inflation/deflation by their action on the size and shape of the ribcage, assisted when breathing is deepest by the *accessory muscles* of respiration, including neck, chest and **abdominal muscles.** *See also* **apnoea, dyspnoea, ventilation**.

**breathing frequency (f)** the number of breaths per minute. Also known as *respiratory rate.* At rest, varies among individuals from about 10 to 20 per minute. In exercise, can rise to 40–50 per minute.

**breathlessness** *see* **dyspnoea**.

**bronchial tree** the air passages leading from the trachea to the lung alveoli, via a left and a right main *bronchus*, the branches from these to the lobes of the lungs, and within the lungs the progressively smaller *bronchioles*, *terminal bronchioles* (~0.2 mm diameter) and finally the *respiratory bronchioles* which open into the alveolar ducts and the alveoli. All branches except the final, smallest ones have circular smooth muscle in their walls, which can change the diameter, varying the resistance to airflow. Cartilage stiffens the walls down to the bronchioles, forming complete rings in the trachea, becoming less complete in the bronchi and their branches. *See also* **airway(s)**, *appendix 1.3 fig 4.*

**bronchodilator** any agent which dilates the bronchioles, by relaxing the smooth muscle in their walls. Used in sport by those with asthma to relieve wheeze or breathlessness. *See also* **beta-agonists**; *appendix 6.*

**bronchospasm** sudden constriction of the bronchial tubes due to contraction of the involuntary smooth muscle in their walls. In sport, commonly the result of activity in those with **asthma**.

**Bruce protocol** a protocol for exercise tests in which the intensity is increased incrementally at 3-minute intervals. Normally a treadmill test, with increments of gradient and speed, but can be adapted for a static **cycle ergometer.** Used commonly in the assessment of patients with known or suspected heart disease. The modified Bruce protocol has two initial stages at a lower intensity than in the standard test, allowing assessment of those who are symptomatic at lower levels of activity or less fit as a result of other diseases, such as arthritis or respiratory disease. Named after the American 'Father of Exercise Cardiology' Robert A. Bruce.

**bruise** a discoloration of the skin due to extravasation of blood into the underlying tissues.

**bucket handle tear** describes a type of tear of a **meniscus** (semilunar cartilage) in the knee joint, that extends around the curve of the meniscus.

**buffer systems** substances which are present in the body fluids and limit pH change by their ability to accept or donate hydrogen ions as appropriate. The major buffer systems are: bicarbonate buffer, consisting of a weak acid (carbonic acid) and the salt of that acid (sodium bicarbonate), hydrogen phosphates, and proteins (including **haemoglobin**).

**buffering agents** substances which when ingested induce alkalosis and so counteract and limit reduction in **pH** during exercise. Important agents include sodium bicarbonate and sodium citrate; the minimum dose for improvement in performance is about $2\,\text{g.kg}^{-1}$ body mass. *See also* **ergogenic aids**; *appendix 4.4.*

**bulimia** literally means 'ox hunger' and refers to gorging or insatiable appetite. *bulimia nervosa* is an eating disorder involving repeated uncontrolled consumption of large quantities of food followed by behaviour designed to lose weight such as self-induced vomiting, purging with laxatives and diuretics, fasting or excessive exercise, together with intense feelings of guilt or shame. Excessive eating is often interrupted by periods of anorexia. Also known as *binge-purge syndrome*. *See also* **binge-eating disorder**.

**bunion** *see* **hallux**.

**buoyancy force** the force due to fluid (liquid or gas) supporting an object, resulting from the different densities of the object and the fluid. Usually acts upwards. Also known as *upthrust*. *See also* **centre of buoyancy**.

**burnout** a syndrome induced by chronic exposure to stressors associated with an activity in which the individual regularly engages. Characterized by physical and emotional exhaustion, anxiety, depression and impaired performance. May be related to work or, in the context of sport, to prolonged, intensive training or overfrequent competition. *See also* **overtraining**.

**bursa** a fibrous sac lined with synovial membrane and containing a small quantity of synovial fluid. Bursae are found between tendon and bone, skin and bone, and muscle and muscle. Their function is to facilitate movement by reducing friction between these surfaces. *bursae pl*.

**bursitis** inflammation, with swelling, of a bursa. *olecranon bursitis* of the bursa over the point of the elbow; *prepatellar bursitis* (*syn* housemaid's knee) of the bursa in front of the patella, frequently associated with excessive kneeling; *retrocalcaneal bursitis* of the bursa at the back of the heel between the calcaneum and the Achilles tendon near to its insertion, causing a swelling at both sides of the tendon. *See also* **knee joint**, **trochanteric bursitis**.

**buttocks** these rounded projections are formed mainly by the three *gluteal muscles*. They arise from the surface of the ilium of the hip bone and cross the back of the hip joint to be inserted into the femur. The *gluteus maximus*, the largest, is crucial in the maintenance of the upright posture, as an extensor at the hips, and also in running, climbing and walking up steps. It also assists in keeping the leg straight at the knee, via a fibrous band attached to the tibia. The two smaller muscles (*g. medius, g. minimus*) mainly take part in abduction and rotation at the hip. *See appendix 1.2 fig 4A.*

**B-vitamins** group of water-soluble vitamins, essential for the formation of coenzymes that are vital for a range of cellular processes. *See also* **vitamins**; *appendix 4.2.*

# C

**caffeine** occurs naturally in the leaves, seeds or fruits of more than 60 different plants, including coffee beans, kola nuts (cola) and tea leaves, and is also added to some foods and soft drinks; there is also a closely related substance in cocoa beans (chocolate). Caffeine is often said to be the most widely used drug in the world. It is one of the commonest ingredients in fat-loss supplements; it can help relieve some types of headache, so is an ingredient in a number of pain relievers. By virtue of its stimulant action in the brain, it is used in sport to improve alertness, concentration and reaction time and to delay central fatigue. By promoting lipolysis, and therefore fat oxidation, caffeine acts as an aid to endurance but its diuretic action may enhance fluid loss and thus reduce hydration. *See also* **ergogenic aids**, **fatigue**, **lipolysis**, **methylxanthines**; *appendix 4.4.*

**calcaneum (calcaneus)** the heel bone which articulates with the talus above it and the cuboid bone in front. The **Achilles tendon** attaches to the back of the calcaneum. *See also* **foot**; *appendix 1.2 figs 1–3.*

**calcium** the most abundant mineral in the body. Combined with phosphorus in bones and teeth. The two together represent about 75% of the body's total mineral content. *ionized calcium (Ca$^{2+}$)*, about 1% of the 1200 mg total calcium, plays a crucial role in all physiological functions including muscle action, blood clotting, transmission of nerve impulses, activation of several enzymes, synthesis of the active form of vitamin D, and transport across all cell membranes; its level in the blood is regulated by exchange with Ca in bone and by variation in renal excretion, under hormonal influences. Calcium is one of the most frequently inadequate nutrients in the diet of both athletes and non-athletes. Female dancers, gymnasts and endurance competitors are among those most prone to calcium dietary insufficiency. *See also* **bone, coagulation, excitation-contraction coupling, hormones** *(table appendix 5)*, **micronutrients, minerals, parathyroid gland, tetany.**

**calcium (Ca) pump** one of many similar molecular complexes embodying ion-binding sites and an ATPase in the surface membrane of many cell types, including smooth and cardiac muscle, and in the membrane of the **sarcoplasmic reticulum (SR)** in skeletal muscle. The pumps actively transport calcium ions (Ca$^{2+}$) out of the cytoplasm; those in the surface membrane return them to the extracellular fluid, and those in SR membrane return them to within the SR. All use energy derived from hydrolysis of ATP.

**calculus** the use of small changes to calculate derivatives of equations. Includes differentiation (calculation of gradients) and integration (calculation of areas). Invented in the 17th century by Newton and Leibnitz independently.

**calf** the twin 'bellies' of the **gastrocnemius** are prominent in the upper half of the calf, e.g. when standing on tip-toe; this and the flatter *soleus* in front of it (known together as the *triceps surae*) form the main bulk of the calf muscles; their tendons join to attach to the calcaneum via the **Achilles tendon.** Accessory to the gastrocnemius is the *plantaris.* Deeper muscles include the flexors of the toes, with long tendons passing into the foot. *See appendix 1.2 fig 6B.*

**callus** the collagenous tissue which forms around a healing bone at the site of injury.

**calorie** a unit of energy, defined as the energy in the form of heat that will raise the temperature of 1 gram of water by 1 degree Celsius. Values are more often quoted in kcal (kilocalories): 1 kcal = 1000 calories = 4.2 kJ. In food, 1 g of carbohydrate or protein provides about 4 kcal and 1 g of fat, 9 kcal of energy. Energy is also provided by alcohol, at 7 kcal per gram. *calorie restriction* is the commonest treatment of obesity and overweight: an essential part of any weight control programme. Obsession with weight loss may result in disordered eating. *See also* **anorexia**, **bulimia**.

**calorimetry** technique used for the measurement of energy expenditure. *direct calorimetry* evaluates energy expended over a given time by measuring heat emitted from the body. Heat loss is detected by using room-sized chambers. *indirect calorimetry* when foods are oxidized in the body, oxygen is used and carbon dioxide is produced in proportion to the heat generated. Energy expended over a given time can be estimated from oxygen consumption alone. For greater accuracy and information about the relative amounts of nutrients (carbohydrate, fat and protein) oxidized, carbon dioxide production is also measured and urea production estimated. *See also* **Douglas bag method.**

**cannabis** *see* **marijuana**.

**capsule** the fibrous tissue that covers a joint. Inflammation of this tissue is known as *capsulitis*.

**carbohydrate (CHO)** the most abundant and economic source of food energy in the human diet, comprising 40–80% of total energy intake in different populations. The recommended ideal is at least 50–55% and a *high-carbohydrate diet* is defined as one providing more than 55% of energy as CHO. Contained in breads, cereals, fruits, vegetables, milk and dairy products, soft drinks, cakes, biscuits and pastry. One gram of CHO provides ~4 kcal of energy. In Western diets about 60% of dietary CHO is in the form of polysaccharides of D-glucose, mostly starch, and about 25% 'free sugars', mainly sucrose. The quantity and quality of carbohydrate consumed have impact on energy balance, digestive function, insulin sensitivity and blood lipids. CHO is present in the blood as **glucose** and *carbohydrate stores* are in the form of **glycogen** in the liver and skeletal muscle and to a small extent in other tissues including, importantly, the brain. *See also* **glycaemic index**; *appendix 4*.

**carbohydrate intake guidelines for athletes** the IOC suggests that athletes with considerable and prolonged energy demands of training should have a high-carbohydrate diet, increasing CHO intake to 65–70% of

## Carbohydrate intake guidelines for athletes

| Purpose | Intake per kg body mass | Intake for body mass of 70 kg |
|---|---|---|
| To accumulate muscle glycogen for endurance events of 1–3 hours at moderate to high intensity | 7–10 g daily | 490–700 g daily |
| To accumulate muscle glycogen for endurance events of 4–5 hours at moderate to high intensity | 10–12 g daily | 700–840 g daily |
| To increase availability before a long session | 1–4 g within 4 hours of start | 70–280 g within 4 hours of start |
| To maintain CHO supply during moderate or intermittent exercise lasting longer than 1 hour | 0.5–1.0 g hourly | 40–70 g hourly |
| To assist recovery of muscle glycogen, when interval between exercise sessions is only a few hours | 1 g immediately after exercise, repeated after 2 hours | 70 g repeated |

dietary energy. However, due to the high total energy intake of athletes, population dietary guidelines that recommend a CHO component of at least 50–55% are in most cases appropriate also for the health needs and fuel requirements of athletes. For athletes, therefore, the recommended CHO intake is usually expressed in grams per day or grams per day per kg body mass, rather than as a percentage of the total.

**carbohydrate-electrolyte solutions** *see* **sports drinks**.

**carbohydrate loading** aims to maximize (supercompensate) muscle glycogen stores. This allows athletes to maintain a chosen pace for longer periods and also enhances the performance of a set amount of work (i.e. set distance) by preventing a decline in pace or work output associated with CHO depletion. The procedure is popular with long-distance runners and other endurance-type athletes; it is an important nutritional strategy for events lasting more than 90 minutes, which would otherwise be limited by the depletion of muscle glycogen stores. In practice, loading is performed in two stages: a glycogen depletion stage and a carbohydrate loading phase, typically spread over 6–7 days, which entail a few days of minimal CHO intake with initially high but then decreasing intensity of training, followed by a few days of high CHO diet and minimal exercise.

**cardiac arrest** cessation of the heart beat. *See also* **cardiopulmonary resuscitation (CPR)**, **sudden death**.

**cardiac arrhythmias** *see* **arrhythmia**.

**cardiac cycle** the events in the **heart** over the period from the beginning of the generation of one heart beat to the beginning of the next. The *electrical* cycle begins with discharge from the sinoatrial node, spreading excitation through the atrial muscle then via the atrioventricular node to the ventricular muscle; after this an isoelectric phase precedes the next cycle. The *mechanical* cycle begins with simultaneous contraction of the right and left atria (assisting filling of the ventricles); contraction of the ventricles (systole), raising pressure within them, which closes the atrioventricular and opens the aortic and pulmonary valves; ejection of blood; then relaxation (diastole) and refilling. *See also* **blood pressure**, **cardiac output**, **electrocardiogram (ECG)**.

**cardiac hypertrophy** thickening of the myocardium, particularly the left ventricle. This may occur physiologically as a result of athletic training and is usually a uniform increase in thickness of the ventricular wall. Pathologically it may be the result of hypertension, secondary to outflow tract obstruction (e.g. **aortic valve stenosis**) or to congenital abnormalities. *See also* **athlete's heart, hypertrophic obstructive cardiomyopathy (HOCM)**.

**cardiac massage** performed to restore/maintain circulation when there is cardiac arrest. For *external cardiac massage* the lower part of the sternum (breastbone) is rhythmically depressed to compress the heart and force out blood into the arteries. More drastically, the chest may be opened, to allow direct manual compression of the heart. *See also* **cardiopulmonary resuscitation (CPR)**.

**cardiac muscle** *see* **muscle**.

**cardiac output (CO)** the volume of blood ejected per minute from each ventricle of the heart simultaneously, i.e. to the lungs via the pulmonary artery, and to the rest of the body via the aorta (although often defined solely as the output from the left ventricle). The product of **stroke volume** (SV) and **heart rate** (HR): at rest, e.g. $70\,mL \times 70$ per minute $= 4.9\,L.min^{-1}$ ($4$–$6\,L.min^{-1}$ varying with body size). Increase in CO in exercise involves increase in heart rate, accompanied by greater filling during diastole (by increased venous return to the heart), maintaining then increasing stroke volume, due to stretch of the ventricular muscle and to enhanced contractility from sympathetic stimulation; also the residual volume remaining in the ventricles after ejection decreases. Maximal CO in exercise increases with athletic training (by hypertrophy of ventricular muscle, with raised SV and lowered HR at rest, allowing a greater increase) exceptionally up to SV $200\,mL \times HR\,200 = 40\,L.min^{-1}$, but a more modest maximum is typical.

**cardiac rehabilitation** a structured, planned programme, originally restricted to patients following myocardial infarction, designed to achieve and maintain the maximum degree of physical and psychological independence of which they are capable. Now extended to include all patients with any cardiovascular disease. The programme is exercise based, with a gradual increase in activity individually tailored to suit clinical status and level of symptoms. Educational (risk factor modification) and nutritional sessions are included for both patient and spouse/partner and the psychosocial aspects such as return to work, resumption of sexual intercourse, etc. are covered.

**cardiomyopathy** a group of diseases of the myocardium associated with cardiac dysfunction. It is classified as dilated, hypertrophic or restrictive. Management includes treatment of the cause (if possible) and treatment of heart failure. Heart transplantation is sometimes required. *See also* **hypertrophic obstructive cardiomyopathy (HOCM), sudden death.**

**cardiopulmonary resuscitation (CPR)** the techniques used to restore and maintain the circulation and ventilation of the lungs following cardiopulmonary arrest. Involves (a) opening and clearing the airway; (b) **artificial ventilation (artificial respiration)**, mouth-to-mouth or mouth-to-nose, using a bag and face mask, or via an endotracheal tube; (c) external **cardiac massage**.

**carnitine (L-carnitine)** a short-chain nitrogen-containing carboxylic acid, mainly located in skeletal and cardiac muscle cells. Over half the daily requirement is provided from meat and dairy products in a balanced diet; the remainder is synthesized in the liver. It has been hypothesized that supplementary ingestion of L-carnitine might upregulate the capacity to transport fatty acids into mitochondria matrix where they are metabolized and so increase their oxidation, thus benefiting both endurance athletes and those wishing to reduce their body fat. Research has not supported these claims. *See also* **ergogenic aids**; *appendix 4.4.*

**carotid arteries** the principal arteries on each side of the neck, providing a major part of the blood supply to the head and neck. Where each *common carotid artery* divides into external and internal branches, there is a dilatation, the *carotid sinus*; nerve endings in its walls (**baroreceptors**) are sensitive to stretch caused by rising arterial blood pressure, and via connections to the brain stem lead to reflex slowing of the heart rate and thus a corrective fall in pressure (baroreflex). The *internal carotid artery* enters the base of the skull to reach the brain; the *external carotid artery* provides branches that supply the extracranial tissues of the head and neck. *See appendix 1.3 fig 2.*

**carotid bodies** small clumps of tissue close to the carotid arteries, containing **chemoreceptors** that respond rapidly to a fall in oxygen, decrease in pH and/or increase in carbon dioxide in the arterial blood. Via neural connections to the brain stem, they mediate reflex responses (*chemoreflexes*) including an increase in ventilation, which correct or compensate for these changes. *See also* **hypoxia**.

**carpal bones** *see* **scaphoid bone, wrist, wrist joint**.

**carpal tunnel syndrome** nocturnal pain, numbness, weakness of the thumb and tingling in the area of distribution of the median nerve in the hand. Due to compression of the nerve as it passes under the fascial band on the front of the wrist. Most common in middle-aged women.

**Cartesian co-ordinate system** *see* **co-ordinates**.

**cartilage** a dense connective tissue capable of withstanding pressure. There are several types according to the function each has to fulfil. There is relatively more cartilage in a child's skeleton but much of it has been converted into bone by adulthood. *cartilaginous adj.* *See also* **knee joint, meniscus**.

**catabolism** *see* **metabolism**.

**catastrophe theory** a set of mathematical theorems employed in the modelling of discontinuities in the physical world, that result when gradually changing and interacting variables reach a critical point. Applied in sport psychology to the understanding of sudden decrements or increments in performance, incorporating changes in cognitive anxiety, physiological arousal and self-confidence.

**catecholamines** substances that mediate the effects of activity of the sympathetic nervous system. Released into the blood as hormones from the adrenal medulla, and act as neurotransmitters at sympathetic nerve endings and within the central nervous system. The main ones are **adrenaline** (epinephrine), **noradrenaline** (norepinephrine) and **dopamine**. *See also* **adrenoceptors**, **hormones**; *appendix 5*.

**cauliflower ear** colloquial term for an *auricular haematoma* – a collection of blood within the pinna (external ear). Usually the result of trauma, especially common in boxing and rugby. The close adherence of the skin to the underlying cartilage of the pinna leads to painful stretching of the tissue, which may need surgical drainage and pressure to prevent further accumulation and later deformity.

**causality** *see* **locus of causality**.

**cavus foot** *see* **pes cavus**.

**cell** the basic structural unit of living organisms. A human body would typically have $\sim 10^{14}$ cells of different types, ranging in diameter from about 1 to 100 microns. The outer *cell membrane* (*syn plasma membrane*) is a double layer of lipid with embedded protein molecules. These include: molecules that embody enzymes involved in transport across the membrane; receptor molecules which selectively bind hormones, drugs and other agents, mediating their signal to the cell; and others with water-filled pores that allow exchange across the cell membrane of water, ions and small molecules, related to concentration and electrical gradients. The enclosed *cytoplasm* contains the intracellular fluid and a great number and variety of structures, some surrounded by their own membrane, including the *nucleus* containing the **chromosomes** that carry the **genes**, and **mitochondria** in all cells where oxidative

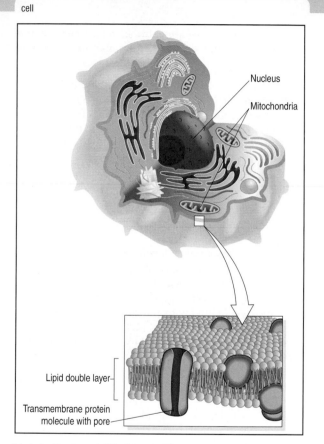

Nucleus

Mitochondria

Lipid double layer

Transmembrane protein
molecule with pore

A typical cell and a part of its plasma membrane.

metabolism occurs. *See also* **membrane potential, potassium, sodium, sodium-potassium (Na-K) pump**.

**cellulitis** diffuse inflammation of the skin and connective tissue. In sport cellulitis is usually the result of a traumatic break in the skin, often with secondary infection.

**central fatigue** contribution of the central nervous system to the overall condition of **fatigue** in physical activity. Mainly significant in prolonged exercise, such as marathon running, where voluntary effort declines before muscle glycogen is exhausted and other peripheral indicators (heart rate, blood lactate, blood glucose, etc.) do not suggest particular stress. There is evidence that elevated **serotonin** (5-HT) and/or reduced **dopamine** levels in the brain are involved.

**central nervous system** the **brain** and the **spinal cord**. *See also* **autonomic nervous system, peripheral nervous system**; *appendix 1.1 figs 1–4*.

**centre of buoyancy** imaginary point calculated by adding up the moments of the buoyancy forces of all segments of a body or object.

**centre of gravity (CoG)** imaginary point calculated by adding up the moments of the weights of all segments of a body or object. Usually the same as centre of mass (CoM) (except where gravity varies within a body or object, as for example in a tall building – gravitational force would be very slightly different over the height of the building, so the CoG and the CoM would be very close but not in exactly the same place).

**centre of mass (CoM)** geometric centre of a body or object. Its position can be calculated by the *segmental method* from the position of the CoM of each body segment and the mass of each segment. Usually the same as centre of gravity.

**centre of percussion** imaginary point on a pivoted object or body where translational forces are equal and opposite to rotational ones. Also known as the *sweet spot*. For example, if a shot with a cricket bat is hit from the centre of percussion then it 'feels good' because the translational forces and rotational forces are balanced.

**centre of pressure** imaginary point calculated by adding up the moments of the fluid (liquid or gas) pressure, or drag, of all segments of a body or object.

**centrifugal** literally, *'centre-fleeing'*. *centrifugal force* apparent (inertial) force on an object and *centrifugal acceleration* apparent (inertial) acceleration of an object, imagined by a moving observer who is rotating. For example, if a hammer thrower is rotating, all objects in his surroundings appear to him to be moving, i.e. to have centrifugal acceleration, whilst the hammer itself appears to stay still, yet he is having to apply a centripetal acceleration to keep it moving in a circle. Therefore, by Newton's first law there must be a balancing (centrifugal) acceleration, but this is imaginary since due only to the rotation of the thrower himself, whilst the hammer is not actually stationary.

**centripetal** literally, *'centre-seeking'*. *centripetal acceleration* a real acceleration towards the centre of a circle (or curve) due to change in the directional component of velocity. *centripetal force* a real force towards the centre of a circle (or curve) equal to centripetal acceleration multiplied by mass.

**cerebral haemorrhage** bleeding within the cerebral hemispheres of the **brain**. In sport cerebral haemorrhage may be caused by a **head injury** and can result in a deteriorating level of consciousness and possibly death. *See also* **Glasgow Coma Scale (GCS)**.

**cervical spine** the seven cervical vertebrae, through which the cervical part of the **spinal cord** passes from the brain to the thoracic part of the spine. Damage to the spinal cord at a high cervical level, where the phrenic nerves to the diaphragm originate, can paralyse breathing. Cervical damage in sport may result in **quadriplegia**, seen in sports such as rugby (collapsed scrum), trampolining and horse riding. *See also* **spinal injury**; *appendix 1.1 figs 2–5.*

**charley horse** the name given in sport to a **haematoma** of the quadriceps muscle as a result of trauma. Rarely it may develop areas of ossification, which prolong rehabilitation and may require surgery.

**chemoreceptors** neural receptors that respond to some local chemical change. Usually refers to those which influence the respiratory and cardiovascular control centres in the brain stem: the *medullary chemoreceptors,* sensitive to pH changes in the cerebral extracellular fluid, and the *arterial chemoreceptors* which continually sense and respond to changes mainly in blood oxygen, carbon dioxide and pH, leading to appropriate reflex adjustments via afferent nerves to the brain stem control centres (e.g. increase in ventilation if arterial oxygen tension tends to fall and/or carbon dioxide to rise). *See also* **breathing, hypoxia**.

**chest injury** in sport may be superficial, such as damage to the sternum or ribs, or more seriously to the internal organs, particularly the lungs, which can result in a **pneumothorax**.

**chiropody** *see* **podiatry**.

**chiropractic** a technique of spinal manipulation, based on the principle that defects in vertebral alignment may result in various problems caused by functional changes in the nervous system.

**choking** in sport psychology, a sudden inability to perform at one's normal standard. Associated with high levels of competitive sport **anxiety**.

**cholesterol** a sterol which is essential for the formation of cell membranes and for the synthesis of **steroid hormones** and bile acids. Some is ingested in foods such as egg yolk, but most is made in the liver. Circulates in the blood combined with high-density and low-density lipoproteins (HDL and LDL). HDL-cholesterol removes excess cholesterol from cells and transports it to the liver for excretion; LDL-cholesterol delivers cholesterol to cells of all organs and tissues. An abnormally high concentration of total and particularly LDL-cholesterol increases uptake of cholesterol by the cells of arterial walls, promoting atherosclerosis.

**choline** is promoted as an **ergogenic aid** to increase strength and/or decrease fat. No valid studies have confirmed these effects. *See also* **ergogenic aids**; *appendix 4.4.*

**chondritis** inflammation of cartilage.

**chondromalacia patellae** painful condition resulting from the softening of the patellar articular cartilage. Also known as *patellofemoral pain*. Common in young athletes (causing discomfort with exercise) where its origin is suggested to be an alteration of the **Q-angle** due to malalignment of the lower limbs. Seen in overpronation of the foot and valgus deformity at the knee. Treatment involves attempts to restore the normal Q-angle via a quadriceps strengthening programme.

**chromium** *see* **minerals**; *appendix 4.3.*

**chromosomes** carriers of genetic material in the nucleus of body cells. Each consists mainly of an elongated macromolecule of **deoxyribonucleic acid (DNA).** In human cells there are 23 pairs of chromosomes, each with a 'string' of hundreds to thousands of **genes**; one of each pair is derived from the germ cell (ovum or sperm) of each parent. One of the pairs are the *sex chromosomes,* known as 'XX' in the female, 'XY' in the male; splitting of the pairs in the formation of the germ cells in the gonads provides either an X or a Y chromosome in each sperm, so that combination with an X at fertilization determines the gender of the offspring.

**chronic fatigue syndrome (CFS)** state of severe physical and mental lassitude, related neither to excessive exertion nor to any apparent medical condition, although it may follow a viral infection. Defined as persistent fatigue continuing for at least 6 months (but often extending for much longer), accompanied by a specific set of symptoms including muscle and/or joint pains, which may last for up to 24 h after even mild exertion. Also known as *myalgic encephalomyelitis (ME)*.

**chylomicrons** *see* **lipoproteins**.

**cinematography** in biomechanics, the use of cine film for analysis of human movement, now less common than video analysis.

**circadian rhythm** physiological variations over 24 h, generated by a 'clock' in the brain (nerve centres in the hypothalamus, with input from the eyes); normally synchronized to the light–dark cycle, but effective even in conditions without cues from light or time. Influenced by the hormone *melatonin* from the pineal gland. Circadian means 'about a day'. Variables affected include body temperature, alertness and sleepiness, urine output, cortisol secretion. *See also* **jet lag**.

**circuit training** programme of mixed resistance, aerobic and flexibility exercises performed in sequence at a series of stations.

**circulation of the blood** the flow of blood from the left side of the **heart** through the *systemic circulation* via the branching arterial system to the capillary beds in all tissues except the lungs, and returning in the veins to the right side of the heart; thence in the *pulmonary circulation*, via the pulmonary artery and its branches to the alveolar capillaries in the lungs, and carrying oxygenated blood back to the left side of the heart via the pulmonary veins The pulmonary circulation is characterized by operating at lower pressure than in the systemic circulation. *See appendix 1.3.*

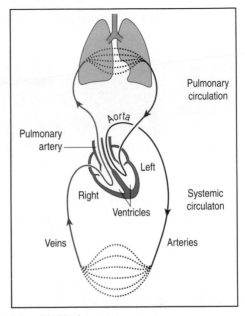

The circulation of the blood.

**circumplex model** any of a variety of models that have been applied to the understanding of **personality**, **affect** or other psychological domains whereby variables are arranged in two-dimensional space into a circular array and along two orthogonal axes. Elements that lie close together on the circumference of the circle are more related than elements that lie further apart and elements lying in opposite positions on the axes are negatively related. For example, a popular model of exercise-

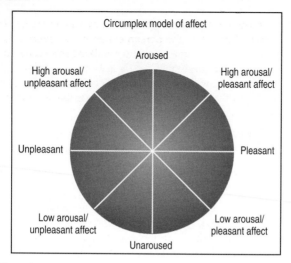

Circumplex model of affect.

induced affect conceptualizes affect as varying along two dimensions: valence (pleasant *vs* unpleasant feelings) and activation (aroused *vs* unaroused). Individuals can be located within the circumplex according to the combination of these two dimensions.

**citrate** *see* **buffering agents**.

**citric acid cycle (citrate cycle)** *see* **Krebs cycle**.

**claudication** (from *claudare*, Latin, to limp) limping, with pain, caused by interference with the blood supply to the legs, the result of atheromatous narrowing, blockage or, less often, spasm of an artery. More common in cigarette smokers and diabetics. Known as *intermittent claudication* when the person experiences severe pain in the legs (calves or thighs) after walking for a time but is able to continue after a short rest. Randomized clinical trials have shown that a graduated exercise programme will increase the distance walked before the symptoms are first felt.

**clavicle** the collar bone. Can be fractured in contact sports or with a fall on the outstretched arm. *See appendix 1.2 fig 1.*

**closed kinetic chain** exercise in which a distal body segment is not free to move.

**closed loop control** in motor control, a movement in which sensory feedback is involved in its planning, execution and modification. For example, when catching a ball, visual information concerning its trajectory is used to guide one's grasp. *See also* **open-loop control**.

**club foot** *see* **varum, varus**.

**coaction effects** *see* **social facilitation**.

**coagulation** *see* **blood coagulation**.

**cobalamin (vitamin $B_{12}$)** obtained from seafood, meat and milk products. Intestinal absorption of vitamin $B_{12}$ requires the presence of the protein known as intrinsic factor, secreted by the stomach. Red blood cell formation depends on vitamin $B_{12}$ and in the absence of *intrinsic factor*, $B_{12}$ deficiency causes pernicious anaemia. Vitamin $B_{12}$ is promoted as an **ergogenic aid** to enhance DNA synthesis and increase muscle growth in strength training, but research indicates no effect.

**cocaine** a powerful local anaesthetic obtained from the leaves of the coca plant. It is a controlled drug which is highly addictive and subject to considerable criminal misuse. Toxic, especially to the brain; may cause agitation, disorientation and convulsions. *crack cocaine* a highly potent and addictive form. Cocaine is on the **WADA** list of banned substances in sport.

**coccyx** the last bone of the vertebral column. Composed of four or five rudimentary vertebrae, cartilaginous at birth, ossification and fusion not being complete until the age of 25–30. *coccydynia* pain in the region of the coccyx; in sport, usually the result of a fall. *coccygeal adj. See appendix 1.2 fig 2.*

**coefficient of friction** *see* **friction**.

**coefficient of restitution** dimensionless (no units) number representing the ratio of separation velocity to approach velocity after impact of two bodies or objects. Dependent on elasticity of the objects. For example, during impact of a golf ball on a golf club face, ball and club deform and then rebound, which means that the ball increases its velocity. Likewise with a ball and racquet strings.

**coenzyme Q10** also known as *ubiquinone*, a non-essential lipid-soluble nutrient found predominantly in animal foods and at low levels in plant foods. In the body it is located primarily in the mitochondria, especially in skeletal and cardiac muscle. As a component of the electron transport chain, it is important for ATP formation. It is also believed to have an **antioxidant** function, protecting DNA and cell membranes from oxidative damage. For athletes, coenzyme Q10 supplements are claimed to enhance energy production through the electron transport chain, and to reduce the oxidative damage of exercise. Research does not support the claim, reporting either no effect or in some cases an ergolytic rather than ergogenic effect. *See also* **ergogenic aids**; *appendix 4.4.*

**cognition** the psychological processes by which individuals acquire and process information, generally applied to thought processes and memory. *cognitive psychology* the branch of psychology concerned with the study of cognition.

**cognitive anxiety** *see* **anxiety.**

**cognitive behaviour therapy (CBT)** a form of psychotherapy combining elements of cognitive therapy and behaviour therapy which aims to modify dysfunctional patterns of thinking and self-talk in order to resolve a variety of mental and social health problems. Also known as *cognitive behaviour modification*.

**cognitive dissonance** a subjective state of psychological tension induced when a person holds two or more cognitions that are inconsistent. For example, a person might hold the cognition that they enjoy smoking whilst at the same time believing that smoking is harmful to their health. It is proposed that such dissonant states motivate one of three kinds of behaviour to reduce the dissonance: changing one of the cognitions (for example, by changing the behaviour associated with it, such as giving up smoking); dismissing the importance of one of the cognitions (for example, by telling oneself that smoking is not that bad for one's health); or by adding a justifying cognition (for example, by telling oneself that one does not smoke too much).

**cognitive interview** a structured interview designed to facilitate recall of an event by the use of a variety of memory-enhancing techniques.

**cognitive restructuring** *see* **reframing**.

**cognitive skills** *see* **mental skills**.

**cognitive stress** *see* **anxiety**.

**cognitive therapy** a form of psychotherapy designed to modify dysfunctional beliefs and thinking styles based on the assumption that mental health problems such as depression are the result of faulty or distorted perceptions of oneself or the world. *See also* **cognitive behaviour therapy**.

**cold, exposure to** *see* **body temperature**, **hypothermia**.

**colinear forces** forces that have the same line of action.

**collagen** *see* **connective tissue**.

**collar bone** *see* **clavicle**.

**Colles' fracture** a break at the lower end of the radius following a fall on the outstretched hand. The backward displacement of the hand produces the 'dinner fork' deformity. A common fracture in older women and associated with osteoporosis (first described by Abraham Colles, an 18th-century Irish surgeon).

**collision sport** individual or team sports during which the participants use their bodies to deter or block opponents, thereby relying on the physical dominance of one athlete over another.

**coma** a state of unrousable unconsciousness, of which the severity can be assessed by testing the reflex responses to various stimuli. *comatose adj. See also* **Glasgow Coma Scale (GCS)**, **recovery position**.

**coma position** *see* **recovery position**.

**compartment syndrome** effects of increased pressure due to swelling of groups of lower leg muscles confined by fibrous sheets of fascia which restrict expansion within the different compartments. *acute compartment syndrome* swelling leading to ischaemia and potential necrosis of muscle tissue. May be caused by bleeding following injury. Treatment involves alleviation of the pressure with elevation and anti-inflammatory medication; may require release of pressure by surgical incision of the fascia. *chronic exertional compartment syndrome* often comes on with a particular predictable amount of strenuous activity, when increased muscle volume raises compartment pressure, impeding blood flow and causing pain which is relieved by rest. Many causes include repetitive overuse, muscle hypertrophy due to training, and foot conditions which alter lower limb biomechanics. *anterior compartment syndrome* pain on the front of the lower leg, down the outer side of the tibia, when (mainly) the ankle dorsiflexor (tibialis anterior) and toe extensors are affected. *lateral compartment syndrome* pain on the outer side of the leg when the plantarflexors/everters (peroneus muscles) are affected. *posterior compartment syndrome* pain in the calf when the muscles in the superficial (mainly the gastrocnemius and soleus) or the deep compartment (tibialis posterior and toe flexors) are involved.

**competence** the ability to perform a task effectively; *perceived competence* a person's perception of their general abilities within a given domain, such as in sport in general.

**compliance** (1) in psychology, the extent to which a person follows a prescribed behavioural regimen, such as exercise, *see also* **adherence**; (2) with reference to the lungs, the ease of inflation, diminished in chronic obstructive lung disease.

**compound fracture** *see* **fracture**.

**computed tomography (CT)** used in sports medicine to image the internal structure of joints (e.g. meniscal tears) or to ascertain the extent of brain damage following a head injury.

**concentric contraction** *(concentric action)* the 'true' form of contraction of a muscle in which it shortens against a load (which may be only that of gravity on the relevant body part), and so does positive work. Hence *concentric exercise:* that in which the principal agonists act concentrically. *See also* **muscle contraction.**

**concurrent forces** forces that act at the same point.

**concussion** a temporary impairment of consciousness caused by a blow to the head, followed by **amnesia** for the impact and for a variable period after it. Most common in contact sports, such as boxing or rugby, or where a fall is likely, such as horse riding. *See also* **Glasgow Coma Scale (GCS).**

**conditioning** (1) the process of learning through which a response becomes dependent on the occurrence of a stimulus. *classical conditioning* the process of learning through which an initially neutral stimulus comes to elicit a *conditioned (or conditional) response* following repeated pairings with an unconditioned (or unconditional) stimulus. For example, in Pavlov's experiments with dogs, after repeated pairings with an unconditioned stimulus (food) the sound of a bell (a neutral stimulus) becomes a conditioned stimulus to evoke a conditioned salivation response. *operant conditioning* the process of learning through which the frequency of a response increases as a result of the provision of a reward or reinforcement for its occurrence. (2) In sport and exercise usage, 'conditioning' often refers broadly to physical training, particularly **muscle conditioning.** *See also* **unconditioned response**, **unconditioned stimulus**.

**connective tissues** tissues with a variety of functions including support, protection and partitioning around and within body structures. Different types vary from delicate networks to tough bands and sheets. All have cells within some type of matrix, which they form, and which may be mainly fibrous, cartilaginous, bony or fluid. Bundles of white *collagen fibres* (containing the protein *collagen*), strong and only slightly extensible, provide a supporting network in organs and tissues everywhere in the body (except the central nervous system) and in the sheaths and membranes that surround or separate them, form the basis of tendons and ligaments and are components of **cartilage** and **bone**. Extensible *elastic fibres* (containing the protein *elastin*) form networks, e.g. in the walls of arteries and in the lungs, and are a component of flexible cartilage (such as in the nose and ears); *reticular fibres* form delicate networks, e.g. in the skin deep to the epidermis, and in the walls of small blood vessels. The cells associated with all these fibres are known as *fibroblasts* or, when inactive, *as fibrocytes*. **adipose tissue** is a connective tissue with a fibrous stroma, widely distributed internally as well as subcutaneously; its cells, *adipocytes*, are closely related to fibrocytes; likewise the *osteocytes* in bone and *chondrocytes* in cartilage. Also classified as connective tissue are the various cells in the tissue interstices (e.g. macrophages) and in the blood.

**conscientiousness** one of the **big five** personality factors characterized by a tendency to be organized, thorough and reliable.

**conservation of energy** general principle that the total energy of a system (object or body) and its surroundings does not change, but varies in its different components.

**constructivism** in the philosophy of science, the doctrine that people actively construct their reality on the basis of their beliefs and expectations. Also known as *constructionism*. **constructivist** a person who espouses constructivism.

**contact force** the force due to contact between two objects or bodies.

**contact sport** sport in which forceful contact between opponents is an integral and frequent factor, e.g. boxing, rugby.

**contraceptive, oral** medication to prevent pregnancy, known commonly as 'the pill'. Used in sport to manipulate the menstrual cycle to avoid menses during competition or to control irregular or heavy periods.

**contraction of muscle** *see* **muscle contraction**.

**controlled processing** information processing that requires conscious attention, especially as in the execution of a novel or difficult task. *See also* **automatic processing**.

**contusion** a common injury in sport, the result of direct contact without the skin being broken. If superficial, it will result in visible bruising. If deep, a **haematoma** will develop within the affected tissue, commonly muscle.

**coordinates** numbers specifying the position of an object or body. *Cartesian coordinates* are specified on axes that are orthogonal (at right angles) to each other (usually X, Y and Z or i, j and k). *polar coordinates* are specified by an angle (degrees) and a distance from a fixed point.

**coplanar forces** forces acting in the same plane.

**core stability** the ability to control the movement and position of the muscles of the central 'core' of the body which are responsible for posture and limb movement. These include the muscle groups of the lower back and abdomen. Good core stability will allow the sportsman/woman to maximize their sporting performance and minimize injury risk. A well-conditioned core will control and increase the power of muscle movement, resulting in more efficient and coordinated limb movement and limiting potential injury by excessive or abnormal loads. Core stability is improved through a regular and repeated exercise programme, which does not require any equipment.

**core temperature** *see* **body temperature**.

**Cori cycle** recycles **lactate** produced by muscle during anaerobic glycolysis. The lactate is released to the blood, taken up by the liver and converted back to glucose, which is released again to be used by muscle.

**coronary artery disease** also known as *coronary heart disease* or *ischaemic heart disease*. Includes angina pectoris and myocardial infarction. A deficient supply of oxygenated blood to the myocardium causes central chest pain of varying intensity that may radiate to arms and jaw. The blood vessels are usually narrowed by atheromatous plaques. Commonest cause of **sudden death** in sport in those over 45 years. *See also* **angina pectoris**, **cardiac rehabilitation**.

**corroborating evidence** generally, any evidence which tallies with the predictions of a hypothesis or theory. For the strict proponent of **falsificationism**, however, only a prediction unique to the theory concerned corroborates it.

**cortex** from the Latin meaning 'bark' – the outer layer of an organ, e.g. of the adrenal glands, the kidneys, parts of the brain (cerebral cortex, cerebellar cortex). *adj* **cortical**.

**corticosteroids** the **glucocorticoid** and **mineralocorticoid** hormones secreted by the adrenal cortex. *See also* **adrenal glands**, **aldosterone**, **hormones** *(table)*, **steroid hormones**.

**cortisol** *syn hydrocortisone see* **glucocorticoids**.

**couple** two moments applied in the same rotational direction to a rotating object or body. Also known as *force couple*.

**cramp** specific form of spasm: involuntary, sustained and painful muscle contraction, particularly in the legs, often associated with fatigue and usually relieved by stretching. *exercise-associated muscle cramp (EAMC)* occurs mainly during or after prolonged or high-intensity running; formerly blamed on salt and/or water deficiency or overheating, but more recently attributed to fatigue-enhanced input from muscle spindles that overactivates spinal motor neurons, whilst suppressing the **Golgi tendon organs** which are normally inhibitory. *nocturnal cramp* occasionally disturbing sleep, particularly in older people; remains unexplained.

**cranial nerves** twelve pairs of nerves (sensory, motor or mixed) that originate in the brain stem; includes those serving the 'special senses' of hearing and balance, vision, taste and smell.

**creatine (Cr)** nitrogenous organic compound, held primarily in skeletal muscle. Obtained from a normal diet (mainly in meat and eggs) and also synthesized from amino acids in the liver. In resting conditions, about 60% is in the phosphorylated form, creatine phosphate (CrP). Cr + CrP constitute the *creatine pool*. Creatine is the fastest selling **ergogenic aid** among athletes; *creatine supplementation* aims to increase the CrP energy reserve, delaying creatine phosphate (CrP) depletion and hence reducing requirement for anaerobic glycolysis; also facilitating CrP resynthesis between bouts of high-intensity exercise, enhancing performance during multiple repeats. When supplementation is combined with resistance training, leads to greater gain in muscle mass. A typical protocol involves daily Cr intake of 20–25 g for 5 days, then continued daily supplementation with 2–3 g. The response varies between individuals, with uptake inversely related to the initial muscle concentration, and ~30% appearing to be 'non-responders'. *See also* **ergogenic aids**; *appendix 4.4.*

**creatine kinase (CK)** *syn creatine phosphokinase (CPK)* enzyme which catalyses transfer of phosphate group from creatine phosphate to ADP, producing ATP and creatine. Occurs as three isoenzymes, originating in brain, skeletal muscle and cardiac muscle. *creatine kinase test* estimates the myocardial isoenzyme in the blood: an increased level indicates acute myocardial infarction. If the test follows strenuous exercise, especially if it had a large eccentric component, distinction from the skeletal muscle isoenzyme is critical. *See also* **muscle enzymes**.

**creatine phosphate (CrP)** provides muscle with a reservoir of 'high-energy' phosphate for the rapid rephosphorylation of ADP to ATP during high-intensity exercise. Other functions of CrP are the buffering of hydrogen ions produced during anaerobic glycolysis, and the transport of ATP, generated by aerobic metabolism, from mitochondria to cytoplasm where it can be utilized in contraction and other cellular processes. Also known as *phosphocreatine (PCr)*.

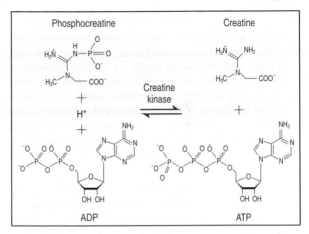

Phosphocreatine / Creatine

Creatine kinase reaction.

**creatinine** breakdown product of creatine in muscle, released into the blood and filtered out by the kidneys; measurements in blood and urine are used as an indicator of renal function. Blood level of creatinine is related to muscle mass.

**crepitus** the creaking or grinding noise heard over an injured or damaged joint (such as in **osteoarthritis**).

**critical power** if the tolerable duration of high-intensity exercise is plotted (horizontal axis) against a direct or indirect measure of power output (e.g. running speed: vertical axis), starting at the top end (maximum aerobic power, $\dot{V}O_{2\,max}$), a power output will be found at which endurance extends into a plateau. This is termed the critical power and in a trained endurance athlete, may last several tens of minutes.

**cross-bridge (XB)** in full *(actin-)myosin cross-bridge* in **muscle**, strictly refers to the molecular structure consisting of a **myosin** head-group bound to an **actin** molecule. Widely, though loosely, also used for the head-group alone, particularly when seen as an ultrastructural component in a striated muscle fibre. *cross-bridge cycle* cycle of force-generating attachment/detachment interactions between myosin head-groups and actin, powered by the hydrolysis of ATP. *See also* **length–tension relationship**, **muscle contraction**, **myosin**; *appendix 1.2.*

**crossover concept** refers to the intensity during graded exercise at which the contribution of fat to ATP production becomes matched by that of carbohydrate. At intensities above this point, carbohydrates become increasingly more important. (Term introduced by Brooks & Mercer 1994.)

**cruciate ligaments** two intracapsular ligaments of the knee, forming an X-shape, linking the femur to the tibia, strong but not elastic, which are crucial for the stability of the **knee joint**. The *anterior cruciate ligament* runs upwards, backwards and laterally from the front of the upper end of the tibia to attach to the medial aspect of the lateral femoral condyle; it limits forward movement of the tibia relative to the femur and tightens with extension at the knee. It is short and thick with a poor blood supply. The *posterior cruciate ligament* arises from the posterior intercondylar area of the tibia and runs forwards, upwards and medially to attach to the anterolateral surface of the medial femoral condyle. It limits backwards movement of the tibia relative to the femur and tightens with flexion at the knee.

*cruciate ligament injury* (especially anterior) can result in a rapid accumulation of blood in the knee joint (hae-marthrosis) and is often associated with damage to other structures, especially the medial meniscus. Treatment depends on the sport involved, the degree of instability and of other damage. In sportspeople complete rupture usually requires surgical repair, resulting in a lengthy (up to 9 months) rehabilitation programme, before return to sport. Disruption of only the posterior ligament may result in significant instability but may be hard to diagnose clinically. *See also* **drawer sign**, **Lachman test**.

**cryotherapy** the use of cold in the treatment of sporting injuries. Part of the **RICE** regime. Local application of cold will reduce bleeding and swelling and limit tissue damage, resulting in an earlier return to activity.

**cycle ergometer** a fixed cycling machine used in fitness testing to estimate the exercise intensity (power output) from the rpm and the resistance to pedalling, which can be adjusted to vary the intensity.

**cytochromes** heme-containing proteins in the electron transport chain that can be alternately in an oxidized or reduced state. *See also* **oxidative phosphorylation**.

**cytoplasmic energy state** *see* **phosphorylation potential**.

# D

**dead space** in human anatomy and physiology, refers to the respiratory passages (airways) leading to the alveoli of the lungs, so named because the air breathed in and out of this space does not reach the alveoli and so takes no part in gas exchange with the blood; *dead space ventilation* the volume of gas breathed in and out of the dead space per minute, normally about one-third of the total **ventilation** (minute volume) at rest, becoming a smaller fraction as tidal volume increases in exercise.

**deceleration** a change in motion of an object or body usually understood as the rate of reduction in speed (although it can also refer to a change in direction). A negative acceleration.

**decompression illness** the adverse effects of uncontrolled return to normal ambient pressure following exposure to high pressure when surfacing from a dive or, less commonly, exposure to rapid reduction in pressure in ascent from sea level in unpressurized aircraft. Symptoms range from pains in the joints, chest and back, weakness or sensory loss, to paralysis and loss of consciousness; severe neurological symptoms can be life-threatening. There are two main causes: (1) damage to the lungs by expansion of the gas in them if a diver does not freely exhale when surfacing. Gas can leak into the circulating blood (air embolus) or into the pleural cavity (pneumothorax); (2) release in the tissues (e.g. around joints or in the spinal cord) of bubbles of nitrogen that was dissolved in body fluids whilst at the higher pressure. Avoided or minimized by using computed tables to control speed of ascent and frequency of pauses, in relation to the duration and depth of the dive. All types of decompression illness require oxygen breathing as a first aid measure, and urgent treatment for all but the mildest by recompression to the initial higher pressure in a *hyperbaric chamber,* so that nitrogen is redissolved in body fluids, then more gradually released and exhaled as pressure is allowed to fall. *See also* **diving**.

**deep friction massage** the use of massage to the deep soft tissues, which aims to break up scar tissue.

**defibrillation** the application of a direct current (DC) electric shock to arrest ventricular fibrillation of the heart and restore normal cardiac rhythm.

**degenerative disease** disease characterized by deterioration in quality or function of a tissue or organ. In sport and exercise, acceleration in the deterioration of a joint (e.g. knee osteoarthritis) is seen following injury.

**dehydration** in general, the process of removal or loss of water from a substance or body. For related terms used in the context of human fluid balance, *see also* **hydration status**.

**delayed-onset muscle soreness (DOMS)** appears 24–48 h after exercise: may follow severe unaccustomed exercise, particularly that involving **eccentric action** of the muscles.

**deltoid muscle** the muscle which covers the shoulder joint. Arises from the shoulder girdle, in continuity from the outer third of the front of the clavicle, the acromion of the scapula above the shoulder and the spine of the scapula behind it. From here the fibres converge to be inserted into the 'deltoid tuberosity' on the outer side of the humerus. A powerful abductor of the arm.

**density** the ratio of mass to volume. Measured in kilograms per cubic metre ($kg.m^{-3}$).

**dental injury** common in contact sports such as boxing and rugby.

**deoxyribonucleic acid (DNA)** a long macromolecule in the nucleus of animal and plant cells, which stores genetic information in its component **genes**, and instructions for their *expression* in controlling function and development. Each strand is closely linked to another in a *double helix*. There is also a small amount of *mitochondrial DNA* which carries only maternal genetic material, being transmitted in ova but not in sperm.

**depression** a mood disorder characterized by feelings of profound sadness. May be classified by severity, by the presence of somatic symptoms and by the presence or absence of psychotic symptoms. Cognitive symptoms include hopelessness, helplessness, guilt, low self-esteem and suicidal thoughts. *endogenous depression* not resulting from a reaction to a particular negative experience. *reactive depression* resulting from a reaction to a particular negative experience (such as bereavement, physical illness or loss of employment), also known as *exogenous depression*. Research has shown that a structured exercise programme can have a mood-enhancing effect similar (and complementary) to that seen with the use of antidepressant medication. *See also* **antidepressants**.

**derivative** the result of the calculation (usually with calculus) of the change of one variable with respect to another. Also alludes to the number of 'steps' of calculus required (e.g. acceleration is the second derivative of displacement with respect to time). *See also* **differentiation**.

**depolarization** reduction of the normal voltage difference between the inside and the outside of a cell. *See also* **action potential**, **membrane potential**.

**desensitization** (1) in psychology, a form of behaviour therapy in which an anxiety-provoking stimulus is repeatedly paired with a relaxation response, either in the imagination or in real life (the latter known as *in vivo desensitization*) in order to eventually eliminate the anxiety response and replace it with the relaxation response. In *systematic desensitization* a hierarchy of increasingly anxiety-provoking stimuli is established and each stimulus is paired with the relaxation response in turn, beginning with the least feared and working towards the most feared. Also known as *reciprocal inhibition therapy*; (2) in medical practice, treatment of a hypersensitive response to an allergen, by deliberate exposure to a very small, and then a gradually increasing, dose; (3) with reference to repeated dose of a drug, a progressive decline in its effect.

**dexamethasone** *see* **glucocorticoids**.

**diabetes** a condition characterized by excessive urine output and consequent excessive thirst and fluid intake. Most commonly refers to *diabetes mellitus*, a disease due to failure of pancreatic secretion of **insulin**, or to failure of its function in controlling glucose metabolism; the blood glucose level is raised (hyperglycaemia) and there is glucose in the urine. Diabetics who exercise need to achieve optimal blood glucose control and to be aware of the potential for exercise-induced hypoglycaemia.

**diaphragm** the musculotendinous partition between the thoracic and abdominal cavities, penetrated by the lower end of the oesophagus, aorta, vena cava and other vessels and nerves. Attached around its periphery to the ribcage and the vertebral column. The main muscle of breathing, controlled by rhythmic impulses from the brain stem via the phrenic nerves. Contraction flattens it, expanding the thorax, reducing the pressure inside the lungs and causing inspiration; in relaxation, it rises again to a 'dome', allowing passive expiration (this *diaphragmatic or abdominal breathing* is the normal pattern at rest: the abdomen protrudes as the diaphragm is lowered). Lavish blood supply and high oxidative capacity enable the diaphragm to sustain the major increase in the work of breathing during exercise, but at high intensity its demand for blood competes with that of the exercising muscles. Fatigue of the diaphragm (and of other respiratory muscles) has been shown to contribute to exercise

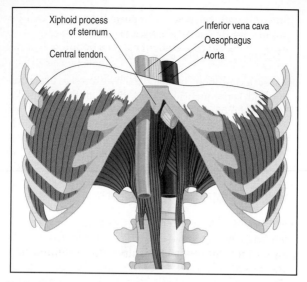

Xiphoid process of sternum
Central tendon
Inferior vena cava
Oesophagus
Aorta

The diaphragm.

limitation. Unique among skeletal muscles in maintaining its activity continuously for a lifetime under involuntary control, yet which can, within limits, be voluntarily overridden. *See appendices 1.3 fig 4, 1.4 fig 1.*

**diastole** the phase between beats when the heart muscle is relaxed, and the chambers are filling. *See also* **cardiac cycle**, **electrocardiogram**, **venous return**.

**dietary fibre** *see* **non-starch polysaccharides (NSP)**.

**dietary reference values (DRVs)** in the UK a set of tables that estimate a range of nutritional requirements for different groups of healthy individuals in the population. Three values may be used: *estimated average requirement (EAR)* about half of a population group will need more than the EAR and half will need less; *reference nutrient intake (RNI)* an intake of two standard deviations above EAR; this is enough or more than enough for at least 97.5% of people in a group, including those with high requirements; *lower reference nutrient intake (LRNI)* an intake of two standard deviations below the EAR and sufficient only for a small number of people (about 2.5%) in a group who have low needs. *See also* **balanced diet, energy requirement, recommended daily allowance**; *appendix 4.*

## Dietary reference values and intakes for UK adults

| | Recommended DoH 1991 | National Diet and Nutrition Survey 2003 |
|---|---|---|
| Energy intake (kcal) EAR | | Mean ± SD |
| Men | 2550 kcal/day | 2313 ± 582 |
| Women | 1940 kcal/day | 1632 ± 418 |
| % Total energy intake | | |
| Carbohydrate | | |
| Men | 50% | 47.7 ± 6.0% |
| Women | 50% | 48.5 ± 6.7% |
| Fat | | |
| Men | 35% | 35.8 ± 5.6% |
| Women | 35% | 34.9 ± 6.5% |
| Protein | | |
| Men | 15% | 16.5 ± 3.6% |
| Women | 15% | 16.6 ± 3.5% |
| Alcohol | | |
| Men | *5% | 6.5 ± 7.2% |
| Women | *5% | 3.9 ± 5.1% |

*Average intake, not recommendation

**dietary supplementation** *see* **carbohydrates**, **ergogenic aids**; *appendix 4.4.*

**dietetics** the interpretation and application of scientific principles of nutrition to feeding in health and disease.

**diet-induced thermogenesis** the energy required to digest and assimilate the food; measured as an increase in body heat production after eating. It typically represents only about 10% of total daily energy expenditure and is related to the type and amount of food ingested. Also known as *thermic effect of food*. Fats have relatively little thermic effect and proteins the most.

**dieting** any type of eating plan that aims at reducing body mass and body fat, and requires one to eat and drink sparingly or according to prescribed rules. Weight or fat reduction in athletes is generally motivated by a desire either to achieve a predesignated weight in order to compete in a specific weight class or category (e.g. horse racing, boxing) or to optimize performance by improving power to weight ratio (e.g jumping events, distance running).

**difference threshold** in psychophysics, the smallest difference between two sensory inputs that can be detected. Also known as *difference limen*, *discrimination threshold* or *just noticeable difference* (*jnd*). *See also* **absolute threshold**.

**differentiation** in mathematics, the use of calculus to compute the change of one variable with respect to another. Equal to the gradient (slope) of a graph of the one plotted against the other.

**diffusing capacity** of the lungs: the volume of a gas that moves across from the alveoli into the blood per minute, per unit partial pressure difference for that gas over the lungs as a whole. Depends, for any gas, on the total area and average thickness of the alveolar–capillary interface. Of most interest for oxygen, since it determines the efficacy of oxygen intake, but usually estimated in terms of the diffusing capacity for carbon monoxide which is more straightforward to measure. Increased in exercise as greater lung expansion both enlarges the area and decreases the thickness of the gas exchange surface.

**digestion** the processes which break down ingested food to substances that are absorbed from the alimentary canal into the blood or lymph. Catalysed by the digestive enzymes in the saliva, gastric juice, pancreatic juice and those secreted from the lining of the small intestine. These 'juices' together add up to a total of about 10 litres per day entering the gut. Apart from those that occur in the lumen of the gut, some further digestive processes are effected by the enterocytes, the cells in the lining of the small intestine. Depends also on other chemical processes, including for example emulsification of fats by **bile** from the liver.

**digitization** the conversion of an analogue variable to a digital one, i.e. a continuous variable into a set of numbers. Used in biomechanics to describe the derivation of co-ordinate data from video (or cine) pictures, e.g. plotting the **co-ordinates** of markers on the body.

**disability** inability to participate in activity at a standard level.

**disc, intervertebral** *see* **intervertebral disc**.

**dislocation** displacement of the articular surfaces of a joint, so that apposition between them is lost and the bony components no longer form a working joint. The cause can be congenital, spontaneous or traumatic, and dislocation may be recurrent. In sport, dislocations of fingers and the shoulder are the most common, as the result of collision with either an opponent or an object such as the ground or goal post. Replacement in position ('reduction') may be spontaneous but if not, it should be attempted early and only by a skilled operator.

**displacement** (1) change in position of a body or object, including size (magnitude) and direction of change, i.e. a vector quantity. *linear displacement* the distance and direction between the start and end point. Contains a measure of distance (e.g. metres) and a measure of direction (e.g. an angle in degrees to the horizontal) – effectively the distance and direction 'as the crow flies'. *angular displacement* the angle between the start and finish positions in a rotational movement, including a direction (e.g. clockwise or anticlockwise). Measured in degrees or radians. (2) the volume of fluid (usually water) that is moved when a body or object is immersed in it. (Displacement must be distinguished from 'distance moved' which includes only magnitude and not direction.)

**disposition** a relatively enduring tendency to behave or respond to situations in a typical way. *dispositional adj.*

**dissociative strategy** in sport psychology, a strategy used by athletes in which they focus attention externally in order to distract themselves from feelings of pain or fatigue. Also known as *dissociation*. *See also* **associative strategy**.

**distal (to)** in anatomy, further away from some reference point. For example, in a limb, further from the trunk: the wrist is distal to the forearm; the abdominal aorta divides *distally adj.* into the two iliac arteries. Opposite of **proximal.**

**distractor** in experimental psychology, a stimulus that diverts a participant's attention away from another stimulus that they are required to detect or respond to.

**disuse atrophy** loss of muscle mass due to inactivity. May follow a period of immobilization, e.g. bed rest or with a plaster cast. Prolonged disuse results in fibrous tissue replacing muscle tissue, limiting the extent of full rehabilitation.

**diuretics** substances contained in food and drink (e.g. caffeine), or given as medication, that increase the secretion of urine by the kidneys (*diuresis*). Used in medicine as a treatment for high blood pressure. In sport the use of diuretics for two main purposes is banned: as a means of losing fluid, and thus weight, in sports such as boxing and weight lifting, which have weight categories or in an attempt to increase the production of urine and thus the excretion of a banned drug, to avoid detection. *See appendix 6.*

**diving** (1) diving in swimming pools carries the potential hazard of neck injury, if the dive is too steep relative to the depth of the water; (2) in *scuba diving* the diver breathes compressed air from a cylinder, through a face mask and a closed system of tubes ('self-contained underwater breathing apparatus'). Pressure increases by 1 atmosphere (1 bar) per 10 metres of depth. Below 30 m the 'intoxicating' effect of *nitrogen narcosis* is a danger, avoided by the use of helium–oxygen mixtures. Hypothermia is also a hazard in cold climates; (3) in *breath-hold diving* the duration of immersion can be increased if the dive is preceded by vigorous hyperventilation. This depletes carbon dioxide in the body so that it will take longer to rise to the level which would normally trigger the break-point, but oxygen in the lungs and the blood can be depleted to the point of threatening consciousness. *See also* **barotrauma**, **cervical spine**, **decompression illness**.

**dopamine**  a neurotransmitter, especially within the brain, in pathways related to the co-ordination of movement and to behaviour and emotion; deficiency of dopamine in the brain is associated with Parkinson's disease. Its secretion from the brain into the hypophysial portal blood vessels inhibits prolactin secretion from the anterior pituitary. Also, in the adrenal medulla it is a precursor of adrenaline and noradrenaline, and is itself released as a neurohormone.

**doping**  the use of banned substances or methods (as defined and listed by **WADA**) in sport to attempt to gain an unfair advantage. Considered to derive from the South African word 'dop' for a stimulant drink first given to racehorses. The WADA list is an agreed table of both synthetic and naturally occurring substances considered to offer an advantage when taken during training and competition. Sportsmen and women take performance-enhancing substances for a number of reasons. These include the physical effects of the drug itself (anabolic steroids will allow the athlete to train harder, faster and for longer), the pressure on the athlete to succeed (from coach, family, sponsors, media and general public) and the direct effect on athletes themselves (to boost confidence, lessen anxiety, etc.). *See also* **banned substance**; *appendix 6.*

**dorsal** at or towards the back of the body (opposite of **ventral**), referring to the embryological history of the surfaces. In the '**anatomical position**' the palms face forwards and dorsal applies to the back of the hands and arms.

**dorsiflexion** movement at the ankle joint that points the foot up towards the leg, or movement of the toes that lifts them away from the sole of the foot (compare **plantarflexion**).

**double-blind study** comparison of the effect of a drug or other intervention in a group of subjects with that of a placebo (an inactive 'fake' substance or procedure) in a second similar group, when neither those taking part as subjects nor the investigators observing the effects are aware of the group to which any subject has been allocated, until after completion of the study.

**Douglas bag method** for measurements of pulmonary ventilation and respiratory gas exchange and hence estimation of energy expenditure (indirect calorimetry). The subject breathes via a mouthpiece or face mask and one-way valve, so that the expired gas is collected in a large bag over a recorded period of time; the volume is then measured and the gas analysed for oxygen and carbon dioxide content; the differences from inspired air allow calculation of the rates of $O_2$ uptake and $CO_2$ output. Described in 1911 by Oxford physiologist C.G. Douglas.

**drag force** a retarding force, acting opposite to the direction of motion of a body or object. Often caused by air resistance or friction. *form drag* the resistance force caused by the shape of a body or object which is moving through a fluid medium. *surface drag* the force, opposing the direction of motion, that is due to the interaction between the surface of an object and the medium through which it is passing (or that is moving past it). *propulsive drag force* the force used by sportspeople to propel themselves, usually by pushing against a fluid medium (e.g. swimmers or rowers).

**drawer sign** a clinical sign that describes the movement of the tibia relative to the femur and is positive if the relevant **cruciate ligament** is torn. The cruciates provide the primary stability of the knee joint. Disruption of the anterior cruciate will allow excess anterior movement of the tibia relative to the femur and posterior movement is a sign of posterior cruciate damage. For the *anterior drawer test*, with the subject's knee flexed to 90°, the hamstrings relaxed and the foot stabilized, the examiner firmly grasps the leg below the knee and pulls it so as to move the tibia forward; for the *posterior drawer test*, with the knee flexed to 80° and the foot stabilized, the examiner attempts to move the tibia backwards.

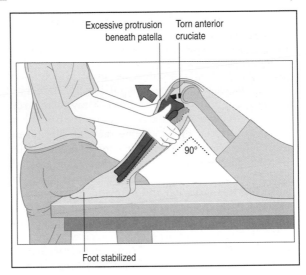

Excessive protrusion beneath patella  Torn anterior cruciate

90°

Foot stabilized

The anterior drawer test.

Excessive movement, compared to the other knee, indicates rupture of the ligament. *See also* **knee injury**.

**drinks** *see* **hydration status, sports drinks, water balance**.

**drive theory** a theory of learning developed by American psychologist Clark Leonard Hull (1884–1952) which proposes that deficits in physiological needs create a state of arousal that motivates the organism to engage in a behaviour to satisfy the need in order to reduce the arousal. For example, hunger motivates the organism to seek food. The linking of the drive state with the response that leads to the reduction in arousal produces learning of that response.

**dual emission X-ray absorptiometry (DEXA)** a scanning technique that is currently the most widely used method of measuring bone mineral density. The subject lies on a table and the scanner directs X-ray energy from two sources (increasing the accuracy) at the bone being examined. The greater the bone mineral density, the greater the signal picked up by the photon counter. DEXA scanning is more accurate than other methods (e.g. plain X-ray): quick, non-invasive, exposes the subject to less radiation and is relatively inexpensive. Estimation of bone mineral density is a good predictor of fracture risk and DEXA can be used to screen those most at risk (postmenopausal women, previous fracture victims, smokers and those on long-term corticosteroids). DEXA can also be used for a three-compartment assessment of body composition, estimating lean body mass, fat mass and bone mass. *See also* **osteoporosis**.

**dynamic contraction** muscle shortening which results in movement.

**dynamic exercise** exercise in which recurrent and substantial body movements predominate.

**dynamic flexibility** flexibility displayed during movement.

**dynamic friction** *see* **friction**.

**dynamics** the branch of mechanics concerned with the effects of forces on the motion of physical bodies. *See also* **acceleration**, **force**.

**dynamic strength** generally, strength displayed during movement; quantitatively expressed in terms of limb or trunk torque at a specified angular velocity, almost always during concentric muscle action.

**dynamometry** measurement of external force production by a human subject in a specific exercise such as knee extension or hand grip; may be performed either statically or dynamically, the latter in either concentric or eccentric mode, at a specified angular velocity. *See also* **grip dynamometer**, **isokinetic**.

**dysmenorrhoea** painful menstrual periods. *spasmodic* or *primary dysmenorrhoea* starts most often within a year or two after the periods begin, when ovulation has become established. *congestive* or *secondary dysmenorrhoea* occurs later and is associated with pathological conditions, such as fibroids or endometriosis. Painful periods can interfere with training programmes or affect performance in sport. Sportswomen often use the combined oral contraceptive pill to regulate or manipulate the timing of their periods (to avoid competitions) and control dysmenorrhoea and its symptoms. Moderate physical exercise can be helpful for relieving period pain, and may help prevent it.

**dysphoria** an unpleasant moodstate including feelings of anxiety, discomfort or uneasiness.

**dyspnoea** breathlessness, laboured breathing, to the point of discomfort or distress. *dyspnoeic adj.*

# E

**ear** the structures concerned with hearing and also with
**balance** and posture. (1) The *external ear* leads to the
tympanic membrane (eardrum) which separates it from
(2) the *middle ear*, where the chain of 'ossicles' transmits
sound vibrations to (3) the *inner ear* containing the sense
organs for hearing (the *cochlea*) and for movements
of the head (the **vestibular apparatus**). Afferents
from these pass into the brain in the *auditory nerve*.

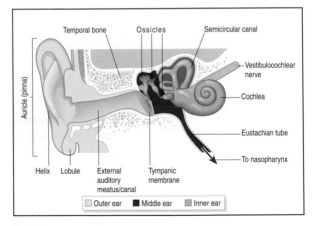

The ear.

The cavity of the middle ear is connected to the pharynx via the **Eustachian tube**.

**ear injury** usually refers to injury of the *external ear*, most commonly seen in contact sports such as rugby (especially in forwards) and boxing, and due to direct trauma. Lacerations and bruising are the most common. *See also* **cauliflower ear**.

**eating disorders** the key functional requirements for the clinical definition of an eating disorder are that the behaviour must no longer be under personal control and/or must cause significant adverse changes in psychological, social or physical functioning. The most severe eating disorders are anorexia nervosa and bulimia nervosa. *See* also **anorexia**, **bulimia**.

**eccentric action** active resistance by a muscle to lengthening, e.g. that of quadriceps during controlled descent of a hill or stairs. Also referred to, paradoxically and unwisely, as 'eccentric contraction' or even 'lengthening contraction'. Unlike a spring in the equivalent situation, a muscle expends energy even during such passive extension, as both excitation and cross-bridge cycling must continue, although this is a fraction of the energy cost of concentric actions generating the same force at the same absolute velocity. *eccentric exercise* involves the principal muscles in eccentric action. Because most (though not all) muscles can produce higher forces in this mode of action than in isometric or concentric exercise, greater training effects are widely considered to result, though greater muscle damage and **delayed-onset muscle soreness (DOMS)** may ensue in unaccustomed subjects. *See also* **force–velocity relationship**, **muscle contraction**, **work**.

**eccentric force** a force applied at a distance away from an axis of rotation, therefore a force causing a rotational moment (torque). Applies to all muscle actions at joints, whether the muscle itself is acting eccentrically or concentrically. *See also* **concentric contraction**, **eccentric action**.

**echocardiography** the use of **ultrasound** as a diagnostic tool for studying the structure and function of the heart. Used in sport primarily as a screening tool for the potential causes of **sudden death**. Echocardiography is non-invasive but requires expensive equipment and a trained operator. *See also* **hypertrophic obstructive cardiomyopathy**.

**efferent** 'going away'. Describes nerves that carry impulses away from the central nervous system, or from relay stations outside it, to effector organs or tissues, e.g. motor nerves to muscle, secretory nerves to glands. Also describes blood or lymph vessels in which flow is away from some point of reference, e.g. efferent arterioles leaving the glomeruli of the kidney; efferent lymph vessels draining lymph glands. Opposite of **afferent**.

**efficiency** the ratio of energy (or work) output by a body or device to the energy input required. *mechanical efficiency* the ratio of mechanical energy output (or work output) to the energy input.

**effusion** extravasation of fluid into body tissues or cavities, such as a pleural effusion, or into joints where it causes swelling. In sport a joint effusion is a sign of significant damage to the joint. A knee filled with blood, rather than with joint (synovial) fluid, is called a *haemarthrosis*, an injury requiring immediate care (e.g. cruciate ligament damage in the knee).

**ego involvement** a state in which the individual's goal is to demonstrate ability relative to that of others. *ego-involved* adj. *See also* **task involvement**, **performance goal**.

**ego orientation** a dispositional tendency to feel most successful in an activity only when one demonstrates one's ability relative to that of others, such as when one outperforms an opponent. *See also* **achievement goal orientation**, **task orientation**.

**elastic potential energy** the energy due to changes in the distance between molecules of a body or object, usually when it is compressed (e.g. a spring) or stretched (e.g. an elastic band). In animal (human) movement, important sources of such energy are muscles and tendons.

**elasticity** the ability of a material to be compressed or stretched, and to return to its original state.

**elastin** *see* **connective tissues**.

**elbow joint** 'hinge joint', allowing only flexion and extension, between the lower end of the humerus and the upper ends of the ulna and radius. The prominent medial and lateral epicondyles of the humerus provide attachment for the major ligaments on the two sides of the joint: on the inside to the margin of the concave notch on the ulna, and on the outside to the ligament

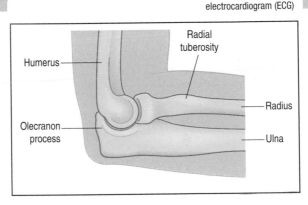

Right elbow joint, lateral view.

around the head of the radius. *elbow injury see* **tennis
elbow**, **golfer's elbow**; *appendix 1.2*.

**elderly** *see* **ageing**.

**electrocardiogram (ECG)** a recording of the electrical activity of the heart muscle during the **cardiac cycle**, as
transmitted to electrodes placed at specific sites on the
chest. The normal heart produces a waveform which
consists of five deflections known as PQRST, relating
to consecutive events in the atria and ventricles. *ambulatory ECG (Holter monitoring)* recording over 24 h to
detect any transient ischaemia or arrhythmias; the person continues with their normal activities, keeping a
record of their time and nature. *exercise (stress) ECG*
may be performed during increasing levels of exertion,
such as on a treadmill, to detect any abnormalities caused
by physical stress. Used for the diagnosis or prognosis
of heart disease or to monitor cardiac rehabilitation.

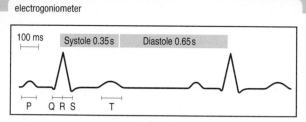

ECG at rest at heart rate 60 per minute.

In sport, used primarily as a simple and inexpensive screening tool for potential causes of **sudden death;** ECG is recorded continuously during treadmill and **cycle ergometer** fitness testing.

**electrogoniometer** a device for measuring angles (usually joint angles) directly, giving an electrical output (often interfaced to a computer). *electrogoniometry* the use of this device.

**electrolyte balance** the state of appropriate concentrations of ionized solutes in the body fluids. Exercise-induced disturbances in electrolyte balance are mainly related to either increase or decrease in concentration of sodium [Na$^+$], the most abundant cation in the extracellular fluids. Increase in plasma [Na$^+$] (*hypernatraemia*) is associated with depletion of blood volume by severe sweat loss and is common in athletes at the end of long-distance races. Exercise-associated decrease in plasma [Na$^+$] (**hyponatraemia**) is not uncommonly seen after prolonged activity such as a marathon where runners, aware of the importance of adequate fluid intake and rehydration, overcompensate with low-sodium drinks or excessive plain water (*water intoxication*). This can result in significant hyponatraemia, leading at worst to cardio-vascular collapse and death. *See also* **hydration status, potassium, sodium, sports drinks**.

**electrolytes** substances in solution in the ionized state, carrying an electrical charge (anions negative, cations positive). Applies to those in the body fluids, where dissociated sodium chloride is the major electrolyte in extracellular fluids ($Na^+$ and $Cl^-$), and potassium ($K^+$), with organic anions, in intracellular fluids. Other physiologically important cations are calcium and magnesium, and the anions bicarbonate and phosphate. Normal electrolyte concentrations are essential for normal cellular function. Movements of ions are crucial in the maintenance of potential differences across cell membranes and, for example, in the generation and transmission of nervous impulses, neuromuscular and synaptic transmission, and all secretory function. *See also* **minerals**; *appendix 4.3.*

**electromyography (EMG)** technique of recording electrical activity of muscle either percutaneously, with adhesive pad electrodes (more common but can only be applied to superficial muscles), or intramuscularly, through fine wires, usually of platinum, insulated except at their tips (records from a smaller domain within a muscle, but not necessarily a superficial one). EMG is used in both normal and pathophysiology to study the timing of muscle activation, as well as its extent, to which the resultant force generation is approximately proportionate. *electromyogram* the trace that is recorded. *integrated EMG* electronically processed modification of the direct signal from the electrodes. As muscle action potentials

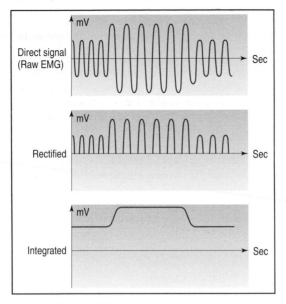

Electromyogram (diagrammatic).

pass under the electrodes they will each go positive and negative by turns, making a 'biphasic' (AC) signal; to integrate this, the signal is first rectified and then smoothed with a time constant such that the trace produced looks similar in form to a mechanical record of the resulting contraction.

**electron transport chain** a group of specific carrier molecules in the inner mitochondrial membrane that transfer electrons from hydrogen to oxygen. Electrochemical energy generated via electron transport is transferred to ADP to reform ATP. *See also* **oxidative phosphorylation**.

**electrotherapy** the use of electrical energy in the treatment of injury, relief of pain or other therapeutic applications to stimulate tissue healing and restore function. Though the exact mechanism of action remains unclear, electrotherapy is used in **physiotherapy** to enhance natural healing. Electrical stimulation has been shown to block transmission of pain and promote endorphin release. Different forms of electrotherapy, each producing different frequencies and waveforms, include **transcutaneous nerve stimulation (TENS)**, *short-wave diathermy* and *interferential electrotherapy*. The various forms are used, as appropriate, to treat injury to different tissue types and at different stages.

**elevated post-exercise oxygen consumption (EPOC)** *see* **oxygen debt**.

**elite athlete** world-class performer in any physical sport.

**emotion** a short-term positive or negative affective state. Typically differentiated from mood in that an emotion is of shorter duration and evoked in response to a specific event, such as anger.

**emotional intelligence** ability to effectively manage one's emotional life and to read and respond appropriately to other people's emotions.

**endocrine** related to internal secretions: *adj* describing (1) glands or organs that produce and secrete hormones directly into the blood stream; (2) tissues not in the form of discrete glands that produce and secrete hormones into local body fluids or into the blood stream; (3) the secretions of such glands or tissues; (4) the whole-body system or function that involves the production, secretion and action of hormones. *See also* **hormones**; *appendix 5*.

**endogenous** made within the body.

**endorphins** group of opioid peptides made in nerve cells in the brain and released from their axons as neurotransmitters or neurohormones, which bind to and activate opioid receptors of other cells (where opioid drugs also act). The first to be identified in brain tissue (1970s) were named *enkephalins*; many more were later identified. They are released in strenuous exercise and in stressful or painful situations. Subgroups have varied and widespread actions, diminishing the sensation of pain, inducing euphoria (e.g. 'runner's high') and interacting with the immune system.

**endurance** in general, the ability to perform physical work for a long time; quantitatively, the maximum duration for which an individual can sustain a specific activity, preferably also at a specified intensity. Used in isolation, the word usually implies whole-body endurance, considered in terms of many minutes or hours (*long-term endurance*) which is principally limited by cardiovascular fitness and muscle glycogen storage. *local muscular endurance* the ability of specific muscles to maintain power output or tension, influenced by similar factors but with local vascularity predominating over central cardiorespiratory performance. *anaerobic endurance syn short-term endurance* the ability to sustain whole-body work at 'supramaximal' intensity (i.e. above $\dot{V}O_{2\max}$), measured in terms of tens of seconds.

**endurance capacity** loosely, equivalent to endurance. Also used to mean aerobic power or $\dot{V}O_{2\,max}$.

**endurance training** prolonged training at relatively low intensity, aimed at enhancement of cardiorespiratory function, together with aerobic capacity of the exercised muscles.

**energy** the capacity to do work. Includes kinetic, gravitational, potential, elastic potential, heat, sound, chemical, nuclear. Measured in joules (J) or calories.

**energy balance** the condition when energy intake equals energy expenditure, so that there is neither increase nor decrease in body mass. *See also* **energy requirement**.

**energy charge** the ratio: $[ATP] + \frac{1}{2}[ADP]/[ATP] + [ADP] + [AMP]$ proposed by Atkinson in 1977 as an index of cellular energy status. *See also* **adenosine mono-, di- and triphosphates (AMP, ADP, ATP), phosphorylation potential**.

**energy expenditure** the amount of energy, measured in kilocalories or kilojoules, that an individual uses in a given time. *24-h energy expenditure* can be divided into three components: basal metabolic rate (BMR), energy expenditure of physical activity or thermic effect of activity (TEA), and the thermic effect of food (TEF). *See also* **diet-induced thermogenesis, metabolic equivalent, metabolic rate**.

**energy requirement** the energy intake that balances energy expenditure and thus in adults provides body mass stability. In children additional energy is needed for growth; also during pregnancy, for the growth of the uterus and the fetus, and in lactation for production of milk. In **elite athletes**, requirement is higher than in sedentary individuals since they easily expend 4100–8300 kJ/day 1000–2000 kcal/day) in sport-related activities. *See also* **balanced diet**.

**energy systems** those related to metabolic processes which yield energy for synthesis of ATP. These processes include **creatine phosphate** hydrolysis; **glycolysis**, which involves breakdown of blood-borne glucose or of muscle glycogen to either pyruvate (in aerobic conditions, when aerobic metabolism is possible) or lactate (when aerobic metabolism is not possible) and produces ATP by substrate-level phosphorylation reactions; **oxidative phosphorylation**, which involves oxidation within mitochondria of products of carbohydrate, fat, protein and alcohol metabolism to carbon dioxide and water.

**enzymes** proteins made in cells that act as catalysts, ensuring speed and completion of all intra- and extracellular chemical processes. Each enzyme catalyses a specific biochemical reaction involving a specific substrate, most but not all within the cells themselves. Others are secreted by cells for external action, e.g. the digestive enzymes released into the gut. Enzyme names usually reflect their function or their substrate, e.g. dehydrogenases catalyse the removal of hydrogen in oxidative reactions and ATPases, the conversion of ATP to ADP. *rate-limiting enzymes* those acting within a complex chain or cycle, but having very much greater sensitivity than others to excitatory and inhibitory influences, thus effectively controlling flux in the whole pathway. *isoenzymes (isozymes)* multiple forms of enzymes that catalyse the same reaction, but with some different properties. *See also* **muscle enzymes**.

**epicondyles** bony eminences on the sides of the lower end of the femur and of the humerus, which provide attachment for tendons around the knee and elbow joints. *epicondylitis* inflammation of the muscles and tendons around the elbow. Can occur if either the lateral (outer) structures or the medial (inner) structures are subjected to excess or repetitive stress. *lateral epicondylitis (tennis elbow)* is associated with racquet sports and weight training. *medial epicondylitis* (**golfer's elbow**, javelin thrower's elbow) an overuse injury associated with poor lifting techniques.

**epilepsy** a condition resulting from disordered electrical activity in the brain and manifesting as *epileptic seizures* or 'fits'. A *generalized seizure* or *grand mal* is the commonest form of epilepsy, with loss of consciousness and generalized convulsions. In *absences* or *petit mal* there is only a brief alteration in consciousness. When the electrical disturbance is limited to a particular focus in the brain there is a *partial seizure,* e.g. twitching of a limb, known as *Jacksonian epilepsy.* Other types include psychomotor seizures, with changes in mood, perception and memory as well as physical symptoms, such as nausea. All types can usually be controlled by appropriate drugs. There is some concern as to whether those with epilepsy should take part in sport and leisure activities but with a few exceptions and precautions, the majority should be encouraged to do so. However, particular care should be taken in uncontrolled epilepsy, especially with water-based sports (seizure while in the water) and those at heights, including horse riding (seizure leading to a fall). Scuba diving is not recommended. Boxing is not considered safe but other contact sports are possible, especially with appropriate head protection. Cyclists should always wear a helmet.

**epiphysis** the end of a growing bone. Separated from the shaft by the epiphyseal cartilage, which becomes ossified to form a solid bony connection when growth ceases. Before this is complete, the junction with the shaft can be confused with a fracture line on X-ray. *epiphyses* pl, *epiphyseal* adj.

**equilibrium** (1) in mechanics, a state when the force and moments on a body or object at rest or moving with constant velocity are balanced (i.e. the net force and net moment are zero); (2) in chemistry, the condition when there are no net changes in the concentrations of reacting substances and their products.

**ergogenic aids** agents that can enhance work output, particularly as it relates to athletic performance; taken as dietary supplements, with the aim of improving performance beyond that associated with the typical balanced diet; they primarily serve to increase muscle mass, muscle energy supply and the rate of energy production in the muscle, but the effects claimed for many of them are not supported by sound evidence. *See appendix 4.4.*

**ergolytic agent** one that decreases work output. Sometimes what is thought to be ergogenic for physical performance may actually be ergolytic. For example, depression of nervous system function by alcohol can profoundly impair performance in sports which require balance, hand-eye co-ordination, fast reaction time and in general any rapid processing of information.

**error scores** in motor control and learning studies involving the performance of multiple trials to attain a criterion such as hitting a target or producing a given force, error scores are used to quantify the deviations of attempts around the target. *absolute error* the mean deviation of the attempts from the target, disregarding the direction of the errors, used as a measure of accuracy; *constant error* the distance from the target to the mean of the attempts, taking into account the direction of the error, used as another measure of accuracy; *variable error* the standard deviation of scores, used as a measure of consistency.

**erythrocytes** the *red blood cells*, the main component of the microscopic 'formed elements' in the circulating blood, about $5 \times 10^6$ per mm$^3$($5 \times 10^{12}$ per litre). Contain the pigment **haemoglobin** which is essential for the uptake of oxygen in the lungs and its transport to the tissues; also for exchanges with the blood plasma involved in carbon dioxide transport and in blood buffering systems. *See also* **bone**, **erythropoiesis**, **haematocrit**, **leucocytes**, **oxyhaemoglobin dissociation curve**.

**erythropoiesis** the formation of red blood cells (*erythrocytes*) from stem cells in the bone marrow. Regulated by the hormone *erythropoietin* from the kidneys, where increased secretion is stimulated by reduced oxygen tension in the blood; a recombinant human form is used therapeutically to treat some types of anaemia.

**essential amino acids** *see* **amino acids**.

**essential fatty acids (EFA)** *see* **fatty acids**.

**euhydration** *see* **hydration status**.

**Eustachian tube** a canal connecting the pharynx with the cavity of the middle ear, opened by the act of swallowing, which allows equalization of the air pressure on the two sides of the eardrum. *Syn pharyngotympanic tube*. First described by Eustachi, 16th-century Italian physician/anatomist. *See also* **ear** *(fig)*.

**eustress** any kind of stress that is experienced as positive or that promotes well-being.

**eversion** with reference to the foot, tilting of the sole outwards. *eversion injury* damage to the medial structures of the **ankle joint**, by outward turning of the foot; the relative strength of the medial (deltoid) ligament may result in a fragment of bone being pulled off (avulsion fracture) rather than tearing of the ligament, and also accounts for it being less common than **inversion** injury.

**excess post-exercise oxygen consumption (EPOC)** estimates the post-exercise elevation in resting metabolic rate. The duration and rate of EPOC depend on duration and intensity of the preceding exercise, training status, environmental circumstances, gender and other variables. Although the contribution of EPOC to daily energy expenditure is negligible, it may contribute to the regulation of energy balance and play a role in body mass reduction or maintenance.

**excitation–contraction coupling** the link between excitation of muscle membrane and initiation of force generation at **cross-bridges**, producing **muscle contraction.** In all types of muscle this involves a rise in cytoplasmic calcium concentration [$Ca^{2+}$] but mechanisms for this rise differ substantially. In healthy skeletal muscle the **sarcoplasmic reticulum (SR)** is the sole effective source of $Ca^{2+}$ which (within normal physiological function) can only be released from the SR by a muscle **action potential (AP)**, triggered via the motor nerve. In cardiac muscle, the AP is spontaneously initiated in cardiac **pacemaker** cells rather than by nerves, and $Ca^{2+}$ release from the SR is triggered by $Ca^{2+}$ itself, entering the cell from the extracellular fluid during the AP. In certain smooth muscle masses, neural control mechanisms analogous to those of skeletal muscle operate but more commonly, hormones and/or other chemicals are involved; the $Ca^{2+}$ comes from both the SR and the extracellular fluid, as it does in cardiac muscle, but mediated largely by different mechanisms.

**exercise dependence** a dependency on engaging in exercise characterized by excessive amounts of exercising, often to the exclusion of other normal life activities, and feelings of guilt and negative moodstates when the exercise schedule is not adhered to. Also known as *exercise addiction* and *compulsion to exercise*.

**exercise-induced asthma** *see* **asthma**.

**exercise tolerance test (ETT)** also known as *exercise stress test.* An electrocardiogram (ECG) is recorded while the subject is walking on a treadmill or using a cycle ergometer. Patients with suspected or confirmed heart disease are studied using standard protocols, which allow subsequent results to be compared. Continuous ECG recording and interval blood pressure measurements are made throughout the test. Changes may be seen in the ECG that are characteristic of heart disease. This allows initial diagnosis to be confirmed, progress monitored and a risk stratification made for individual patients. *See also* **Bruce protocol**.

**exhaustion** *see* **fatigue**.

**expectancy–value theory** in psychology, the theory that behaviour is a function of the interaction between a person's expectancies about the outcomes of actions and the value they place on those outcomes. For example, a person might engage in regular exercise because they believe that exercise is good for their health and they also value good health.

**extension** a movement at a joint that increases the joint angle, e.g. straightening the leg at the knee or the arm at the elbow, moving the hand backwards at the wrist; or one involving several joints that brings dorsal surfaces nearer together, e.g. extending the neck to tilt the head backwards or curving the spine backwards. *extensor muscles* those with this action, e.g. triceps acting at the elbow, quadriceps at the knee. Opposite of **flexion**. *See appendix 1.2 fig 3*.

**external rotation** a movement at a joint that causes rotation of a limb or part of a limb around its long axis away from the midline of the body, e.g. external rotation at the elbow turns the forearm outwards, bringing the palm of the hand to face forwards, or the whole arm can be externally rotated at the shoulder; the whole leg can be externally rotated from the hip but the knee does not allow external rotation of the lower leg alone. Opposite of **internal rotation**. *See appendix 1.2 fig 3.*

**extrasystole** a premature beat in the pulse rhythm, due to initiation of the cardiac impulse at an abnormal focus. This *ectopic beat* is followed by a prolonged pulse interval.

**extraversion** one of the **big five** personality factors characterized by a tendency to be sociable, outgoing and assertive. *extravert* a person who manifests extraversion. *extraverted adj.*

**extrinsic injury** one which results from factors external to the body. Extrinsic factors include equipment, footwear, opponents or environmental factors (such as the sporting surface and weather), poor training methods (such as dramatic changes in intensity or duration or excessive load), poor technique and lack of warm-up.

**extrinsic motivation** *see* **motivation**.

**eye injuries** sport is the commonest context for injury to the eyes, most commonly those such as football, rugby, boxing where opponents' fingers or elbows may come into contact with the eyes or those where small balls or the implements for hitting them may do the damage (squash, hockey, golf). Wearing protective glasses can reduce the incidence of injury.

# F

**facial injury** injuries to the structures in and around the face including the facial bones; abrasions and lacerations, septal and auricular haematomas and other injuries around the nose, ears and eyes. Sport accounts for up to 25% of facial injuries. They can result from direct contact with another person, with equipment such as a squash racquet, a goalpost or the ground. Common in contact sports such as rugby and boxing. The incidence can be reduced by the use of protective equipment, e.g. hockey goalkeeper's face protector.

**falsificationism** view, propounded by the philosopher Popper and coming to prominence in the English-speaking world in the 1950s, that the hallmark of good science is to challenge every hypothesis or theory ('conjecture') by actively identifying and testing predictions which follow only from it, not from competing theories, one criterion of a good theory being that it gives rise to many such explicit, unique and so 'vulnerable' predictions. Failure of the prediction will then falsify or refute the theory; on the other hand, success of a prediction can be regarded as **corroborating evidence** but not as irrefutable proof, which is never possible. *aka refutationism*; contrasts with *verificationism*.

**fast muscle fibres** *see* **muscle fibre types**.

**fat** true or neutral fats belong to the broad category of **lipids**; they consist of one molecule of glycerol combined with three fatty acids to form a triglyceride (*syn* **triacylglycerol**). *dietary fat* may be of animal or vegetable origin. Vegetable fats with polyunsaturated and monounsaturated **fatty acids** are liquids (oils) whereas the animal fats, e.g. on a lamb chop, contain more saturated fatty acids and are solid. 'Fats' is sometimes used loosely to include other lipids. *See also* **body fat**.

**fat-free (body) mass (FFBM/FFM)** *see* **body composition**.

**fatigue** reduction in ability to sustain a physical or mental function as a consequence of the intensity and/or duration of the effort. Fatigue can last for periods ranging from a few tens of seconds to several days, its duration broadly correlating with that of the fatiguing activity, e.g. recovery from a 60 m sprint takes only a few minutes but few people would wish to run competitive marathons less than 7–10 days apart. *See also* **central fatigue**, **glycogen**, **muscle fatigue**.

**fatty acids** the main components of fat, consisting of straight hydrocarbon chains with the number of carbon atoms ranging from 4 to more than 20, although chains of 16 and 18 are the most prevalent. All fat-containing foods, and all fat or lipid in the human body, consist of a mixture of different proportions of (1) *saturated fatty acids (SFA)* which have only single bonds between carbon atoms, all the remaining bonds being attached to hydrogen. SFA occur primarily in animal products like beef, lamb, pork, chicken, cream, milk, butter. Coconut and palm oil, hydrogenated margarine, commercially prepared cakes, pies, and biscuits are also rich in SFA; (2) *monounsaturated fatty acids (MUFA)* which have one double bond along the main carbon chain. They are present in canola oil, olive oil, peanut oil and oil in almonds, pecans and avocados; (3) *polyunsaturated fatty acids (PUFA)* which have two or more double bonds along the main carbon chain. Safflower, sunflower, soybean and corn oil are rich in PUFA. *See also* **essential fatty acids**, **free fatty acids**, **omega-3 fatty acids**.

**female athletic triad** the combination of an **eating disorder**, **amenorrhoea** and **osteoporosis**. The signs may be hidden by the athlete, making the diagnosis difficult, though early recognition can be achieved through risk factor assessment and screening questions. Risk factors include being a competitive athlete, taking part in sports in which low body weight is an advantage (such as gymnastics) or endurance sports (such as distance running). More common in those whose sport takes up all of their free time, and who may be under pressure from parents or coach. Features include amenorrhoea for more than 3 months, fainting, loss of weight to more than 10% below ideal. Decreased bone mineral density can result in recurrent premature osteoporotic stress fractures, with normal density never regained. There is also low self-esteem, anxiety, excessive exercise and a preoccupation with food and weight management. Treatment requires involvement of the athlete, her parents, coach, doctor and nutritionist, and includes appropriate diet, exercise modification and psychological support and counselling.

**femoral** referring to the thigh.

**femur** the thigh bone – the longest and strongest in the body. Articulates proximally with the pelvis at the hip and distally with the tibia at the knee. Fractures of the femur can result in significant blood loss and clinical shock. *See appendix 1.2 figs 1, 2.*

**ferritin** an iron-protein complex, which acts as a store for iron. Found mainly in the liver but also in the spleen and bone marrow. Serum ferritin measurement is used as a marker of total body iron. *See also* **anaemia**.

**fibre** *see* **connective tissue, muscle fibre, nerve fibre, non-starch polysaccharides**.

**fibrillation** unco-ordinated contraction of muscle, referring usually to heart muscle. *atrial fibrillation* chaotic atrial rhythm with irregular transmission to the ventricles, causing irregular heart beat. *ventricular fibrillation* ineffective ventricular activity with failure of cardiac output. A common cause of sudden death following myocardial infarction.

**fibula** (Latin *clasp*) the smaller and outer of the two bones of the lower leg; articulates with the lateral condyle of the tibia at its upper end, and with the tibia and talus at its lower end. It is non-weight-bearing but assists in stabilizing the ankle. *See appendix 1.2 fig 1.*

**finger injury** *see* **dislocation, mallet finger, trigger finger**.

**fitness test** test performed to assess an individual's physical ability to undertake a specific activity, e.g. after recovery from injury.

**flexibility** the range of movement around a joint; dependent on a number of factors, including the size and shape of the bones, the ability of tendons to stretch, the condition of the ligaments, normal joint mechanics, soft tissue mobility and extensibility of the muscles. Good flexibility is beneficial in sport especially, for example, gymnastics and should be part of a sports-specific training programme and warm-up. However, flexibility training needs to be balanced with strength training to maintain joint stability. *flexibility assessment* can be made directly by measuring the angle of joint displacement using a goniometer, but this requires a skilful operator to achieve consistent results. More indirect measurements include the sit-and-reach or standing toe-touch tests. *See also* **hypermobility**.

**flexion** a movement which decreases the joint angle between two ventral surfaces of the body, e.g. bending the elbow or knee, tilting the head forwards. *flexor muscles* those with this action, e.g. biceps, hamstrings. Opposite of **extension**. *See appendix 1.2 fig 3*.

**flow** (1) the volume of a fluid (liquid or gas) moving per unit time, e.g. *blood flow* to or through a region of the body, expressed in mL per minute; (2) in psychology, a state of complete involvement and focus on a task that occurs when there is a perfect match between one's skills and the demands of the task.

**flow-volume loops** graphical representation of the relation between inspiratory and expiratory airflow and the change in volume of the lungs; used in the assessment of lung function with respect to patency or obstruction of the airways, e.g. in the assessment of **asthma**.

**fluid balance** *see* **hydration status, water balance**.

**fluid dynamics** the study of motion (strictly accelerating motion) in or of a fluid medium (liquid or gas).

**foot** as well as supporting the weight of the body, the foot works as a lever to move the body forwards. The many joints between the bones of the foot allow it to change shape to accommodate different and uneven surfaces. The skeleton of the foot consists of: the seven *tarsal bones*, including the heel bone (calcaneum) and the talus which articulates with the leg bones at the **ankle joint**; beyond these, the five *metatarsals* and, in the toes, the *phalanges*. There are layers of small muscles in the sole, and tendons from the lower leg traverse the ankle to reach their various insertions in the sole and on the dorsum (upper part) of the foot. *See appendix 1.2 fig 6.*

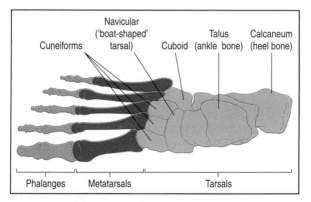

Bones of the right foot, from above.

**footballer's ankle** also known as *anterior impingement of the ankle*. Occurs as a result of repeated injury to the joint capsule and ligaments. Overstretching allows excessive movement of the bones with local inflammation and the development of bony outgrowths at the front of the ankle where the capsule is attached. These may break off, becoming 'loose bodies' within the joint, resulting in pain and tenderness across the front of the ankle and on bending the foot up and down.

**force** an interaction between two bodies, objects or agents which changes (or tends to change) motion either by contact or by action at-a-distance. May be a 'push' or a 'pull'. Note that a force changes the state of motion (including change from zero) but does not itself maintain an existing state of motion. *net force* the mathematical result of all the forces applied to an object or body, taking into account the size and direction of the forces. Measured in newtons (N). *See also* **inertial movement**.

**force couple** *see* **couple**.

**forced-choice** a test or experimental procedure where a respondent has to select a response from a limited set of alternatives.

**force development, rate of** the slope of a force–time graph, usually obtained from a force transducer (e.g. a force plate). May give information about how fast a muscle can develop forceful contraction. Can also be calculated as **mass** $\times$ **jerk**. Measured in newtons per second (N.s$^{-1}$).

**forced expiratory volume (FEV)** the volume that can be forcefully expired after a full inspiration, *aka forced* *vital capacity*. Measurement of the volume expired in the first second (*FEV₁*) as a fraction of vital capacity (*FEV₁/VC*) is used in the assessment of airways obstruction, e.g. in **asthma**. *See also* **lung volumes**.

**force plate** a device for measuring the force between a body or object and the ground (the *ground reaction force*). Often constructed from strain gauges or piezoelectric transducers. Also known as a *force platform*.

**force–velocity relationship** the relationship between force and velocity in a contracting muscle or isolated muscle fibre. In **concentric contraction** force is zero at maximum velocity and maximal at very low or at zero velocity (the latter being an **isometric contraction**). Between these extremes the *force–velocity curve* is approximately hyperbolic, as described by A.V. Hill in 1938. By contrast, in **eccentric action,** the form of the curve varies substantially between different muscles and in no case can it be adequately approximated mathematically. Thus in isolated, artificially stimulated muscles the force resisting extension rises well above the level in **isotonic contraction** as extension velocity increases, before falling off again at even higher velocities (*fig A facing*) but in intact muscles the resisting force is less than this, to the extreme that the knee extensors (presumably because they act at a joint which is vulnerable in the face of high gravitational stress) show an almost flat curve in untrained people (*fig B facing*), and only a modestly convex one in those who are strength trained. Commonly plotted with force on the ordinate and velocity on the abscissa, even though this might

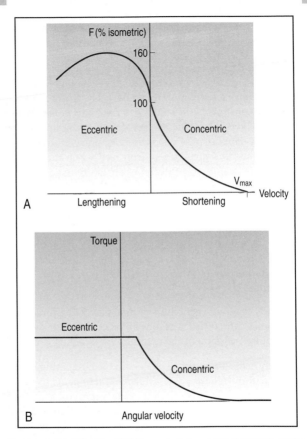

Force–velocity relationship. (A) F–V curve including region of eccentric activity. (B) Torque–angular velocity curve for human knee extensors in both concentric and eccentric actions, obtained by isokinetic dynamometry.

more properly be called the 'velocity–force' relation. *See also* **torque–angular velocity relation**.

**fracture** breach in continuity of a bone as a result of injury. Known as a *closed fracture* when there is no break in the skin or *open (compound)* when there is a wound linking the broken bone to the outside of the body; *comminuted* when a bone is broken into several pieces, splintered or crushed; *complicated* when there is injury to surrounding organs and structures; *depressed* when the broken bone presses on an underlying structure, e.g. brain or lung; *impacted* when one part of the broken bone is driven into the other; *incomplete* when the bone is only cracked or fissured, called a *greenstick* fracture in children. A *pathological* fracture can occur in abnormal bone (e.g. with a cancerous deposit) as a result of force which would not break a normal bone; also known as a *spontaneous* fracture when there is no appreciable violence.

**free body diagram** a method of analysis of the force and motion characteristics of a body or object by drawing a simplified version of the external forces acting on it.

**free fatty acids (FFA)** those present in the circulating blood and within cells; *aka non-esterified fatty acids (NEFA)*. Circulating FFA arise from **triacylglycerol** molecules of adipose tissue and triacylglycerol-rich lipoproteins. During endurance-type exercise a considerable amount of the energy released by contracting skeletal muscle is derived from oxidation of both circulating FFA and that provided by triacylglycerol stored in muscle. Theoretically, increasing FFA availability and utilization may reduce reliance on muscle glycogen and therefore delay onset of fatigue. There is therefore interest in strategies designed to enhance FFA oxidation (e.g. high-fat diets, caffeine, carnitine supplementation).

**free radicals** *see* **reactive oxygen species**.

**Freiberg's disease** osteochondritis (disturbance of bone and cartilage formation) of the head of the metatarsals (especially the second). Aetiology is unknown: both traumatic and vascular causes have been suggested. Most common in athletic girls aged 10–15. Presents with pain and local tenderness. Changes may not be evident initially on X-ray, but can be visualized on MRI. (First described in 1914 by Albert Freiberg, American surgeon.)

**friction** the force between the surfaces of two objects in contact, at least one of which is moving (or tending to move) relative to the other. *kinetic friction* friction due to motion of one object relative to another; also known as *dynamic friction. coefficient of friction* dimensionless (no units) number representing friction between two bodies or objects. Calculated as the force parallel to the object or surface (tangential force) divided by the force perpendicular to the object or surface (normal force).

**frozen shoulder** also known as *adhesive capsulitis*. Condition of unknown aetiology, which results from shrinkage and scarring of the capsule in a previously normal joint. Symptoms include pain (lasting months) with stiffness, inflammation and significant restriction of movement (lasting months to years), making everyday activities, such as dressing and brushing hair, difficult. Most common in those aged 50 + and may result from injury or be associated with a number of conditions, e.g. heart disease, thyroid disease or diabetes. Treatment includes adequate pain control and a daily exercise programme; **corticosteroid** injections and manipulation under anaesthetic are sometimes used.

**fructose** (also called *laevulose* or fruit sugar) is a six-carbon hexose. Fructose is the sweetest of simple sugars, present in fruits and honey. Some fructose is absorbed directly into the blood from the small intestine and the liver converts it to glucose; for this reason it is now being added to some energy drinks to provide a greater rate of carbohydrate uptake than can be achieved with glucose.

**fulcrum** the axis or pivot about which a lever system rotates (or could rotate).

**functional equivalence** the hypothesis that mental imagery functions in the same way as the physical perception. Thus, for example, if asked to scan between different objects within a mental image, it takes people longer to scan between objects close together than between objects further apart, just as it would if they were scanning between real objects in perception.

**functional residual capacity (FRC)** volume remaining in the lungs at the end of an unforced expiration, typically 2–3 litres at rest but decreases as tidal volume increases in exercise. *See also* **lung volumes**.

# G

**gait** style of locomotion, usually referring to walking or running. *See also* **step length**, **stride**, **support**, **swing**.

**gamekeeper's thumb** *see* **skier's thumb**.

**gamesmanship** in sport, the use of unfair tactics or methods, which are not strictly against the rules of the sport, in order to obtain an advantage over one's opponent(s), such as feigning injury or engaging in other time-wasting strategies in order to delay the game.

**gamma-(γ)-aminobutyric acid (GABA)** inhibitory neurotransmitter in the central nervous system, with a general calming effect, promoting relaxation.

**gamma (motor) system** the component of the motor nerve outflow from the spinal cord which innervates 'intra-fusal' muscle fibres (the fibres within **muscle spindles**). The *gamma (γ) motor neurons* have smaller cell bodies and narrower-diameter axons than **alpha (α) motor neurons**, which innervate the main working fibres of the muscle (extrafusal fibres).

**ganglion** (1) in anatomy: a small mass of nerve cells, outside the central nervous system, where synaptic connections relay afferent or efferent nerve impulses. **ganglia** *pl.*

*dorsal root ganglia* contain the cell bodies of sensory neurons, providing relay into the spinal cord, and there are equivalent afferent relays to the brain stem for sensory components of cranial nerves. *autonomic ganglia* provide efferent relay from nerve fibres from the central nervous system to the sympathetic and parasympathetic neurons that innervate relevant tissues throughout the body; (2) in pathology: a fluid-filled fibrous tissue sac that develops on a tendon sheath, especially around the wrist. A ganglion is usually painless but they can increase in size to become tender, unsightly or large enough to restrict movement; treatment is not usually required but they can be surgically removed if troublesome.

**gas exchange** in the animal kingdom, the uptake of oxygen and excretion of carbon dioxide, exchanged between the body and the environment *aka* **respiratory gas exchange.** In human physiology *pulmonary gas exchange* refers to the diffusion of oxygen from the gas phase in the lung alveoli, through the thin alveolar-capillary membrane, into solution in the pulmonary capillary blood, and of carbon dioxide in the opposite direction, both driven by partial pressure gradients. *See also* **blood gases**.

**gastric** *adj* referring to the stomach.

**gastrocnemius** the most superficial of the muscles of the back of the lower leg. It arises from the medial and lateral femoral condyles by two heads which join to form the inferior border of the popliteal fossa behind the knee. Together with its smaller accessory, the *plantaris*, and the *soleus* muscle (arising from the shaft of the tibia), it converges onto the **Achilles tendon**, to be inserted into the middle of the back of the calcaneum. It acts to plantarflex the foot and raise the heel when walking. Gastrocnemius and plantaris also act as weak flexors at the knee. *See appendix 1.2 fig 6B.*

**gender** (1) in general use, synonym for biological sex; (2) the socially constructed views of feminine and masculine behaviour within individual cultural groups. *gender identity* a person's sense of their biological sex. *gender role* the set of behaviours, attitudes and other characteristics normally associated with masculinity and femininity within a given culture or social group; for example, certain sports are stereotypically viewed as reflecting a masculine role (e.g. basketball) whereas others reflect a feminine role (e.g. netball).

**general adaptation syndrome (GAS)** the three-phase physiological response of the body to a stressor described in 1952 by the endocrinologist Hans Selye, of the University of Montreal. Comprises alarm, resistance/adaptation and exhaustion. The alarm phase is the short-term immediate response involving activation of the sympathetic nervous system. The resistance/adaptation phase involves the activation of the body's defences against the stressor. If the stressor continues and cannot be adapted to, the exhaustion phase ensues in which resistance to the stressor and ability to resist disease collapses.

**genes** agents of heredity, each located at a specific site as part of the DNA macromolecule of a specific **chromosome**, in the nucleus of body cells. *genotype* an individual's complete genetic endowment (specific *genome*) in

the form of DNA, which largely, but not entirely, determines the individual's unique characteristics, known as
the *phenotype*. *See also* **performance genes**.

**gene therapy** *see* **performance genes**.

**genetic potential** theoretical optimum performance capability which an individual could achieve in a specific
activity, after an ideal upbringing, nutrition and training.
In real terms it may be assumed that the finalists in a world
championship are among the human beings whose performance comes closest to their genetic potential. Also
known as *genetic endowment*. *See also* **performance genes**.

**genetic profiling** *see* **performance genes**.

**genu valgum (*bow legs*)** abnormal outward curving of the
legs resulting in separation of the knees. Associated
with hypermobility. *See also* **genu varum**.

**genu varum (*knock knee*)** abnormal incurving of the legs
so that there is a gap between the feet when the knees are
in contact. Associated with hypermobility. *See also* **genu
valgum**.

**ginseng** name commonly used for several species of
*Panax* herbs. A naturally occurring substance, not
banned in sport, ginseng has been suggested to have
performance-enhancing properties, though these have
not been scientifically proven. In addition, several preparations of ginseng have been found to be contaminated with banned substances. Side effects include
insomnia, depression and high blood pressure.

**gland** an organ or structure whose cells produce a secretion:
*exocrine,* delivered via ducts to the skin surface or an

internal surface, e.g. in the gut, or *endocrine,* passed into the blood stream. *See also* **digestion**, **hormones**, **sweating**.

**Glasgow Coma Scale (GCS)** reliable and universally recognized method for assessment of conscious level following head injury (described by neurosurgeons Teasdale & Jennett 1974). Three types of response are measured: *best motor response* (score 1–6), *best verbal response* (score 1–5) and *eye opening* (score 1–4). The lowest score is 3 (1 in each category). A GCS of 8 or less indicates severe injury, 9–12 moderate injury and 13–15 a mild injury.

**glucagon** polypeptide hormone secreted by alpha cells of the islets of Langerhans in the pancreas. Secretion is stimulated by a decrease in blood glucose level. It elevates blood glucose by promoting glycogenolysis and gluconeogenesis in the liver and also mobilizes free fatty acids from adipose tissue, having opposite actions at these sites to those of **insulin**. The ratio of insulin to glucagon secretion appropriately decreases in exercise.

**glucocorticoids** the group of **corticosteroid** hormones (mainly *cortisol syn hydrocortisone,* of which *cortisone* is the precursor) produced by the adrenal cortex, under the control of **adrenocorticotrophic hormone** (ACTH) from the anterior pituitary. Their major actions on nutrient metabolism have the net effect of promoting glucose and free fatty acid availability as fuels. Also vital for normal cellular processes as diverse, for example, as excitation–contraction coupling and the health of connective tissues. Synthetic steroids such as *prednisolone* and *dexamethasone* have similar actions and are used in the treatment of, for example, asthma and rheumatic conditions. Banned in sport due to their powerful anti-inflammatory action and effect of producing euphoria and masking pain. (Not to be confused with **anabolic steroids**). *See also* **adrenal glands, hormones**; *appendix 5.*

**gluconeogenesis** synthesis of glucose from non-carbohydrate precursors mainly in the liver and to a smaller extent in the renal cortex. Precursors include pyruvate, lactate, glycerol and the *glucogenic amino acids* derived from skeletal muscle. The *glucose-alanine cycle* involves the conversion of alanine, formed in muscle, to glucose in the liver; activity of the cycle is increased during the postabsorptive state and in starvation or prolonged exercise, slowly mobilizing glycogen stores and using protein for the maintenance of normal blood glucose concentration. Gluconeogenesis and export of glucose from the liver are promoted by the hormone **glucagon**, and inhibited by **insulin**.

**glucose** a hexose (monosaccharide) found in certain foods, and in the circulating blood and cells of all animals; of major importance as a source of energy in all tissues, and essential for some. Ingestion of carbohydrates provides glucose for replenishment and for accumulation of liver and muscle glycogen. When there is overconsumption of carbohydrate, excess glucose is used in the formation of triglycerides which are stored in adipose tissue. Glucose metabolism is mainly controlled by the hormones **insulin** and **glucagon**. The **glucocorticoid** hormones from the adrenal cortex and **growth hormone** from the anterior pituitary are also involved. *See also* **blood glucose**.

**glucose-electrolyte drinks** *see* **sports drinks**.

**glucose transporters** a family of membrane proteins that transport glucose across cell membranes down its concentration gradient, into most cells but out of the liver and kidney cells when gluconeogenesis occurs.

**glutamine** the amide of amino acid glutamate, synthesized in skeletal muscle. Glutamine is one of the major fuels of the gut lining, and of the cells of the immune system. It is also a precursor for the gluconeogenesis that occurs in the kidneys after an overnight fast or in starvation. Glutamine supplementation is popular among athletes attempting to maintain a healthy immune system during training. *See also* **glucogenic amino acids**, **ergogenic aids**; *appendix 4.4.*

**gluteal muscles**. *see* **buttocks**; *appendix 1.2 figs 4A, 6B.*

**glycaemic index (GI)** a ranking of foods based on the extent and rate of the postprandial rise in **blood glucose** that they cause, compared to the response to a reference food (either glucose or white bread); the higher the GI, the greater and more rapid the rise. Intake of carbohydrate (CHO)-rich foods with lower GI has been shown to be beneficial in improving glucose control, particularly in people with type 2 diabetes. Consideration of GI may also be relevant to athletic performance. High-index CHO-rich meals have been reported to enhance the storage of muscle glycogen during recovery from prolonged exercise. On the other hand, some evidence favours consumption prior to exercise of low rather than high GI CHO-rich foods, since high GI may elicit an inappropriate surge of insulin and/or attentuate fat oxidation, leading to faster depletion of glycogen and onset of fatigue. *See also* **carbohydrate intake guidelines for athletes**.

**glycerol** three-carbon carbohydrate; known as the 'backbone of triacylglycerol'. Blood glycerol concentration mainly depends on the rate of lipolysis of triglycerides in adipose tissue. Glycerol is an important source of glucose during periods of fasting or starvation. In sport, consumption of glycerol may be used for hyperhydration, as it reduces renal water clearance, increasing fluid retention and total body water. *See also* **gluconeogenesis, hydration status**.

**glycogen** branched polysaccharide formed of glucose subunits. Glycogen accumulation in liver and skeletal muscle is the principal way of storing ingested carbohydrate. The liver normally contains ~100 g (energy value 400 kcal) and skeletal muscle ~400 g (1600 kcal) of glycogen. It is also stored in the brain. The body's upper limit for glycogen storage is ~1050 g. It is known that aerobic endurance performance is directly related to the initial muscle glycogen and that perception of **fatigue** during prolonged exercise parallels the decline in these stores. *See also* **carbohydrate, carbohydrate loading, glycogenesis**.

**glycogen loading** *see* **carbohydrate loading**.

**glycogenesis** the formation of glycogen from glucose by the action of the enzyme *glycogen synthetase* in liver and muscle. Very active after depletion of muscle glycogen in exercise, making rapid restoration possible, provided that there is adequate consumption of carbohydrates. Even more ample carbohydrate supply can allow *glycogen supercompensation* – elevation in muscle glycogen content above normal. *See also* **carbohydrate loading**.

**glycogenolysis** removal of a glucose molecule from glycogen, by the action of the enzyme *glycogen phosphorylase*, present in liver, kidneys, muscle and brain. The products are a glycogen molecule that is one glucose residue shorter than before and glucose-1-phosphate. This in turn is converted to glucose-6-phosphate, from which free glucose can be released from the liver and kidneys (but *not* from skeletal muscle or brain) by the action of glucose-6-phosphatase. *See also* **glucose, glycolysis**.

**glycolysis** a catabolic pathway that breaks down glucose 6-phosphate, derived from glucose or glycogen, and in the process generates energy which leads to production of ATP. In aerobic conditions, pyruvate is the end-product. In conditions when oxygen cannot be utilized *anaerobic glycolysis* involves the additional step of reducing pyruvate to lactate. *See also* **aerobic exercise, anaerobic exercise**.

**goal orientation** *see* **achievement goal orientation, task orientation, ego orientation**.

**golfer's elbow** also known as *medial epicondylitis* or *javelin thrower's elbow*. An inflammatory condition affecting the common origin of the flexor tendons of the forearm which results in pain and tenderness on the inside (ulnar side) of the elbow at the medial epicondyle of the humerus. Most commonly the result of overactivity of the wrist flexors, especially with increasing intensity or duration of activity or poor technique. Treatment includes rest, anti-inflammatory medication, physiotherapy and corticosteroid injection. Prevention of recurrence depends on identifying training or technique errors which can be corrected.

**golfer's toe** an inflammatory condition of the big toe, which is thought to be the result of overextension of the toe of the back foot on the follow-through. Continued overuse can lead to arthritis.

**Golgi tendon organs** tension sensors in tendons that send afferent impulses to the central nervous system, causing reflex inhibition to counterbalance whatever neural influences, voluntary and reflex, are stimulating the contraction. Thus they guard against excessive tension generation (with potential tearing of muscle or tendon). In less extreme circumstances, which are more common and probably more important, tendon organs interact with muscle spindles to control limb stiffness. First described in 1898 by Camillo Golgi, Italian histologist and Nobel prize winner.

**gonad** organ that produces the *gametes (germ cells)*: ovary and testis.

**gonadotrophins** hormones secreted by the anterior pituitary, under the influence of the hypothalamus, which control the development and secretory function of the ovaries and testes. In pregnancy, ovarian function is under the influence of the placental secretion of *human chorionic gonadotrophin (HCG)*, which also acts on the fetal testis. *See also* **hormones**; *appendix 5*.

**goniometer** a protractor-like device, commonly with a 180° range, used to measure a joint's position when stationary, at any point over its whole range of movement. Used in practice to assess flexibility, perhaps as part of a musculoskeletal screen.

**graded exercise test** used to assess physiological responses to exercise, with its intensity increasing in incremental stages. *See also* **exercise stress test**.

**gravitation, law of** relates the attraction between two bodies or objects to their masses and the distance between their centres of gravity squared. First proposed by Isaac Newton.

**gravitational acceleration** acceleration caused by the gravitational attraction between two bodies or objects which depends on their masses and the distance between them squared.

**gravitational potential energy** the energy due to the position of a body or object in a gravitational field. Often calculated as weight multiplied by vertical height above some base (arbitrary) datum. Also known as *potential energy*.

**gravity** the force due to the attraction between two bodies or objects which depends on the product of their masses and inversely on the square of the distance between their centres of gravity.

**greenstick fracture** a fracture where the bone does not break completely, is essentially intact, but splinters like a 'green stick'. Occurs in children due to the flexibility of immature bone, commonly in sport with a fall on an outstretched arm.

**grip dynamometer** instrument for measuring the maximum isometric force with which an individual can squeeze two handles together between palm and fingers. Also known as *handgrip dynamometer*.

**groin pain** is most common in dynamic sports where quick turns are made, such as football, martial arts and skiing. The cause can be difficult to identify. Sporting causes include strains of the muscles in the area (e.g. the adductors, gluteal muscles, iliopsoas), bursitis, osteitis pubis and hernias. Abduction of the leg against resistance is restricted by pain. Because there are more serious causes of groin pain, a full clinical examination must be carried out if the pain is persistent. Treatment can be difficult and requires a formal rehabilitation programme to prevent a chronic condition. *See also* **groin strain**.

**groin strain** an injury which results from overstretching of the adductors in the groin, especially common in football. Requires a rehabilitation programme for both flexibility and strengthening. *See also* **groin pain**.

**ground reaction force** *see* **force plate**.

**group cohesion** a group's tendency to stick together in its pursuit of common goals. Also known as *team cohesion*.

**group dynamics** the ongoing social interactions and processes within a group.

**group environment** the task-related or social aspects of a group that can facilitate or undermine group cohesion.

**group integration** the beliefs that individual group members hold about the cohesiveness of the group as a whole.

**group therapy** any of various forms of psychotherapy in which individuals are treated together in groups.

**growth curve** a graph of change-in-height against age, which shows the greatest rate of change in infancy, flattening off until the *growth spurt* which on average reaches a peak at about age 12 in girls and 14 in boys.

**growth hormone (GH)** *aka human growth hormone (HGH)*, *somatotrophin*. Hormone secreted by the **anterior pituitary** under the control of GH releasing hormone (GH-RH) and GH release-inhibiting hormone (GH-RIH) (*aka somatostatin*) from the **hypothalamus**. As well as being vital for normal growth and development (e.g. stimulates the growth of the long bones), GH is involved throughout life in metabolism and utilization of all the macronutrients, e.g. it increases protein synthesis and raises blood glucose level. GH acts directly on some body cells (e.g. on adipocytes, promoting triglyceride breakdown) but mostly indirectly, via the anabolic *insulin-like growth factors (IGF) syn somatomedins* which it causes the liver and other tissues to release, crucial, for example, for the muscle hypertrophy resulting from training. For this reason supplements rich in **arginine**, which is believed (but without conclusive evidence) to promote GH secretion, are frequently taken by body builders. Any exercise of sufficient intensity stimulates GH release; its level in the blood has been shown to rise within the first 15 minutes and it is important throughout in maintaining lipolysis and lipid metabolism. Synthetic GH is commercially available, but banned in sport.

**gumshield** *see* **protective equipment**.

**gymnast's back** injury to the back, including fractures, due to excessive hyperextension during gymnastic activity.

**habit** (1) a tendency to behave in a certain way; (2) a well-learned behavioural response associated with a particular stimulus or situation, typically evoked without conscious intention.

**habituation** the reduction in the strength or frequency of a response to a stimulus due to repeated exposure to the stimulus.

**haemarthrosis** the presence of blood in a joint cavity. This may be the result of trauma or occur spontaneously, as in haemophilia. In sport haemarthrosis is most commonly seen in the **knee joint** where it is always indicative of significant injury such as cruciate (70% have an anterior cruciate tear) and/or collateral ligament injury, intra-articular fractures, meniscal tears or patellar dislocation. Blood accumulates in the joint within 1–2 h in a haemarthrosis compared to the slower (24 + h) accumulation in a joint effusion. Early referral to a knee specialist is recommended because of the potential for intervention to prevent chronic joint damage.

**haematocrit** the proportion by volume of blood occupied by erythrocytes (red blood cells, RBC): on average 45%, i.e. 45 mL of red cells in 100 mL of whole blood.

Exercise-induced increase in haematocrit, together with measurement of haemoglobin concentration, allows estimation of change in plasma volume. Also known as *packed cell volume (PCV)*. *See also* **altitude acclimatization**.

**haematoma** a swelling, composed of extravasated blood, which is usually traumatic in origin. One of the most common injuries in sport and one which benefits from early treatment with ice, compression and elevation.

**haemoconcentration** decrease in the volume of plasma relative to the volume of cells in the blood (increase in **haematocrit**). Consequence of dehydration.

**haemoglobin** the iron-containing protein with the property of binding oxygen, contained in red blood cells. *See also* **oxyhaemoglobin dissociation curve**.

**haemophilias** a group of inherited conditions in which blood coagulation is defective, resulting in an increased tendency to bleed, both spontaneously and as a result of trauma. For this reason, participation in contact sport is not advised.

**haemopoiesis** *see* **bone**, **erythrocytes**, **erythropoiesis**, **leucocytes**.

**haemorrhage** loss of blood from a ruptured blood vessel. In sport, usually the result of trauma. Significant bleeding may result from either an externally obvious injury (e.g. fractured tibia, lacerations) or less obvious internal trauma (e.g. ruptured spleen, lung trauma) and may result in shock. *See also* **shock**.

**haemothorax** a collection of blood in the pleural cavity around the lung(s).

**hallux** the first, great or big toe. *hallux rigidus* is a stiff and painful toe resulting from osteoarthritis of the metatarsophalangeal joint. In *hallux valgus* the toe bends at this joint towards the second toe, and the joint bulges from the side of the foot. Can result in permanent displacement (possibly with a degree of external rotation) greater than 10%. Additional friction from poorly fitting footwear can result in a bursa, and the prominence of bone-plus-bursa is known as a *bunion.*

**hamstring muscles** the group that forms the bulk of the back of the thigh, made up of three muscles: *semimembranosus, semitendinosus* and *biceps femoris;* their tendons cross behind both the hip and the knee joints, so their action is to extend the hip and flex the knee. Their function is important in standing, walking and running and therefore vital in sport. Injury is common in sport, especially where sprinting or sudden acceleration is required when the muscles are under greatest tension, and is usually felt as a sudden sharp pain in the back of the thigh. *hamstring strains* are graded 1, 2 or 3 (complete rupture) depending on severity. Rehabilitation should include not only treatment of the soft tissue damage but also attempts to ascertain and where possible correct any underlying aetiological factors such as inadequate warm-up/stretching, poor low back flexibility and biomechanical abnormalities, e.g. an abnormally tilted pelvis. *See appendix 1.2 fig 6B.*

**hand** a complex musculoskeletal structure, allowing the complexity of movements required. The *carpal bones* at the wrist articulate with the five *metacarpals*, and each of these in turn with the first of the three *phalanges* of each digit. There are many small muscles attached between the various bones, which contribute to finger and thumb movements together with the long tendons of the forearm muscles which span the wrist in their tendon sheaths. *hand injury* is most common in sports such as basketball, rugby, cricket, volleyball, handball, etc. Injuries include ligament sprains, fractures and dislocations. *See appendix 1.2 fig 1.*

**hand grip** *see* **grip dynamometer**.

**hardiness** in a psychological context, a dispositional tendency comprising a cluster of attitudes, beliefs and behavioural and mental skills that are held to promote resilience to the negative effects of stress on health and well-being.

**Harvard step test** *see* **step test**.

**Hawthorne effect** an improvement in performance due to changes in environmental conditions regardless of the nature of the changes. Named after an electricity company's plant in the US where a series of studies was conducted in the 1920s into the effects of variations in environmental conditions on workers' performance and productivity. In experimental design the term is often used to describe a threat to validity whereby participants' performance on a task improves due to them feeling that the experimenter shows concern for them.

**head injury** potentially the most serious injury in sport. Injury risk is greatest in contact sports (such as boxing, rugby, football and American football) or in sports which involve a fall from height (horse riding, trampolining, gymnastics) or movement at speed (cycling, motor sports). The risk of a head injury is brain damage via either internal bleeding or a shearing force. Management of head injuries in sport requires appropriately trained personnel who adhere to the relevant guidelines especially regarding referral to hospital and advisability or otherwise of return to play. *See also* **amnesia**, **coma**, **concussion**, **Glasgow Coma Scale (GCS)**.

**health education** the provision of information to the public or individuals to reduce ill health and enhance positive health by influencing beliefs, attitudes and behaviour.

**health promotion** any initiatives, by any public or private agency, to prevent ill health and promote positive health through a variety of strategies ranging from the implementation of public health policies to encouraging individual changes in health behaviours.

**hearing** *see* **ear**.

**heart** four-chambered organ, receiving venous blood from the **systemic circulation** into the *right atrium*, passing it on to the *right ventricle* to be pumped through the lungs in the **pulmonary circulation**; oxygenated blood in the *pulmonary veins* enters the *left atrium* and thence to the *left ventricle*, to be pumped out in the aorta to all systemic arteries. Valves control the direction of flow. The *myocardium* (cardiac muscle) forms the walls of the chambers which are lined by the *endocardium*. The heart is contained within the membranous *pericardium*. *See also* **cardiac cycle**; *appendix 1.3. See fig overleaf.*

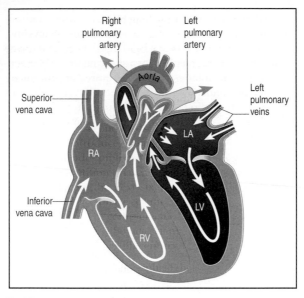

Blood flow through the heart.

**heart attack** also known as *myocardial infarction*. Results from a sudden occlusion of one of the coronary arteries, which supply the heart muscle (myocardium). Usually due to the formation of thrombus (blood clot) at the site of a pre-existing narrowing of the artery (*coronary thrombosis*). Common symptoms include the sensation of tightness or heaviness in the chest, which can radiate to the arm or neck, breathlessness, sweating and nausea. Requires immediate hospital admission due to risk of cardiac arrest. In sport, this is the commonest cause of sudden death in those over 45 years. Risk factors include cigarette smoking, high blood pressure, obesity, physical inactivity and raised cholesterol levels. Exercise programmes are recommended in the prevention of heart disease and used in the rehabilitation of patients following a heart attack. *See also* **cardiac rehabilitation**.

**heart failure** the condition when the heart's ability to pump blood around the body is diminished. Common causes include ischaemic heart disease, hypertension, disorders of the heart muscle or congenital heart disease. Symptoms include breathlessness (especially at night or on exertion) and leg swelling (oedema). Diagnosis is based on the history and clinical examination with additional investigations including a chest X-ray, ECG and echocardiography. Modern drug treatment starts with **diuretics** and ACE inhibitors. *See also* **angiotensin**, **cardiomyopathy**, **coronary artery disease**.

**heart murmur** a sound additional to the normal **heart sounds,** heard on auscultation of the heart. Many murmurs are of no significance (innocent, *physiological murmurs*), particularly in young children, or due to increased blood flow through the heart during exercise, or in pregnancy. *pathological murmurs* may be due to abnormalities in the heart's structure or turbulent flow through a heart valve abnormality (congenital or acquired: in adults most commonly following rheumatic fever). Symptoms may include breathlessness, palpitations, chest pain or fainting but many murmurs are asymptomatic and are identified, for example, during routine medical examination. All sports participants found to have a murmur should undergo full cardiovascular assessment, including **echocardiography**, to exclude any cause which might increase the risk of **sudden death** during exercise. Management is of the underlying cause and surgery may be indicated in certain conditions, especially for significantly narrowed heart valves. *See also* **heart sounds**, **medical screening**.

**heart rate (HR)** the number of heart beats per minute, ranging typically from a *resting heart rate* of 60–75 (but can be less than 50, especially in trained endurance athletes) to a *maximal heart rate* in exercise that depends on fitness and age (average guide: 220 minus years of age). Regulated by the balance between sympathetic and parasympathetic influences on the **pacemaker** (sinoatrial node). *See also* **cardiac output**.

**heart rate reserve (HRR)** maximal minus resting heart rate ($HR_{max} - HR_{rest}$): the *Karvonen formula*.

**heart sounds** The two sounds heard on listening to the heart with a stethoscope (*auscultation*) during normal cardiac contraction. The first (heard best at the apex) is due to the closure of the two atrioventricular valves (mitral and tricuspid); the second (heard best at the base of the heart) marks the closure of the aortic and pulmonary valves. Two components of the second sound can be heard separately (split heart sound) as a normal feature. Additional heart sounds (third or fourth) may be a sign of cardiac disease. *See also* **cardiac cycle**.

**heat acclimatization** the process of improvement in tolerance to heat as a result of repeated sessions of exercise in a hot environment, resulting in a measurable improvement in physiological response. The body's response includes increase in the rate of **sweating** but decrease in sodium in the sweat, preserving salt by the action of **aldosterone**; increase in skin blood flow and overall control of **body temperature** as environmental conditions (air temperature and humidity) change. In addition, acclimatization will reduce the incidence and severity of **heat illness**. *See also* **acclimation**.

**heat illness** the term used to describe the spectrum of conditions which result from the effects of excessive heat, whilst *hyperthermia* refers to any elevation of the body (core) temperature above normal. Heat problems are influenced by humidity, which reduces heat loss by evaporation. Young children have less ability to lose heat by sweating and are therefore more susceptible. *heat cramps* muscle cramps with general fatigue that occur after exercise, associated with profuse sweating and the resulting salt loss. Treatment is removal from the hot environment, plus salt and water replacement. *heat exhaustion* is the most common heat illness in sport. Symptoms are often vague and include faintness, loss of co-ordination, profuse sweating, headache, nausea, dizziness and thirst. It is related to alterations in fluid/electrolyte balance and changes in blood volume. Treatment is removal from the hot environment, external cooling, elevation of the legs, fluid replacement and careful monitoring of airway, breathing and circulation (*ABC*). *heat syncope* occurs with postural pooling of blood and a decrease in venous return resulting in relative cerebral hypoperfusion. It occurs most commonly with a sudden rise in temperature or humidity. Salt and water depletion are less common than in the other types of heat illness. *heat stroke* is rare but can be fatal; it is at the end of the spectrum of heat illness when the body temperature continues to rise as heat loss by sweating fails due to dehydration; the result is collapse, possible seizures, coma and death. It is a medical emergency and should be treated as such with immediate admission to hospital.

**heel bursitis** *see* **bursitis**.

**heel-raise** *see* **orthotics**.

**hepatic** pertaining to the liver.

**hernia** the abnormal protrusion of part of an internal organ through an aperture in the surrounding structures, most commonly part of the intestine through a defect in the abdominal wall musculature. Weakness of the muscle may be due to injury or previous surgery; obesity or heavy lifting add to the risk. If the protrusion becomes stuck in the narrow gap (incarcerated hernia) the blood supply may be compromised (strangulated hernia) and surgery is required. Common types of hernia include *abdominal, femoral* and *inguinal*. In sport the groin is a common site of pain or discomfort, and the term *sportsman's hernia* is sometimes used inappropriately for a variety of other conditions that cause it (including musculotendinous injuries and osteitis of the pubic bone). It is important to diagnose accurately the cause of groin pain, as treatment options, including those involving surgery, will differ, and particularly relevant to identify a true hernia, which may be due to a tear in the external oblique muscle for which there are various methods of surgical repair. *See also* **abdominal muscles**.

**hexokinase** *see* **muscle enzymes**.

**Hick's law** a law specifying the linear relationship between choice reaction time and the number of response options available, stating that choice reaction time increases as a function of the logarithm of the number of alternatives. *See also* **reaction time**.

**high-carbohydrate diet** *see* **carbohydrate (CHO)**, **carbohydrate intake guidelines for athletes**, **carbohydrate loading**.

**high energy bond** chemical bond which is readily hydrolysed by an appropriate catalyst, and releases a large amount of energy when the hydrolysis occurs in the cytoplasm of a living cell; this energy release depends as much on the products of the hydrolysis being present at very low concentrations as it does on the properties of the bond itself. Key instances in muscle are the terminal phosphate bonds of adenosine triphosphate and phosphocreatine.

**high-fat diet** one which provides more than 30% of energy as fat. Research into effects on performance indicates that 3–5 days on a high-fat diet leads to deterioration of endurance performance when compared to a carbohydrate (CHO)-rich diet. However, when adaptation to the diets is combined with training for a period of 1–4 weeks, a high-fat diet does not attenuate endurance performance compared to a high-CHO diet. When such regimes are continued and compared for longer than 4 weeks, endurance performance is markedly better on the CHO-rich diet. There is no performance benefit in switching to high-CHO after long-term adaptation to high-fat, compared to having a high-CHO diet all along.

**high-protein diet** one which provides more than 15% of energy as protein. Traditionally, high-protein diets are low-carbohydrate diets. These diets are claimed to be effective for the reduction of body mass and body fat. Extremely high-protein diets are claimed to suppress appetite through reliance on fat mobilization and ketone body formation. In addition, the elevated thermic effect of dietary protein, with a relatively low coefficient of digestibility (particularly in the case of plant proteins), reduces the net calories available from ingested protein compared with a well-balanced diet of equivalent caloric value. The long-term success of high-protein diets remains questionable and they may even pose health risks, including kidney damage, increased blood lipoprotein levels and dehydration. *See also* **low-carbohydrate ketogenic diets**.

**hip joint** a 'ball-and-socket' joint, where the globular head of the femur articulates with the cup-like hollow (the acetabulum) in the hip bone, which is deepened by a fibrocartilaginous rim; the joint is strongly supported by ligaments attached to this rim and the hip bone above, and to the femur where the neck joins the shaft. *hip injury* is important in sport as the initial treatment usually requires non-weight-bearing activity only and then often a prolonged rehabilitation. *acute injuries* can be the result of a fall, direct trauma or twisting; they include fractures, dislocations and soft tissue injuries to muscles and supporting ligaments. *overuse injuries*

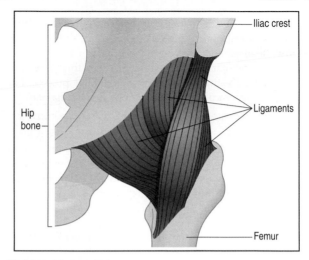

The left hip joint from the front.

result from repetitive weight-bearing activity, such as road running, and include bursitis and tendonitis. *See also appendix 1.2 figs 1, 2.*

**histamine** an amine released in many tissues, with actions dependent on the type of cellular *histamine receptors* including constriction of bronchial muscle (*$H_1$*), stimulation of gastric acid secretion (*$H_2$*) and various actions in nervous tissue (*$H_3$*). In inflammatory conditions, histamine release from mast cells leads to $H_1$-mediated vasodilatation and increased vascular permeability, causing redness and swelling, and initial experiments in vivo with H4 receptor antagonists indicate a role also for the H4 receptor. *See also* **antihistamines**; *appendix 6.*

**hormone** a substance (peptide or steroid) released from secretory cells, mainly those that constitute the endocrine (ductless) glands, into the blood stream; taken up by specific cellular receptors elsewhere in the body and thereby activating some particular cellular process. For sources, chemical nature and actions, *see table appendix 5*.

**hormone-sensitive lipase** enzyme responsible for hydrolysis of triglyceride molecules and therefore release of free fatty acids and glycerol. It functions mainly in adipose tissue and muscle. Activity of the enzyme in both sites is increased during endurance-type exercise, providing free fatty acids for resynthesis of ATP.

**housemaid's knee** *see* **bursitis**.

**human chorionic gonadotrophin (HCG)** *see* **gonadotrophins**.

**human enhancement technologies (HET)** term which may be applied widely to anything which modifies human characteristics or abilities, from antidepressant drugs to gene therapy, but mainly to those used for non-therapeutic purposes to enhance physical or mental performance. An inquiry into HET in sport, with reference chiefly to **doping**, was the subject of a recent UK Government Select Committee Report. *See also* **performance genes**.

**human growth hormone (HGH)** *see* **growth hormone**.

**human immunodeficiency virus (HIV)** the AIDS virus. There are two types: HIV-1 (many strains), mainly responsible for HIV disease in Western Europe, North America and Central Africa, and HIV-2, causing similar disease mainly in West Africa.

**humerus** the bone of the upper arm, articulating at the **shoulder joint** with the scapula, and at the **elbow joint** with the ulna and radius. *See appendix 1.2 fig 1.*

**hydration status** refers to body fluid levels. *euhydration* the normal state of body water content (typically about 40 litres). *hypohydration* reduced total body water which may develop by the process of dehydration due to excessive **sweating** under exercise heat stress. Athletes may lose 2-6% body weight during prolonged exercise. Hypohydration is detrimental to both exercise performance and health and should be prevented by provision of fluids to match water loss. In several sports (e.g. boxing, power lifting, wrestling) athletes may purposely induce dehydration to achieve weight loss prior to competition. *hyperhydration* increased total body water. It has been proposed that prior hyperhydration may improve thermoregulation during exercise heat stress, but studies have had inconsistent results. *See also* **water balance**.

**hydrocortisone** *see* **glucocorticoids**.

**hydrofoil** the shape of a body/object in relation to fluid (water) flow past it.

**hydrotherapy** the use of water in the treatment of medical conditions. The water in hydrotherapy pools is usually warmer than in a swimming pool (allowing better muscle relaxation) and deep enough to allow the patient to exercise out of their depth for non-weight-bearing activity. Thus in sports injuries of the back, groin and lower limb, rehabilitation can begin sooner after injury and proceed at a faster rate. A water-based exercise programme will also allow maintenance and indeed improvement of fitness during the period of the injury, which results in an earlier return to sport.

**hypercapnia** higher than normal partial pressure (tension) of carbon dioxide ($PCO_2$) in the lung alveoli and in arterial blood, due to **hypoventilation** from lung disease, or depression of breathing by drugs. Can occur with inadequate absorption of expired $CO_2$ in breathing apparatus, e.g. in **diving**.

**hyperflexibility** *see* **hypermobility**.

**hyperglycaemia** abnormally high level of blood glucose usually indicative of diabetes mellitus. *See also* **blood glucose, diabetes, insulin.**

**hyperlipidaemia** an abnormally elevated plasma lipid level. A significant risk factor for **coronary artery disease** (ischaemic heart disease) which can be familial or acquired (largely through lifestyle, especially high-fat diet). The condition is asymptomatic and only diagnosed by a screening blood test or following a cardiac event. While treatment requires dietary modification, newer lipid-lowering drugs (statins) have led to much better results and a reduction in morbidity and mortality. *See also* **cholesterol, lipids**.

**hypermobility** excessive movement at a joint, which potentially leads to instability. This is as a result of changes to connective tissue, particularly collagen, which results in laxity of the supporting structures such as ligaments and tendons. There is a spectrum from the more serious, often genetic, conditions to the more common, which cause fewer problems but nevertheless increase the risk of injury. Hypermobility is assessed by the Beighton Score, which measures the degree of abnormal movement at the lower back, knees, elbows and hands. The higher the score (maximum 9), the more hypermobile an individual is. *See also* **flexibility**.

**hypernatraemia** higher than normal concentration of sodium in the blood (over $145\,mmol.L^{-1}$) due to excessive water loss, or inadequate water intake.

**hyperpnoea** ventilation of the lungs at greater than normal resting rate, whether or not appropriate to meet the demand for increased oxygen consumption. To be distinguished from (although it includes) **hyperventilation**, which is defined as an increase in ventilation that reduces the carbon dioxide tension $(PCO_2)$ in the blood.

**hypertension** abnormally high arterial **blood pressure**.

**hyperthermia** *see* **heat illness**.

**hypertrophic obstructive cardiomyopathy (HOCM)** one of a group of diseases of the myocardium associated with cardiac dysfunction. HOCM is an inherited condition (the result of multiple gene defects) in which the muscle of the left ventricular wall (mainly the septum) is thickened, reducing the size of the ventricular chamber, causing possible valve dysfunction and most importantly obstruction of outflow into the aorta. Microscopically, the myocardial cells are not of normal pattern, resulting in disruption of the electrical pathways within the heart, leading potentially to fatal arrhythmias. HOCM is one of the commonest causes of sudden cardiac death in young sportspeople, when growth of the abnormal cardiac muscle is greatest. HOCM may be asymptomatic or it can cause exercise-related dizziness, breathlessness, chest pain and palpitations. Diagnosis depends on ECG and echocardiography. Treatment includes cessation of strenuous activity, but this does not always prevent premature death. *See also* **sudden death**.

**hypertrophy** the enlargement or overgrowth of an organ or tissue due to an increase in size of its constituent cells. For example, the increase in bulk of skeletal muscles with training: the individual cells (muscle fibres) become larger. (To be distinguished from *hyperplasia* in which bulk is increased by cell division.)

**hyperventilation** increased ventilation of the lungs, such that in alveolar gas (and therefore also in arterial blood) the partial pressure of carbon dioxide ($PCO_2$) is lowered and that of oxygen ($PO_2$) is raised, i.e. ventilation exceeds that which would maintain the normal blood gas levels, with the rate of excretion of $CO_2$ exceeding that of its metabolic production until a new equilibrium is reached. Hyperventilation may be deliberate in order to prolong subsequent breath-holding, e.g. for **diving**; it may accompany anxiety or be a feature of psychological disorder. Low $PCO_2$ (**hypocapnia**) can give rise to symptoms. At sea level the raised $PO_2$ has no significant effect (because at normal $PO_2$ haemoglobin is already virtually saturated with oxygen) but in **altitude acclimatization** hyperventilation is a compensatory response (raising the lowered $PO_2$ improves oxygen saturation); also in **acidaemia** (decreasing $PCO_2$ raises pH).

**hypervolaemia** increase above normal of the circulating blood volume. Can occur in athletes in association with hyponatraemia, e.g. marathon runners who drink an excess of plain water.

**hypnosis** an altered state of consciousness and relaxation brought about by suggestion. *hypnotic adj. hypnotize vt. hypnotic susceptibility* the ease with which a person can be hypnotized, also known as *hypnotizability*.

**hypnotherapy** form of psychotherapy that uses hypnosis.

**hypocapnia** lower than normal partial pressure (tension) of carbon dioxide ($PCO_2$) in the lung alveoli and in the arterial blood, hence respiratory **alkalosis**. If severe, can cause dizziness or confusion (by constrictive effect on brain blood vessels, reducing blood flow), disturbances of sensation and tetany (by reducing ionized calcium in the blood). *See also* **hyperventilation**.

**hypoglycaemia** abnormally low **blood glucose** concentration. May be a consequence of severe fasting, but can occur in healthy well-fed people during the late stages of endurance exercise, particularly when consumption of carbohydrate drinks is neglected or, paradoxically, when a one-off intake of glucose elicits an **insulin** surge. Diabetics are at risk of hypoglycaemia from insulin overdose or during exercise (which lowers blood glucose) unless special care is taken with blood sugar control. Blood glucose may also be low following alcohol ingestion with inadequate food intake. Acute severe hypoglycaemia can result in coma, convulsions and brain damage. *See also* **diabetes**.

**hyponatraemia** decreased sodium concentration in the blood ($<135\,\text{mmol.L}^{-1}$). In otherwise healthy people, causes include vomiting, diarrhoea and excessive **sweating**. Also occurs occasionally, for example, as a result of excessive intake by athletes of water relative to sodium in their use of **sports drinks**. *See also* **electrolyte balance**.

**hypotension**  low arterial blood pressure.

**hypothalamus**  region of the brain which links cerebral function to the endocrine system, initiates physiological responses to emotions and regulates eating and drinking behaviour, body temperature and circadian rhythms. Many of these actions are mediated via the **autonomic nervous system**. Secretes specific 'releasing' and 'inhibitory' hormones into local blood vessels that reach the **anterior pituitary** and influence the secretion of its hormones; also the neurohormones *oxytocin* and **antidiuretic hormone** (*vasopressin*) are formed here in nerve cell bodies and travel down axons in the *hypothalamo-hypophyseal tract* to be stored in, until released from, their terminals in the **posterior pituitary**. *See also* **appetite**, **body temperature**, **hormones**, **thirst**.

**hypothermia**  is defined as body (core) temperature below 35°C. Less severe cooling is counteracted by an increase in metabolic rate, and by shivering, stimulated by the sympathetic nervous system. Progressive cooling below 35°C leads to disturbance then loss of consciousness, and is usually fatal between 25° and 20°C, although recovery has been known from still lower temperatures. As well as extremely low ambient temperature, risks include immersion in cold water and exhaustion, e.g. on mountains, or when swimming for survival. More common in climatic conditions where low environmental temperature is combined with wet and windy conditions, adding to the rapidity and extent of the fall in body temperature. Early signs include shivering, confusion, reduced concentration and reaction time (e.g. ball skills in sport) and the inability to keep up (in outdoor sports, hill-walking, etc.). Treatment includes removal from the cold environment, removal of wet clothing and replacement with dry clothes and gradual rewarming. Further heat loss can be prevented by restriction of continued activity. *See also* **body temperature**.

**hypothesis** a provisional or tentative theory, not yet supported by a significant amount of **corroborative evidence**.

**hypotonic solution** *see* **sports drinks**.

**hypovolaemia** decrease in the volume of the circulating blood. Under exercise conditions hypovolaemia can develop when the volume of fluid ingested is insufficient to match the sweat loss. *See also* **hydration status**.

**hypoxaemia** lower than normal oxygen tension ($PO_2$) in the arterial blood, therefore lower than normal saturation of haemoglobin and oxygen content per unit volume. *See also* **oxyhaemoglobin dissociation curve**.

**hypoxia** deficiency of oxygen in the body due to (1) low partial pressure of oxygen in the blood, because of (i) low oxygen in inspired air, e.g. at altitude, (ii) inadequate ventilation due to lung disease or depression of breathing by drugs (in this case accompanied by hypercapnia), (iii) defective transfer of oxygen from lung alveoli to blood; (2) low content of oxygen in the blood due to inadequate or abnormal haemoglobin; (3) failure of the heart and circulation to deliver an adequate oxygen supply to the tissues, even though the content in the blood may be normal; (4) poisoning of cells so that they cannot use the oxygen delivered to them.

**I**

**iceberg profile** in sport psychology, a proposed ideal profile of moodstate for elite performers, characterized by low scores on negative moods (specifically tension, depression, anger, fatigue and confusion) and high scores on positive moods (specifically vigour). Known as 'iceberg' because, according to this proposition, when elite performers' moodstate scores are standardized and plotted they should show an iceberg-shaped profile with negative mood scores lying below the mean and the vigour score lying above the mean.

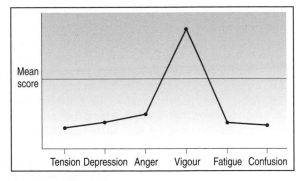

Iceberg profile of moodstates.

**ideal self** a person's conception of how they would ideally like to be.

**idiographic** relating to the study of individuals rather than groups. *See also* **nomothetic**.

**iliotibial band** a band of connective tissue, continuous above with the *tensor fasciae latae* muscle which is attached to the iliac crest, and extending down to be inserted on the outer side of the tibia below the knee. *iliotibial band syndrome* is one of the commonest causes of knee pain in runners, with pain localized to the insertion on the lateral aspect of the tibia where the band rubs on the lateral tibial condyle. Classically caused by road running, especially on cambered surfaces, associated with excessive pronation. The key to treatment is to identify the cause and improve the flexibility and strength of the band.

**imagery** the process of forming symbolic mental representations of objects, events or actions, which may be in any of the sensory modes. In sport psychology the effective and deliberate use of imagery is considered to be one of the fundamental mental skills for sports performers and is used for mental rehearsal, motivation, relaxation and stress management. *external imagery* is that engaged in from a third person perspective as if an external observer were watching the person doing the imaging; *internal imagery* is that engaged in from the first-person perspective of the person doing the imaging. In *kinaesthetic imagery* the person images bodily movements or sensations. In *visual imagery* the person creates a mental picture of an object, event or action, also known as *visualization*. *See also* **psychoneuromuscular theory**.

**immune system** the body's protective measures against threats of damage or disease from invading *antigens* (micro-organisms, foreign proteins, implants or grafts) or in pathological conditions from 'self antigens' (malignant cells, healthy or damaged tissue). *antibodies (immunoglobulins)* are produced, each specific against a particular antigen, and circulate in the blood plasma and tissue fluids. The *immune response* involves interaction of antigen and antibody. *See also* **allergy**, **anaphylaxis**, **immunity**, **lymphatic system**.

**immunity** the protected condition provided by the immune system or by medical interventions. *natural (innate) immunity* includes (1) protective barriers – skin and mucous membranes, and their antibacterial secretions; (2) humoral defences – substances in the body fluids, produced or activated when micro-organisms invade, and promoting the function of (3) phagocytic cells – white blood cells and macrophages. *acquired immunity* (1) active: the result of specific defence mechanisms, each initiated by exposure to a particular antigen and effective against subsequent exposures; includes deliberate *immunization* by injection of a harmless dose of organisms (alive or dead) or their toxins; (2) passive: for urgent treatment (e.g. of tetanus infection or snake bite) transfer of serum or cells from an already immune individual *See also* **lymphatic system**.

**impact force** the force generated at the start of contact or collision. In sport this can be the impact of a jumper as they hit the ground in the long jump. Impact injury can occur in collision with another person or object when the force exceeds the strength and elasticity of the tissues. Includes both fractures and soft tissue injuries.

**impact peak** the high point of the sharp increase seen on a force–time trace due to impact between two bodies or objects (or one body or object and the ground).

**impingement** a term used in sports medicine when soft tissue is trapped, usually between bones, leading to pressure, inflammation, pain and loss of function. Shoulder impingement is common in repetitive overhead sports, especially swimming, where the tendons of the '**rotator cuff**' are trapped between the head of the humerus and the acromion, causing pain when moving the arm forwards and upwards: the *impingement sign*. Treatment aims to alter poor technique and reduce inflammation (rest, ice, anti-inflammatory drugs and steroid injections). Surgery is occasionally required.

**impression management** the act of controlling or regulating information a person gives out in order to influence the impressions formed of them by others.

**impulse** change in momentum produced by a force. *angular impulse* moment applied to a rotating body or object multiplied by the duration of the application (newtons × metres × seconds, N.m.s). *linear impulse* force applied to a translating body or object multiplied by duration of the application (newtons × seconds, N.s).

**incremental exercise** exercise at gradually increasing intensity, usually achieved by stepwise increments at regular intervals, e.g. on a treadmill (*incremental run*) or **cycle ergometer**. Term may also be applied to the

**shuttle test**, where the intervals inevitably decrease as speed increases. *See also* **Bruce protocol**.

**individual zone of optimal functioning (IZOF)** *see* **zone of optimal functioning (ZOF)**.

**induction** the derivation of rules and laws by generalizing from observations. Regarded by most 19th-century and earlier philosophers as the essence of scientific procedure, even though Hume had already, in the 18th century, pointed out that every generalization is logically liable to be invalidated by a contrary future observation. Modern thinking recognizes the subsequent development and testing of explanations for the collected observations as at least an equally crucial aspect of science. *See also* **corroborating evidence**, **falsificationism**, **model**, **verificationism**.

**inertial force** an imaginary force introduced to allow for analysis of the acceleration of bodies or objects from the point of view of an accelerating observer.

**inertial movement** motion without the need for a force. Often occurs when a body segment has been previously accelerated. Consequence of Newton's first law of motion. *See also* **ballistic movement**.

**inertial reference frame** the use of a co-ordinate system (reference frame) that does not move (i.e. is fixed in space).

**inflammation** from the Latin *inflammare*, to set on fire. The term for the pathological process that occurs at the site of tissue damage; a process that enables the body's defensive and regenerative resources to be channelled into tissues which have suffered damage or are contaminated with abnormal material (such as invading microorganisms). It also tends to limit the damaging effects of any contamination, to cleanse and remove foreign particles and damaged tissue debris, and allows healing processes to restore tissues towards normality. Fundamentally important for survival. The classic components of the inflammatory response are heat, redness, swelling and pain.

**information processing** in human brain function, the processes of cognition, including those to do with attention, perception, thinking, remembering, decision making and problem solving. Also parallel meanings in engineering

**information theory** a mathematical theory of the processing, storage and communication of information which is primarily concerned with the amount of information that needs to be conveyed in order to accurately reproduce or describe any given data.

**infrared therapy** the use of infrared radiation to produce local heat. Used by physiotherapists as a local treatment to relieve pain and reduce muscle spasm. The scientific evidence as to its effectiveness is poor: it appears to have no greater benefit than other forms of heat therapy.

**injury** any process causing physical damage. In sport *contact injuries* result from direct contact with another player or object (e.g. goalpost). These include fractures, ligament injuries, head and neck injuries. *overuse injuries* result from either an intrinsic cause, such as biomechanical problems, or an extrinsic cause such as the surface of the playing field. In sport, injuries to the lower limb are most common, especially to the knee. The incidence of injury in sport reflects the need for adequate, appropriately trained medical support.

**inosine** a nucleic acid derivative found naturally in brewer's yeast and organ meats. Not essential in the diet since the body can synthesize it from amino acids and glucose. Metabolically, takes part in formation of adenine, a component of ATP. It has been suggested that inosine supplementation might enhance exercise performance by increasing ATP supply but research studies have found no improvements. *See also* **ergogenic aids**; *appendix 4.4*.

**insertion** with reference to a skeletal muscle, the site of its attachment to bone which during its contraction is relatively mobile, compared to the site of its **origin**. For example, in elbow flexion contraction of the biceps moves the forearm (site of insertion) rather than the scapula (site of origin above the shoulder joint).

**inspiration** the phase of the breathing cycle when air is being drawn into the lungs.

**inspiratory capacity** the maximal volume of air that can be inspired after a normal unforced expiration. *See also* **lung volumes**.

**insulin** a polypeptide hormone produced by the beta cells of the islets of Langerhans in the pancreas, associated mainly with regulation of **blood glucose**, in which it exerts an opposite effect to that of **glucagon**. Involved also in distribution, utilization and storage of protein and fat, as well as of carbohydrate, and in interconversion among them. Insulin secretion is stimulated by a rising blood glucose concentration and by the parasympathetic nervous system. It lowers blood glucose by promoting its transport into cells (notably muscle and fat cells) and diminishing its output from the liver, and it promotes formation of glycogen in liver and muscle. An absolute or relative lack of insulin results in hyperglycaemia (high blood glucose) and presence of glucose in the urine (glycosuria), along with decreased utilization of carbohydrate and increased breakdown of fat and protein: the condition of *diabetes mellitus*. Sporting activity by diabetics tends to reduce blood glucose, so good diabetic control with frequent blood sugar testing and adjustment of insulin dosage is important. *See also* **diabetes**.

**integration** (1) in mathematics, the use of calculus to compute the cumulative addition of one variable with respect to another, displayed graphically as the area under the curve of one variable plotted against another; (2) the summing of different types of information; (3) in physiology, coherent function of interacting systems; (4) in society, for example in medicine or social services, the linking of different approaches or organizations.

**interactive sport** a sport in which a player's performance or actions can directly affect the performance or actions of opposition players, such as tennis as opposed to golf.

**internal force** force occurring inside an object or in the body, e.g. by the action of muscles.

**internal rotation** movement at a joint which rotates the limb, or a part of a limb, inwards, e.g. rotation of the whole arm inwards at the shoulder or rotation of the forearm at the elbow, to bring the palm facing backwards; equivalent movement possible to some extent at the hip but not at the knee. Opposite of **external rotation**. *See appendix 1.2.*

**International Olympic Committee (IOC)** the committee of elected representatives from member countries and sports, which oversees the running and sets the rules of the Olympic Games. The IOC has a Medical Commission, set up in 1966 to oversee doping control. This includes agreeing on the list of banned substances, administering the programme for testing athletes, and implementing appropriate sanctions.

**intervertebral discs** the soft pads between the bodies of the vertebrae which make up the spinal column. Each disc has an inner spongy gelatinous substance (*nucleus pulposus*) surrounded by a protective ring of fibrocartilage (*annulus fibrosus*). The discs contribute to flexibility of the spine and act as shock absorbers. *prolapsed intervertebral disc syn* **slipped disc** protrusion of the nucleus pulposus through its fibrous covering into the spinal canal, due to degenerative changes, heavy lifting or injury in sport. Can press on the spinal cord or on the nerve roots, leading to pain, numbness, paraesthesia or even paralysis. Most common in the lumbar region, causing sciatica if the roots of the sciatic nerve are compressed. Diagnosis is clinical with MRI scanning to confirm. Treatment is initially rest with appropriate analgesia, then a programme of core muscle strengthening to prevent recurrence. Persistent neurological symptoms and signs require investigation and, rarely, surgical treatment with minimally invasive micro-discectomy. In sport the commonest disc injuries are in the lumbar and cervical regions, the latter typically in rugby (scrum collapse or direct injury in a tackle), in judo or in a fall from a height as in trampolining or gymnastics. These injuries highlight the need for adequately trained and experienced medical back-up.

**intestinal absorption** the transfer of the products of digestion, minerals and water (also drugs) from the intestine into the blood or lymph. Food products are absorbed from the small intestine, via its lining of enterocytes (where some further digestive processes take place); hexoses from carbohydrates, and amino acids and peptides from proteins, enter surrounding blood vessels, thence in the portal vein to the liver, which removes some before they reach the general circulation. Lipids enter lymph vessels and these 'lacteals' ('milky' with fat) join other lymph vessels to reach the thoracic duct, thence to the venous blood. Some water is absorbed from the small intestine, but most from the large intestine.

**intestine(s)** the parts of the alimentary tract beyond the stomach. Contents leaving the stomach pass in turn through the *duodenum*, the *small intestine (jejunum and ileum)* and the *large intestine (caecum, colon and rectum)* and finally the *anal canal*. *See appendix 1.4 fig 1.*

**intrafusal fibres** muscle fibres within a **muscle spindle** ('intrafusal': Latin, *within spindle*), invested with afferent ('sensory') nerve endings and located so as to detect length changes in the main working (extrafusal) fibres of the muscle. *See also* **gamma (motor) system, motor neurons**.

**intramuscular haematoma** a collection of blood within a muscle. In sport this is usually the result of direct trauma, e.g. a direct blow to thigh or calf in contact sports or muscle tears in non-contact sports. Treatment is aimed at limitation of bleeding (rest, ice, compression and elevation). The collection of blood causes pain, related to either limitation of movement or the increase in pressure in the tissues. If local pressure compromises the circulation, surgery is required to relieve it and to prevent tissue necrosis by draining the haematoma.

**intrinsic motivation** *see* **motivation**.

**introversion** a personality trait characterized by a focus on one's own inner world rather than the outside world and a tendency to be reserved and to avoid social situations. The opposite of **extraversion**. *introvert* a person who manifests introversion. *adj.* *introverted*.

**inverse dynamics** the calculation of forces and moments by using kinematics and data for mass and moment of inertia, effectively using Newton's second law of motion ($f = ma$) in reverse.

**inversion** with reference to the foot: tilting of the sole inwards. *inversion injury* a common injury to the **ankle joint** in sport. Inversion of the foot usually occurs as a result of 'going over' on the ankle when the foot strikes the ground, especially if uneven or if the person is off balance. Results in damage to the lateral ligament complex, with bleeding, swelling and pain. Importantly affects proprioception and thus balance, necessitating a formal treatment and rehabilitation programme. *See also* **anterior talofibular ligament;** *appendix 1.2 fig 3.*

**inverted-U hypothesis** the proposition that performance on a task progressively improves with increases in **arousal** up to an optimum point, beyond which further increases in arousal lead to progressive decrements in performance. For example, in sport optimal perform-ance is held to occur at a moderate level of arousal. Also known as the Yerkes–Dodson law.

**iodine** necessary in the diet (as iodides) for the production of the the iodine-containing hormones of the **thyroid gland**. Deficiency causes *hypothyroidism*: when severe, in childhood, retarded development (*cretinism*) and in later life *myxoedema.*

**iron** an essential micronutrient; present in the body in the oxygen transport proteins, **haemoglobin** (60–70% of total iron) and **myoglobin** (10% of total iron). Small amounts are present in the plasma, carried by the pro-tein *transferrin,* and it is stored (as *ferritin*) in liver, spleen and bone marrow. A small component (around 2%) is used in metabolic systems (cytochrome C, in mitochondria). Elite and recreational athletes undertak-ing hard training have a higher requirement and turn-over of iron than less active people and quickly deplete iron stores which if untreated can lead to iron deficiency **anaemia**, severely impairing aerobic performance.

**ironic effects** in psychological terms, those that may occur when attempts to suppress a thought increase its acces-sibility to memory so that it is more likely to be brought to mind, especially under conditions of stress or increased mental load. For example, in a racquet sport if a performer focuses attention on not overhitting the ball they will often do just that. Also known as *ironic process*.

**ischaemia** inadequate blood flow to a region, organ or tissue; *ischaemic adj.* Also known as *hypoperfusion*.

**ischaemic heart disease** *see* **coronary artery disease**.

**ischial tuberosity avulsion** detachment of a piece of bone from the tip of the ischial part of the **pelvis**, where the tendons of the hamstring muscles are attached, caused by their sudden strong forced contraction. This produces local pain, which can be severe. Treatment is difficult and chronic symptoms not uncommon.

**isokinetic** without change in velocity. *isokinetic activity* movement of an object, body or body segment, by muscle action, with constant velocity. Sometimes known as *isovelocity motion*: rare in sport. *isokinetic dynamometer* device for measuring moments at a constant velocity. The machine controls velocity (usually angular velocity) and external moment is measured. Sometimes known as *isovelocity dynamometer. See also* **torque–angular velocity relation**.

**isoleucine** *see* **amino acids**.

**isometric contraction** contraction in which a muscle stays at the same length, e.g. when holding a weight steady; *isometric exercise (syn static exercise)* exercise in which this condition obtains. *See also* **force–velocity relationship**.

**isotonic contraction** contraction in which a muscle actively shortens at constant velocity; *isotonic exercise* exercise in which this condition ideally obtains – in practice approximated by constant angular velocity of limb movement (implying exactly isotonic muscle action only in the theoretical case of the joint concerned having constant geometry throughout the movement range, as in a simple hinge). *See also* **force–velocity relationship**.

**isotonic solution** one that has the same **osmolarity** as body fluids. Most commercial sports drinks (6% CHO, $20\,mmol.L^{-1}$ sodium) are isotonic. Isotonic drinks are effective in preventing exercise-induced dehydration and promoting restoration of fluid and electrolyte levels after exercise. *See also* **sports drinks**.

# J

**Jacobson's muscular relaxation** *see* **relaxation**.

**javelin thrower's elbow** *see* **epicondyles**.

**jaw injury** injury to the bones of the face which carry the teeth: the maxilla (upper jaw) and mandible (lower jaw). Jaw injuries include fractures and dislocations and are most common in contact sports such as boxing, rugby, lacrosse and ice hockey. These injuries require immediate assessment as they can lead to difficulty in accessing the airway or even to airway obstruction.

**jerk** the rate of change of acceleration with respect to time.

**jogger's nipple** a painful condition caused by friction of the nipple against clothing, seen particularly in both male and female distance runners. Can be reduced or prevented by the use of lubricating jelly.

**joint angle** angle between two body segments linked by a common joint.

**joint capsule** the fibrous tissue layer that covers a synovial joint, contributing to the 'hinge' of the joint. The capsule comprises two layers: a thick, tough, protective fibrous outer layer and an inner layer, which secretes

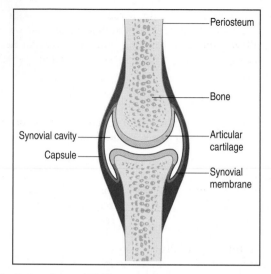

Basic structure of a synovial joint.

synovial fluid, providing nutrition and lubrication to the joint.

**joint injury** damage to a joint (the articulation of two or more bones). Joint injuries are among the most common injuries in sport and range from sprains and supporting ligament injuries to dislocations and fractures. The knee, ankle and shoulder are the most commonly injured.

**joint mobility** the ability of a joint to be moved through its range in different planes. This is dependent on the characteristics of the individual joint itself as well as the supporting muscles and ligaments, the capsule and the anatomy of the articulating surfaces. In some joints, stability is sacrificed in favour of greater mobility, e.g. the **shoulder joint**, where this is achieved by the shallow glenoid articulation with the humeral head. This increases the incidence of dislocation. *See also* **hypermobility**.

**joint pain** *see* **arthralgia**, **arthritis**.

**joint reaction force** the net force between the bone surfaces within a joint, not including muscle forces.

**joint receptors** sensory receptors in joint capsules and associated ligaments, from which information reaching the central nervous system contributes (along with other sensory inputs) to awareness of joint position and movement (proprioceptive sensation), and is necessary also for co-ordinating the action of relevant muscles. To be distinguished from the *nociceptor* nerve endings also present in joint tissues, which give rise to the sensation of pain resulting from overstretching, injury or inflammation.

**joint stiffness** pain and discomfort in a joint, causing difficulty in movement. Can result from medical conditions such as arthritis or from injury, especially when there is protective spasm of the surrounding muscles. Unexplained joint stiffness requires medical assessment and investigation.

**judo elbow** injury to the supporting ligaments around the elbow in judo. Usually the result of holding an opponent with the arms extended.

**jump test** *see* **Sargent jump test**.

**jumper's heel** heel pain felt in jumping sports as a result of the explosive compression forces that occur on landing. The pain is usually felt on the calcaneum deep to the Achilles tendon.

**jumper's knee** *see* **patellar tendonitis**.

**just noticeable difference (jnd)** *see* **difference threshold**.

**keratitis** inflammation of the cornea, the transparent part of the outer coat of the eyeball – the 'window' in front of the the iris and the pupil. Organisms do not usually infect an intact healthy cornea so this is more likely to occur when hygiene is poor, especially if contact lenses are worn. *photokeratitis* (also known as *snowblindness*) occurs as a result of excessive exposure to UV light, as when sunlight is reflected in snow and water sports. It can be very painful, may occur several hours after exposure and may last up to 2 days.

**ketoacidosis** decrease in pH of body fluids due to accumulation of *ketone bodies* (beta-hydroxybutyric acid, acetoacetic acid and acetone), products of the metabolism of fat. A complication of **diabetes**, because of non-availability to the tissues of glucose; also occurs in starvation and (rarely) in alcohol misuse. *See also* **acidosis**.

**kidneys** paired organs in the back of the abdomen. By *filtration* of water and small molecules from the blood flowing through the capillary complex of their *glomeruli*, they extract about 1/5 of the whole blood volume per minute, for passage into the *tubules* where, by selective *reabsorption* back into the blood, the quantity and content of the urine are regulated. By these means, under the influence of **hormones** they excrete waste substances and regulate electrolyte and acid–base balance, as well as blood volume, and the concentration of various substances in the blood. They also secrete *renin* and *renal erythropoietic factor* and are involved in vitamin D metabolism. *See also appendix 5.*

**kinaesthesia** the sense of movement of the body or body parts. Also known as *kinaesthesis.*

**kinaesthetic imagery** *see* **imagery**.

**kinematic feedback** *see* **knowledge of performance**.

**kinematics** the study (and measurement) of motion. *angular kinematics* the study of rotational motion. *linear kinematics* the study of motion which takes place in straight lines (rectilinear) or curves (curvilinear).

**kinetic energy** the energy possessed by a body or object due to movement. Can be translational or rotational (or both). *translational kinetic energy* the energy possessed by an object due to its movement along a straight or a curved line. May be calculated as $\frac{1}{2} mv^2$ where m is the mass of the object and v is linear velocity. *rotational kinetic energy* the mechanical energy possessed by an object due to its rotation about an axis. May be calculated as $\frac{1}{2} Iw^2$ where I is moment of inertia and w is angular velocity. Measured in joules (J).

**kinetics** the study (and measurement) of forces and moments (torques). *linear kinetics* the study of forces but not torques or moments. *angular kinetics* the study of torques or moments but not linear forces.

**knee jerk** reflex extension at the knee in response to tapping the tendon between the patella and the tibia; this stretches quadriceps **muscle spindles**, whence afferents to the spinal cord elicit transient reflex contraction. Tests the integrity and function of the relevant peripheral nerves and lumbar spinal segments. *Syn patellar reflex*. *See also* **tendon jerk reflex**.

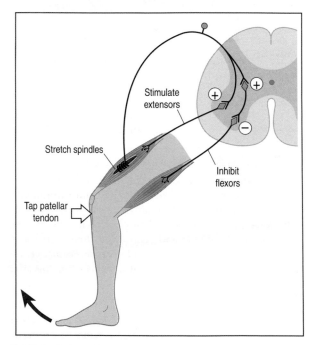

Knee jerk reflex.

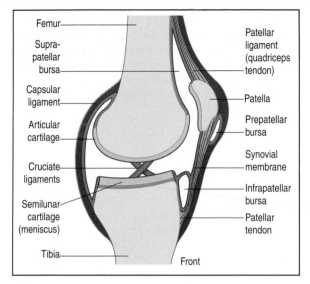

Femur

Supra-
patellar
bursa

Capsular
ligament

Articular
cartilage

Cruciate
ligaments

Semilunar
cartilage
(meniscus)

Tibia

Patellar
ligament
(quadriceps
tendon)

Patella

Prepatellar
bursa

Synovial
membrane

Infrapatellar
bursa

Patellar
tendon

Front

Knee joint. Diagrammatic vertical section from front to back.

**knee joint**  hinge joint between the lower end of the femur
and the upper end of the tibia. The joint most commonly
injured in sport due to its relative instability and mobility. *knee injury* can be complex, involving the bones,
ligaments, tendons and cartilages (menisci), and
can result from both trauma and overuse. *See also* **cruciate ligaments**, **iliotibial band**, **meniscus**, **patella**;
*appendix 1.2.*

**knock knees**  *see* **genu varum**.

**knowledge**  classified in psychology as (1) *declarative
knowledge* awareness of factual information; (2) *proced-
ural knowledge* knowledge of how to perform a task.

**knowledge of performance (KP)** in **motor learning**, feedback or information about the correct production or patterning of a movement, such as when a coach gives a gymnast feedback about the form of a movement. Also known as *kinematic feedback*.

**knowledge of results (KR)** in **motor learning**, feedback about the success of an action with respect to the goal of that movement, such as when an archer *sees* his or her arrow hit the target.

**Krebs cycle** a sequence of reactions within **mitochondria**, constituting the final common pathway for the oxidation of all fuel molecules (glucose, fatty acids and amino acids), in which carbon atoms enter the cycle as acetyl-CoA and emerge as carbon dioxide, and the electrons produced are transferred to the **electron transport chain**. Also provides intermediates for biosynthetic processes. *Syn citrate cycle, citric acid cycle, tricarboxylic cycle*.

**kyphosis** an excessive backwards curvature of the thoracic spine. May be congenital or related to poor posture, especially in adolescent girls, resulting in discomfort. An exercise programme can usually correct postural kyphosis. *Scheurmann's kyphosis* results from a developmental defect that causes wedging of the vertebrae; it is more common in boys, is diagnosed on X-ray and requires surgical correction.

**labyrinthitis** inflammation of the inner ear resulting in disturbance of balance and co-ordination. Dizziness, nausea and loss of balance, especially on head movement, are the commonest symptoms and these will impair performance in sport until they settle. Most commonly caused by a viral infection. Recovery may take some weeks and exercise should be avoided until symptoms have resolved completely. *See also* **ear, vestibular apparatus**.

**Lachman test** an alternative to the anterior **drawer test** in assessment of the integrity of the anterior **cruciate ligament** (ACL), useful as it removes the limitation of the anterior drawer when the hamstrings contract, but is sometimes difficult to perform in athletes with well-developed musculature or where the examiner has small hands. With the patient on a couch, the examiner holds the thigh firmly and flexes the knee to around 20°. The tibia is then drawn forwards to assess cruciate integrity compared to the uninjured knee. The test is graded on the magnitude of movement and whether there is a firm or soft endpoint.

**lactacid oxygen debt** component of **oxygen debt** required to eliminate lactic acid after intense exercise; constitutes the slow phase of return to resting condition.

**lactate** the anion of lactic acid and its salts, although the term 'lactate' is commonly, but incorrectly, used interchangeably with 'lactic acid' itself. At rest and during prolonged moderate exercise, lactate level in the blood is low ($0.7$–$1.4$ mmol.L$^{-1}$). In short-term, high-intensity exercise, lactate production in muscles, and its efflux from them, exceeds its rate of removal from the circulating blood, causing a steep increase in the concentrations of lactate and of hydrogen ions [H$^+$] both in muscle itself and in the blood. Lactate measured in blood therefore reflects the balance between release from exercising muscles and uptake (by the liver, cardiac muscle and any skeletal muscle fibres which are not themselves under anaerobic stress). Contrary to earlier assumptions, lactate is not itself deleterious to most physiological processes and can be used as fuel by well-oxygenated cells, including muscle fibres, but accumulation of H$^+$ in muscle fibres can slow glycolysis and interfere with force generation, while in the extracellular fluid it is thought to contribute, at extremes, to the stimulation of pain receptors. The raised [H$^+$] in the blood acts as an additional stimulus to ventilation, but it impairs fat oxidation by reducing release of free fatty acids from adipose tissue. *See also* **anaerobic exercise**, **metabolic and related thresholds**, **monocarboxylate transporters**.

**lactate analyser** instrument for estimating the concentration of lactate in a sample of fluid, most often blood or plasma.

**lactate dehydrogenase (LDH)** *see* **muscle enzymes**.

**lactate threshold** *see* **metabolic and related thresholds**.

**lactic acid** three-carbon molecule formed by reduction of pyruvic acid in last step of anaerobic **glycolysis**; dissociates to form **lactate** and hydrogen ions ($H^+$). *See also* **monocarboxylate transporters**.

**lactic acid system** old term for anaerobic glycolysis, referring to the production of energy by this metabolic pathway in intensive exercise of duration less than about 2 min, or in the first 40 s or so of less intensive exercise before aerobic metabolism has been fully activated. *See also* **anaerobic exercise**.

**lactose** a disaccharide of glucose and galactose; the major sugar in human and bovine milk (*milk sugar*). The least sweet of disaccharides, lactose can be artificially processed and is often present in carbohydrate-rich, high-calorie drinks. Broken down to glucose and galactose in the small intestine by the action of the enzyme *lactase*. In some individuals who have *lactase deficiency*, ingestion leads to accumulation of gas and fluid in the large intestine, with pain and diarrhoea.

**lateral (to)** at or towards the side. In anatomy, describes position of a structure as further from the middle of the body, in the coronal (side-to-side) plane, when in the **anatomical position**. Opposite of **medial**.

**lateral compartment syndrome** *see* **compartment syndrome**.

**laws of motion** *see* **Newton's laws of motion**.

**laxatives** agents that promote evacuation of the bowel, cathartic or purgative. In sports with weight categories, laxatives (sometimes in combination with food and fluid restriction, excessive exercise and use of sauna and diuretics) are used to lose weight quickly prior to weigh-in; this may diminish physical performance or lead to abnormalities of bone metabolism, impairments in cognitive function and increased susceptibility to heat illness. *See also* **bulimia**.

L-carnitine  *see* **carnitine**.

**leadership style** the manner in which a leader typically provides direction and motivates others. *autocratic leadership style* when the leader takes a dominant, directive role; *democratic leadership style* when the leader consults with the team and involves them in the process of making decisions.

**lean body mass (LBM)** *see* **body composition**.

**learned helplessness** a state of apathy and hopelessness in which the individual feels unable to affect outcomes, resulting from repeated exposure to uncontrollable situations.

**learning** is used to mean (1) a relatively permanent change in behaviour as a result of experience, (2) the state of having knowledge or skills, (3) being in the process of acquiring knowledge or skills. *explicit learning* or knowledge is acquired through conscious, deliberate intention to master or understand a task; *implicit learning* or knowledge is acquired passively, without conscious awareness or deliberate effort; *incidental learning* or knowledge of a task is acquired unintentionally during the acquisition of another task.

**learning goal** a goal focused on personal improvement in performance. *See also* **task involvement**, **performance goal**.

**leg length discrepancy** difference in the true length of one leg compared to the other. It may be *structural* (secondary to a pre-existing condition such as **Perthes' disease**) or *functional* as a result of altered lower limb biomechanics. Differences of 0.5–1 cm are not uncommon and usually asymptomatic. Greater discrepancy will produce a compensatory pelvic tilt or secondary scoliosis (lateral curvature of the spine). This compensation, combined with repetitive exercise, can cause problems including discomfort in the back, lower limb (especially knee) pain or Achilles tendonitis. Treatment includes improving pelvic control and **core stability** and the use of **orthoses**. It is important to identify this problem to allow correct treatment, as treatment of the secondary effect alone will not alleviate the symptoms.

**length–tension relationship** the relation between a muscle's length and the isometric tension (force) which it generates when fully activated. During normal muscular activity, particularly at the longer lengths, tension partly depends on passive stretch of the connective tissue within the muscle, acting in parallel with active force generation by the muscle fibres themselves. When this contribution is subtracted, and only the actively generated force considered, the relation between force and length depends predominantly on the number of actin-myosin **cross-bridges (XB)** which can be formed. Diagram A shows the relationship for skeletal muscle in terms of sarcomere length. Diagram B illustrates how this is accounted for by variations in overlap between thick and thin filaments, and therefore in the formation of cross-bridges. Over the range of decreasing sarcomere length (I–II) progressively more XB can form but when the shortest length (IV) is approached, correctly oriented XB formation diminishes as the thin filaments begin to overlap and force declines. Most muscles in the body operate only over the central, high force, part of the curve shown in A. *See also* **muscle contraction, myofibrils, sliding filament mechanism.**

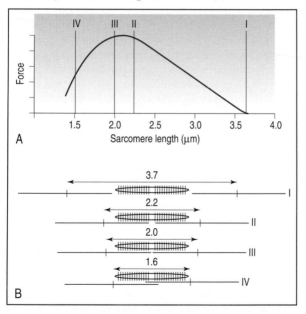

(A) Force generated at different sarcomere lengths. (B) Arrangement of filaments at different sarcomere lengths.

**leptin** a hormone-like protein that is produced by **adipose tissue** and plays a role in regulation of appetite and in fat storage, by acting in the **hypothalamus**. Normally, leptin depresses the urge to eat when food intake is maintaining ideal fat stores. With a gene defective for either adipocyte leptin production or hypothalamic leptin sensitivity, the brain cannot adequately assess adipose tissue status and the urge to eat persists, resulting in overeating. Leptin may also play a role in energy balance regulation in starvation: reduction in leptin production when food is scarce may defend against excess energy expenditure.

**leucine** *see* **amino acids**.

**leucocytes** the *white blood cells (WBC)*. All types are involved in body defences, e.g. as phagocytes or producers of antibodies. Unlike red blood cells, they are nucleated, aerobic and move freely between the blood and tissue fluids. Of a total white cell count of $5–10 \times 10^3$ per $mm^3$, more than 50% are *neutrophils*, which increase in number with many common infections (*leucocytosis*). These together with the much smaller numbers of *basophils* and *eosinophils* have a multilobed nucleus and contain granules with different staining properties. About 35% of WBC are *lymphocytes* with a major role in **immunity**. Less numerous, but largest, are the circulating *monocytes* equivalent to macrophages in the tissues. *See also* **blood cells**, **lymphatic system**. *See fig overleaf.*

**leukotrienes** endogenous chemicals (lipids), derived from arachidonic acid, active in the inflammatory process

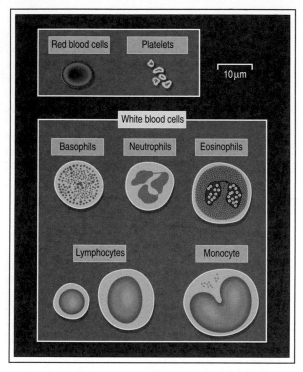

Cells of the blood.

and some allergic responses, and one of the triggers of asthma. Leukotriene receptor-blocking drugs have been developed as part of the treatment regime for asthma and are particularly useful where exercise-induced symptoms are prominent or when there is associated rhinitis.

**lever system** system which has a rigid link (lever) and a fulcrum (or pivot or axis) about which the lever can turn. Can provide increases in force or in range of motion (and velocity) depending on the arrangement of the components and the forces applied. *lever arm* distance from the fulcrum (or pivot or axis) at which a force is applied. *first-class levers* have the force and resistance on opposite sides of the fulcrum. *second-class levers* have the resistance and force on the same side of the fulcrum with the resistance closer to the fulcrum than the force. Very rare in the human body but common in machines (e.g. wheelbarrow). *third-class levers* have the resistance and force on the same side of the fulcrum with the force closer to the fulcrum than the resistance; very common in the human body (e.g. biceps brachii concentric action in elbow flexion). *See also* **mechanical advantage**.

**lie scale** in psychometrics, items included within a test or questionnaire designed to detect whether respondents have responded truthfully to the items the test is designed to tap. An example would be an item that everybody would be expected to endorse if responding truthfully (e.g. 'I sometimes get upset'). If an individual did not endorse this item it would be assumed that they are not responding truthfully.

**lift force** force between a moving object and its surrounding medium that acts at right angles to the direction of travel of the object; may be influenced by its shape, by its angle of orientation to the direction of flow past it of fluid (liquid or gas), or by spin. *See also* **Magnus force**.

**ligament** a strong band of fibrous connective tissue, which binds bones together. Ligaments may form part of the capsule around a joint or be within the joint itself, such as the cruciate ligaments of the knee. Ligaments need to be flexible, to facilitate joint movement, but relatively non-elastic to provide strength and stability and to limit the range and direction of movements at a joint.

**ligament tear** disruption of a ligament, which may be partial or complete. The resultant bleeding causes pain, swelling and loss of function. Ligament tears are graded 1–3 in increasing severity: (1) microtears and stretching but ligament integrity intact; (2) partial disruption with laxity but a discernible endpoint on stressing; (3) complete rupture. Grade 3 tears, though most severe, may be relatively painless if nerve fibres are also torn. Severe or complete tears disrupt joint function and stability. Sometimes a bony fragment is torn off the bone at the ligament attachment – known as an avulsion fracture. Treatment includes **RICE** and anti-inflammatory medication (though 'Rest', i.e. complete immobilization, is now rare, to avoid secondary muscle wasting and loss of function). Surgery may be indicated if return to sport is important, e.g. after complete anterior cruciate ligament rupture. A graduated rehabilitation programme is required with a gradual and progressive increase in strength work, balance and flexibility, before returning to sport or exercise.

**Likert scale** in psychometrics, the most widely used method for generating self-report scales. Named after the American psychologist who devised it in the 1930s. Response categories are assigned increasing numerical values to indicate the strength of the response. Respondents select a value according to the extent to which they agree or disagree with a set of items and their scores are summed or averaged to obtain a total score on the variable being measured. Often referred to as *Likert-type scales*.

**line of action** direction in which a force acts upon a body or object.

**lipid peroxidation** *see* **free radicals**.

**lipids** large group of organic molecules, consisting of carbon, oxygen and hydrogen; some also contain phosphorus and nitrogen, vital in the body for both structure and function. They are insoluble in water but soluble in organic solvents such as alcohol. Includes *neutral (true) fats* (triglycerides *syn* triacylglycerols); the *structural lipids* (phospholipids in cell membranes and lung surfactant; glycolipids in the nervous system); *steroids/sterols* (including **cholesterol**, bile acids and steroid hormones); *prostanoids* with many regulatory functions (prostaglandins, prostacyclin, thromboxanes and leukotrienes). The major lipids circulating in blood are triglycerides, cholesterol, cholesteryl esters, phospholipids and non-esterified fatty acids. *See also* **body fat**, **hyperlipidaemia**, **lipoproteins**.

**lipogenesis** formation of fatty acids from carbohydrate, mainly in the liver. The fatty acids can then be combined with glycerol to form triglycerides (TG) which are incorporated in very low-density lipoproteins (VLDL), passed into the circulation and taken up by adipose and muscle tissue; thus excess of ingested carbohydrate that is not used immediately for metabolic purposes is taken up and stored as TG in adipose tissue and muscle. *See also* **free fatty acids**, **lipoprotein lipase**.

**lipolysis** the enzymatic breakdown of triglyceride molecules, in muscle and adipose tissue, catalysed by the class of enzymes known as *lipases*. During endurance-type exercise, the rate of lipolysis is increased at both sites.

**lipoprotein** a complex of lipids and proteins. Lipoproteins transport **triacylglycerols** (*syn* triglycerides, TG) and **cholesterol** around the body in the blood. Classified into four main groups by increasing density (related inversely to the % TG content): (1) *chylomicrons* the most rich in TG, formed in intestinal cells from the absorbed breakdown products of dietary fat, carried in lymphatic vessels to reach the liver and the general circulation; (2) *very low-density lipoproteins (VLDL)* synthesized in and released into the blood from the liver, rich in endogenously produced TG; (3) *low-density lipoproteins (LDL)*, formed mainly from VLDL after they have lost TG in the tissues. LDL have the highest cholesterol content, carrying this to all tissues. High plasma LDL is associated with increased risk of coronary heart disease, as some cells (particularly macrophages in the arterial wall) may become cholesterol-laden; (4) *high-density lipoproteins (HDL)*, formed in liver and intestinal cells, take up cholesterol from the tissues and transport it to the liver for excretion in the bile. High plasma HDL is associated with reduced risk of coronary heart disease.

**lipoprotein lipase (LPL)** capillary endothelial enzyme that acts on lipoprotein particles (chylomicrons and VLDL) as they pass through capillaries in muscle, heart and adipose tissue, and hydrolyses their triacylglycerol to monoglyceride and fatty acids, which then move into cells. *See also* **lipogenesis**.

**liver** large organ in the right upper part of the abdominal cavity, immediately below the diaphragm, and protected by the lower ribs. Its many vital functions include nutrient metabolism (protein synthesis, formation and storage of glycogen and its breakdown to provide glucose to the blood); production of bile for storage in the attached *gall bladder* and discharge into the gut; detoxification of drugs; regulation of cholesterol. Because of its size and metabolic activity, the liver generates considerable heat. As well as its own arterial blood supply, the liver receives all venous blood from the gut in the *portal vein*, enabling selective uptake of absorbed substances before they reach the general circulation.

**locking** mechanical obstruction within a joint that results in the prohibition of movement throughout its range, e.g. the inability to fully flex the knee or move from a fixed position. In sport the knee is the most common joint to 'lock', often as a result of a loose body or meniscal tear. *false locking* may occur as a result of severe muscle spasm, e.g. of the hamstring muscles, causing limitation of movement at the knee.

**locus of causality** (1) in **attribution** theory, a person's perception of whether the cause of their success or failure at a task is internal (due to personal factors, such as effort and ability) or external (due to external factors, such as luck or chance); (2) in **self-determination theory**, a person's perception of whether the origin of their reasons for engaging in a behaviour is internal (done willingly and out of free choice) or external (done because they are compelled or required to do so, either by external pressure from others or because of self-imposed pressures).

**locus of control** a person's generalized belief or expectation about whether behavioural outcomes (specifically, rewards and punishments) are within their control (the consequence of their own actions) or due to external factors (the consequence of chance, fate or the influence of powerful others). Individuals' generalized locus of control beliefs apply to most of their behaviours, especially in novel situations. Individuals also develop domain-specific control beliefs based upon personal experience, for example *health locus of control* beliefs: whether health outcomes are due to their own behaviour or to external, uncontrollable factors.

**loose body** a small piece of bone or cartilage within a joint, usually the result of wear and tear and/or trauma. Most common in the knee joint. Symptoms include pain, swelling and stiffness and can result in 'locking' of a joint. If symptomatic, can be surgically removed.

**lordosis** exaggerated forward curve of the lumbar spine. There is a normal wide variation in spinal curvature and lordosis is common during the accelerated phases of growth. In sport it is usually the result of poor posture or unequal development of the supporting spinal musculature. Treatment is therefore targeted at correcting posture and improving muscle control, balance and strength.

**low-carbohydrate ketogenic diets** emphasize carbohydrate restriction while generally ignoring total calories and the content of protein, cholesterol and saturated fat. The diet was first promoted in the 1970s by *Atkins* and has appeared in various forms since. These diets generate excess ketone bodies as the by-products of incomplete fat breakdown, with a high level in the plasma that supposedly suppresses appetite. Theoretically, ketones lost in the urine represent unused energy that should also facilitate weight loss. The main mechanism of action, however, may be restriction of the carbohydrate-containing foods, creating a low-calorie diet. These diets have a negative effect on ability to train and compete; they rapidly deplete glycogen stores and also induce significant loss of lean tissue.

**lower reference nutrient intake (LRNI)** *see* **dietary reference values**.

**lung function** *see* **pulmonary function tests**.

**lungs** *see* **breathing, lung volumes, pulmonary circulation, pulmonary function tests, ventilation**; *appendix 1.3 fig 4*.

**lung volumes** measurements made as part of **pulmonary function tests**; the volumes that move in and out during the normal breathing cycle, and with deliberate additional effort, can be measured directly by *spirometry* with the subject breathing through a closed circuit in and out of a cylinder inverted over water, or into a *vitalograph*, or by **pneumotachograph**; the *residual volume* can be measured only indirectly by dilution methods (usually with helium) or by whole body plethysmography. *See also* **ventilation**. *See figure and table overleaf.*

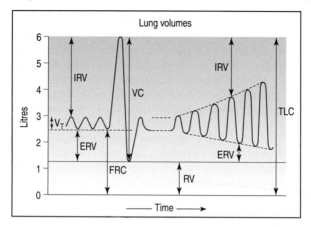

Lung volumes.

## Lung volumes

| | | |
|---|---|---|
| $V_T$ (TV) | Tidal volume | Volume of inspired/expired air moving in and out with each breath |
| IRV ERV | Inspiratory and expiratory reserve volumes | Used when tidal volume increases above that at rest |
| VC | Vital capacity | Volume that can be inspired/expired after full expiration/inspiration |
| $FEV_1$ | Forced expiratory volume in 1s | Volume exhaled in the first second, with maximal effort after full inspiration |
| FRC | Functional residual capacity | Volume remaining in the lungs at end-expiration; decreases as tidal volume increases |
| RV | Residual volume | Remains after a maximal expiratory effort; cannot be exhaled |
| TLC | Total lung capacity | Vital capacity + residual volume |

**lymphatic system** takes part in the movement of body fluids and in the **immune system**. Networks of *lymph vessels (lymphatics)* drain extracellular fluid as *lymph* from all body tissues (except the central nervous system), maintaining balance with fluid that enters the tissues from blood capillaries. After passage through regional *lymph nodes* interpolated in the system of vessels, lymph is returned to the circulating blood via veins in the thorax. The lymph nodes 'filter' the lymph of foreign material, including bacteria, and may become inflamed if draining an area with local infection. *lymphocytes* originate in the bone marrow and pass into the circulation, where they are one of the types of white blood cell (**leucocytes**); they also become widely distributed in organs and tissues, notably the spleen, tonsils and gut lining, as well as in the lymph glands. Lymphocytes are involved, by complex interactions between their different types (*B-* and *T-lymphocytes*) in the production of specific antibodies (*immunoglobulins*). An individual can have a total of up to $10^9$ different antibodies carried in the blood, providing defence against specific antigens.

**macronutrients** the major foodstuffs: carbohydrates, fats and proteins, required in substantial amounts, to provide a sufficient calorie intake, as well as components that are essential to health. *See also* **dietary reference values**, **micronutrients**; *appendix 4.1 fig 1.*

**magnesium** element essential to the life of all body cells, being involved in many enzyme-catalysed processes. The concentration of ionized magnesium [$Mg^{2+}$] in the body fluids is regulated at the correct level for normal excitability of muscle and nerve, including neuronal activity in the central nervous system. Magnesium is present in bone, and its metabolism is linked to that of calcium and phosphate. *See also* **minerals**; *appendix 4.3.*

**Magnus force** the force due to the interaction between the surface of a rotating object or body and the fluid medium (e.g. air or water) in which it is rotating. The force acts at right angles to the axis of rotation and, if the object is translating, to the path of the object. Also sometimes classified as a *lift force*. Examples are top-spin causing downward motion of a ball (e.g. tennis) and sidespin causing sideways motion of a golf ball. (Named after the German physicist who described it in the mid-19th century.)

**malabsorption** impaired absorption of nutrients from the digestive tract. Causes include disease of the small intestine or surgical removal of a major part of it, and lack of digestive enzymes or bile salts.

**malalignment** while each person has a slightly different joint configuration, malalignment is considered to be the abnormal position of a structure relative to another. In sport it can occur, for example, following incomplete treatment of a fracture and results in loss of function with secondary effects, e.g. malalignment of the tibia following a fracture can result in a variety of overuse injuries including pain in the back, lower limb and/or foot, with restriction of activity.

**mallet finger** rupture of the extensor tendon from the distal phalanx as a result of a sudden forced flexion, which results in an inability to extend the joint. It may even cause bony avulsion. Common in catching sports, especially when the ball is caught with a partially closed hand. Treatment is by splinting (Stack splint) with the finger held in full extension for about 6 weeks. Surgery is rarely required. *Syn* **hammer finger, baseball finger**.

**malnutrition** the state of being poorly nourished due to the diet containing inadequate **micro-** and **macronutrients**. Can result in deficiency diseases, such as scurvy (due to lack of vitamin C). Prolonged or repeated weight-loss attempts are likely to cause nutritional deficiencies.

**maltodextrins** water-soluble, easily digestible polymers of glucose with low sweetness. As a convenient source of energy (4 kcal per gram) in combination with sugars added for flavour, they are used in sports drinks, energy bars and nutritional supplement beverages. The malto-dextrins provide a solution of lower osmolality weight for weight than simple sugars such as dextrose, fructose and glucose and so can deliver more calories at the osmolality of body fluids.

**maltose** a disaccharide composed of two glucose molecules, present in beer, cereals and germinating seeds, which makes only a small contribution to the carbohydrate content of a normal diet. Also called *malt sugar*. Broken down by the enzyme *maltase* to two molecules of glucose.

**manipulation** the technique of using the hands to move a body part, particularly to return it to its normal position after displacement, e.g. reduction of a Colles' fracture of the wrist. Manipulation implies a more powerful movement than mobilization and requires skill and experience. Indiscriminate manipulation, especially of the cervical spine, can result in further and serious damage.

**marathon** specifically, a footrace over a road course of 42.195 km (~26 mile 385 yd) nowadays covered by elite performers in less than 2 h 10 min (males) and 2 h 20 min (females). Named after the city of Marathon in ancient Greece, imitating the distance run by a messenger from there to Athens, with news of victory over the Persians, in 490 BC. In general, term applied to any form of very high endurance activity.

**march fracture** a type of stress fracture caused by an increase in physical activity which may so stress a metatarsal (usually the second) as to produce an undisplaced self-healing fracture, with local pain, tenderness and radiographic changes. Management usually involves moderate rest with supportive padding and strapping for a few weeks but sometimes a walking plaster is required. First described in army recruits following prolonged marching.

**march haemoglobinuria** redness of the urine due to presence of haemoglobin following prolonged walking/running. Occurs due to direct trauma to the blood cells in the vessels in the soles of the feet. Requires no specific treatment but can be minimized by decreasing walking/running on hard surfaces or wearing more appropriate footwear.

**march myoglobinuria** reddish-brown urine due to the breakdown of muscle myoglobin following strenuous prolonged walking or running.

**Margaria staircase test** a test of short-term ('burst') anaerobic power in which, after a short run-in, the subject runs as fast as possible up a short flight of stairs of specific dimensions. In each of several versions of the test, the length of run-in, rise of each stair and the steps between which speed is measured (e.g. 8th and 12th) are all specified. Timing is by switchmats on the specified steps. Also known as Margaria–Kalamen test.

**marijuana** *(cannabis, grass, hashish)* one of the so-called social or recreational drugs, obtained from the hemp plant *Cannabis sativa* whose active ingredient is tetrahydrocannabinol. The use of social drugs is increasing in society and sport is no exception. UK government statistics have suggested that 40% of 16–18 year olds had taken social drugs in the 12 months period studied.

Statistics of their use in sport are difficult to obtain and confirm but are likely to be significant given that the majority of sportsmen and women are young. The effects of marijuana include relaxation, euphoria, sedation, disorientation and a lowering of aggression. It is generally accepted that regular use, and these effects, are not compatible with a training regime required for top-level sport. Current **WADA** and **IOC** regulations ban the use of marijuana in competition, but not out of competition. Many believe that in the absence of performance-enhancing effects, an automatic 2-year ban is not justified and that an approach based on education and rehabilitation is preferable, and will assist in maintaining the positive 'role model' example to young people.

**mass** the quantity of material in an object or body. Can be measured in terms of the force needed to accelerate it. Mass is measured in kg and is not to be confused with **weight**.

**massage** the use of several soft tissue manipulations (kneading, stroking, rubbing, tapping, etc.) at different depths, rates and strengths. Massage is used in sport to break down adhesions (deep friction), reduce swelling and oedema, and relax muscles. While massage will aid relaxation and reduce muscle stiffness, there is little scientific evidence of any reduction in injury rates.

**matching hypothesis** the proposition that psychological or behavioural interventions or training programmes should match the presenting problem or personal characteristics of the person being treated or trained. For example, it has been proposed that cognitive-based relaxation techniques should be used to treat cognitive anxiety whereas relaxation techniques designed to reduce physiological arousal should be used to treat somatic anxiety.

**Matveyev's six phases** system of athletic training in which the first period consists simply of general body conditioning, the second adds some sport-specific training, the third introduces competition-specific features, the fourth includes preliminary competitions, the fifth is the main competition phase and the sixth is a recuperation period before the next six-phase cycle is commenced. Normally the phase durations are of the order of months, and the complete six-phase cycle lasts a year. (Named after the Soviet scientist who established the system in the mid-20th century.)

**maximal heart rate** the highest heart rate that can be attained by an individual in strenuous activity, varying with fitness and, in adults, inversely with age. A 'rule-of-thumb' formula for the predicted maximum is '220 minus age'.

**maximal lactate steady state** *see* **metabolic and related thresholds**.

**maximal oxygen consumption (uptake) ($\dot{V}O_{2\,max}$)** the rate of oxygen uptake at the highest work rate an individual can attain and sustain for some minutes, equivalent to **aerobic capacity**. Measured at the peak of incremental exercise or by extrapolation to predicted maximal heart rate, from successive submaximal measurements of heart rate and oxygen uptake.

**maximum voluntary contraction (MVC)** maximum force which a human subject can produce in a specific isometric exercise. In practice, usually taken as the best of three efforts in a single test session.

**maximum voluntary ventilation (MVV)** *syn maximum breathing capacity (MBC)* the greatest pulmonary ventilation in L.min$^{-1}$ that a person can attain by deliberately increasing the depth and frequency of breathing.

**mean arterial (blood) pressure** *see* **blood pressure**.

**mechanical advantage** the difference in forces in a lever system due to the inequalities of the lever arms between the forces and the fulcrum (pivot or axis). *See also* **efficiency**.

**mechanical energy** may be **kinetic energy** (translational or rotational), **gravitational potential energy** or **elastic potential energy**. *conservation of mechanical energy* in the absence of changes in all other sorts of energy, the total mechanical energy of an object or body will remain constant.

**mechanics** the study of forces and motion of bodies and objects.

**medial (to)** in anatomy, describes position of a structure as nearer to the middle of the body, in the coronal (side-to-side) plane, when in the **anatomical position**. Opposite of **lateral**.

**medial epicondylitis** *see* **golfer's elbow**.

**medial tibial stress syndrome** pain down the inner side of the shin, attributed to periostitis of the tibia. Often called *shin splints*, although this term is also used for pain at other sites in the leg. The most likely cause is biomechanical, related to such as poor footwear, previous injury (with altered biomechanics) or conditions of the foot such as overpronation.

**mediating variable** in statistics, a variable that transmits the indirect effects of an independent variable or variables on a dependent variable. For example, the relationship between social support and exercise adherence could be mediated by motivation: social support leads people to be more motivated which in turn leads them to adhere to an exercise programme. *See also* **moderating variable**.

**medical screening** a preventive measure used to identify potential or incipient disease at an early, usually asymptomatic stage, which allays progression and allows treatment. Screening can identify and stratify risk in sport, but the potential benefits must be balanced against the resultant anxiety and the fact that some conditions identified may not be treatable. Routine, organized screening in sport in the UK is uncommon: boxing is an exception with compulsory pre-fight medical examinations and annual CT scanning. Screening is more common in the USA and Italy. In some sports it is compulsory when participants reach a certain level. Screening normally consists of a musculoskeletal assessment (to identify muscle imbalance, degree of flexibility, muscle strength, previous injury, biomechanical abnormalities, etc.) and testing for iron deficiency anaemia in female athletes. Cardiac screening seeks to identify abnormalities which increase the risk associated with participation in sport (especially that of sudden death); this includes a medical questionnaire (personal and family history, symptoms, etc.), clinical examination, ECG and echocardiography. Population screening in sport is indicated and cost-effective when a condition is relatively common, easily identifiable and treatable.

**medium-chain triglycerides (MCT)** triglyceride molecules containing fatty acids with a carbon chain length of 6–10. Used in sports to provide a rapid source of fatty acid fuel. Their fatty acids are absorbed from the gut into the blood (rather than into lymphatics as are long-chain triglycerides) and thus rapidly reach the liver directly via the portal vein. Entering the general circulation, they rapidly raise the **free fatty acids** available to the tissues, where they readily enter cells to be used as a fuel. Being oxidized as easily as glucose, they might therefore have liver and muscle glycogen-sparing effects, delaying the onset of fatigue during endurance-type exercise. However, only a few of the numerous studies on MCT supplements have shown an increase in performance, and most reported some gastrointestinal problems. *See also* **ergogenic aids**; *appendix 4.4.*

**membrane potential** electrical potential difference maintained across a cell membrane, with the inside negative to the outside: $-10\,\text{mV}$ to $-30\,\text{mV}$ in non-excitable cells, and $-70$ to $-90\,\text{mV}$ (the *resting potential*) in quiescent excitable cells (nerve and muscle). Due to unequal distributions mainly of potassium and sodium ions (the cell membrane being partially, but not equally, permeable to both) which in turn determines the relative movements of these ions down their respective diffusion gradients (potassium outwards and sodium inwards). The gradients are themselves maintained by the **sodium–potassium (Na–K) pump** which uses metabolic energy to transport the ions back 'uphill'. *See also* **action potential**, **depolarization**.

**memory** *short-term memory* stores a limited amount of information for a short period of time (up to around 30 seconds); *long-term memory* lasts from over 30 seconds to many years; *working memory* a temporary memory store used for manipulating information in and out of short-term memory.

**menarche** the onset of **menstrual cycles**.

**meniscectomy** removal of part or all of a **meniscus** (semilunar cartilage) from the **knee joint**.

**meniscus** *syn semilunar cartilage pl menisci* flattened crescent-shaped pieces of cartilage inside the **knee joint** (one medial, one lateral), wedged between the articular surfaces (condyles) of the femur and the tibia and thickest around their convexity towards the outside of the joint. Act as shock absorbers and increase joint stability. *meniscal injury* is most common in contact sports as a result of trauma, especially with twisting or rotational stress at the joint – especially medial damage due to the attachment of the medial collateral ligament resulting in combined injury. Most tears occur in the outer border of the meniscus, which has a better blood supply and is thus more easily repaired, but cartilage repair is not favoured by professional sportsmen due to the time (and finance) lost from sport in the extended rehabilitation period. Many opt for removal of the torn

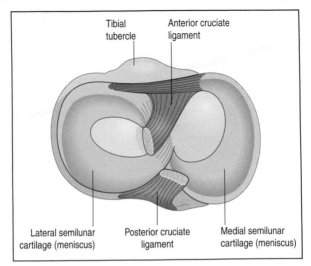

Tibial tubercle

Anterior cruciate ligament

Lateral semilunar cartilage (meniscus)

Posterior cruciate ligament

Medial semilunar cartilage (meniscus)

The upper end of the left tibia showing the semilunar cartilages and the cruciate ligaments (cut).

fragment – *partial meniscectomy* – with its quicker return to action. Surgical treatment aims to minimize the amount of meniscus removed to limit the extent of later osteoarthritis. Sometimes a tear can heal spontaneously. It may result in the development of a cyst or a fragment may break off, forming a **loose body** inside the joint; either of these is likely to require surgical removal.

**menstrual cycle** in women, normally from the **menarche** to the menopause except when interrupted by pregnancy, the 4-week cycle under the control of pituitary and ovarian hormones, that ends with menstruation. The cycle appears to have little or no negative impact on women's athletic performance, despite the physiological changes that occur. Studies of $\dot{V}O_{2\,max}$ during different phases of the cycle have shown no disadvantageous effect on performance despite subjective feelings of bloating and fatigue (seen with **premenstrual syndrome**) and the known effects of oestrogen and progesterone on oxygen utilization. Indeed, studies have shown that world records have been set during all phases of the menstrual cycle. *See also* **amenorrhoea, female athletic triad**.

**mental imagery** *see* **imagery**.

**mental practice** *see* **mental rehearsal**.

**mental preparation** the act of mentally preparing oneself for a performance.

**mental rehearsal** the use of **imagery** to practise an act mentally. In sport psychology, mental rehearsal is considered to be one of the fundamental mental skills for sports performers and is used for learning new skills, practising existing skills, preparing for performance and enhancing motivation. Also known as *mental practice*.

**mental skills** the set of trainable mental abilities and methods that are held to underpin successful learning and performance. The basic mental skills include concentration, goal-setting, imagery and mental rehearsal, relaxation and self-talk. Also known as *cognitive skills* and *psychological skills*.

**metabolic acidosis** *see* **acidosis**.

**metabolic alkalosis** *see* **alkalosis**.

**metabolic and related thresholds** intensities of exercise (expressed as power output or as percentages of aerobic capacity, $\dot{V}O_{2\ max}$) at which specific metabolic and related changes are considered to take place. A plethora of thresholds has been proposed historically. These included many giving the same label to different criteria, or different labels to the same criterion; a number also embodied assumptions about bodily processes, at best unproven and sometimes now known to be false. The table lists six which appear unambiguous, the first five exactly as first described and the sixth slightly modified; however the two that are not related to observable phenomena (anaerobic and aerobic thresholds) are not recommended for further use. The $[Lac]_b$ (blood lactate concentration) values cited are representative approximations for a healthy but untrained young adult; they are used in some laboratories as working indices, but should *not* be taken as definitions of the term concerned. Other usages in the literature include: (1) OBLA as equivalent to LT or AT – confusions possible only if the reference to continuous rise is omitted from the OBLA definition; (2) the $4\ mmol.L^{-1}$ criterion being designated as any one of 'anaerobic', 'aerobic' or 'aerobic/anaerobic' thresholds. *See table overleaf.*

**metabolic equivalent (MET)** expresses the approximate energy cost (in terms of oxygen consumption) of a particular activity relative to the energy expenditure at rest, i.e. at rest MET = 1, equivalent to oxygen consumption of about $3.5\ mL\ O_2\ kg^{-1}.\ min^{-1}$. Scores for over 500 different activities are reported in a comprehensive and

## Metabolic and related thresholds

| Term | Definition | $[Lac]_b$ mmol.$L^{-1}$ |
|---|---|---|
| Lactate threshold (LT, $T_{lact}$) | Minimum work rate at which $[Lac]_b$ is found, at least in the early minutes, to be significantly above (sometimes defined as 1 mmol.$L^{-1}$ above) resting value | 2 |
| Anaerobic threshold (AT) | Work rate at which it has been considered that shortfall in oxygen supply to working muscles causes them to begin drawing on anaerobic pathways. Previously taken as equating to LT but there is now good evidence that fully aerobic muscles release lactate | 2 |
| Ventilatory threshold (VT, $T_{vent}$) | Work rate at which the gradient of the ventilation/work rate plot increases. Attributed to rise in $[Lac]_b$ so used as non-invasive indicator of LT/AT, but precision of the agreement varies with method of determining VT | 2 |
| Aerobic threshold | Work rate considered to be minimum for achievement of aerobic training effects (not that at which aerobic metabolism starts, which is of course zero) | 2 |
| Maximum lactate steady state (MLSS) | Highest work rate which can be maintained without continuous rise in $[Lac]_b$ (see comment under OBLA). Functionally equivalent to critical power (qv) though this is defined in terms of $\dot{V}O_2$, not $[Lac]_b$ | 4 |
| Onset of blood lactate accumulation (OBLA) | Work rate at which a *continuous* rise in $[Lac]_b$ begins. (At and a little above LT, it rises only initially, and falls gradually again after a few minutes.) OBLA is thus theoretically slightly above MLSS, but it is doubtful whether they are distinguishable in practice | 4 |

well-validated list in the *Compendium of Physical Activities*, e.g. walking at 3 mph: 3.3 MET; running at 8 mph: 13.3 MET. The total daily energy expenditure can be calculated, knowing body mass, the time spent in each activity and the relevant MET scores.

**metabolic rate** the rate of energy expenditure during any given state of rest or specified activity. Commonly assessed in terms of respiratory gas exchange (*indirect calorimetry*) by obtaining values for oxygen uptake and carbon dioxide output, and relating these to the equivalent release of energy in kJ or kcal per minute. *basal metabolic rate (BMR)* the rate of energy expenditure which is required at complete rest for all cellular function, to maintain the systems of the body and to regulate body temperature. It is measured before the person rises in the morning after fasting for at least 12 hours, requiring an overnight stay under controlled conditions in the laboratory. BMR is influenced by age, sex, body size and fat-free mass. In most sedentary healthy adults it accounts for approximately 60–80% of total daily energy expenditure, amounting to ~4000–7000 kJ per 24 hours for individuals with body mass within the normal range. In elite endurance athletes during days of competition or training, BMR may represent only 38–47% of total daily energy expenditure. *resting metabolic rate (RMR)* is more commonly measured, since it allows the person to sleep at home, to travel to the laboratory in the morning and to rest there before RMR is assessed. Values for BMR and RMR usually differ by less than 10% and sometimes are used interchangeably. RMR is typically close to 4.2 kJ per kg of body mass per hour or 3.5 mL $O_2$ utilized per kg of body mass per minute. *See also* **Douglas bag method**, **oxygen consumption**.

**metabolism** continuous series of chemical processes in the living body by which life is maintained. Nutrients and tissues are broken down (*catabolism*), releasing energy which is utilized in the creation of new substances for growth and rebuilding (*anabolism*). *metabolite* any substance produced by a metabolic process. *See also* **energy systems**.

**metacognition** knowledge of one's own mental processes. Sometimes applied to the self-regulation of cognitive processes, such as in the application of mental skills.

**metatarsalgia** pain under the metatarsal heads in the foot as a result of abnormal foot shape, intense training or overuse, altered biomechanics or poorly fitting shoes. Stress fracture should be excluded by X-ray, though this can be negative initially. Treatment initially is with rest and analgesia but aims to reverse the cause, avoid overweight and encourage good well-fitting supportive shoes. **orthoses** can be helpful. *Morton's metatarsalgia (Morton's neuroma)* painful neuralgia caused by a neuroma on a digital nerve, most commonly that supplying the third toe cleft. Symptoms include pain and tingling in the two adjacent toes. In sport, most common in those where repetitive weight-bearing is a feature. The condition is exacerbated by ill-fitting shoes, so treatment is targeted to assess footwear and relieve pressure locally. Surgery may be required in resistant cases. (Named after the American surgeon who described it in 1876.)

**methylxanthines** a group of alkaloids that includes caffeine and related substances. Ingested caffeine is rapidly metabolized in the liver to three dimethylxanthines: paraxanthine, theophylline and theobromine; these are released in the plasma and remain in the circulation while caffeine concentration declines. As caffeine and its metabolites are often present at the same time, it is difficult to resolve which tissues are directly or indirectly affected by which compound.

**micronutrients** nutrients needed by the body in relatively small amounts: the **vitamins** and **minerals**. With proper nutrition from a variety of food sources, the physically active person or competitive athlete need not consume vitamin and mineral supplements; such practices usually have no benefits and some micronutrients consumed in excess can adversely affect health and safety. *See appendix 4.2, 4.3.*

**midstance** the point of gait (walking or running) when the **centre of mass** of the body is above the supporting foot.

**mineralocorticoid** *see* **adrenal glands**, **aldosterone**.

**minerals** inorganic substances which are obtained in a well-balanced diet. The substances required in the largest amounts (sometimes known as macrominerals) are sodium, potassium, calcium, phosphorus and magnesium, and many others are essential in smaller amounts. Minerals are essential in all metabolic processes, from maintenance of cell volume and structure to muscle contraction and relaxation, regulation of acid–base equilibrium, protection from oxidative stress, bone metabolism, immune function and haemoglobin synthesis.

No mineral supplements should be required for athletes who are consuming a well-balanced diet but they frequently take them, especially iron, magnesium and chromium. *See appendix 4.3.*

**minute volume** the volume of air entering ($\dot{V}_I$) or leaving ($\dot{V}_E$) the lungs per minute. *Syn **minute ventilation**. See also* **ventilation**.

**mitochondria** intracellular (including intramuscular) organelles in which oxidative phosphorylation of ADP to ATP takes place: the essential 'power houses' of the cell. *See also* **electron transport chain**, **Krebs cycle**.

**mixed venous blood** the blood flowing into the right side of the heart and thence out to the lungs in the pulmonary artery, which is a mixture of venous blood from the whole of the systemic circulation (i.e. from all parts of the body except the lungs). May be sampled by cardiac catheterization, for estimates of whole body **arteriovenous difference**. *See also* **oxyhaemoglobin dissociation curve**.

**model** in the context of scientfic methodology, a simplified representation of a more complex reality. In physiology and related disciplines, the term may be applied to a physical model (e.g. an animal preparation); more widely throughout science it indicates a mental or formal (e.g. mathematical) representation. A good model of either sort enables clear and, ideally, quantitative predictions to be made; testing these predictions will thus provide evidence as to whether the simplified concepts embodied in the model sufficiently approximate the real-world system. *See also* **falsificationism**, **verificationism**.

**modelling** in the context of training, a method whereby a person learns a skill or action by imitating another person (the *model*) demonstrating the skill or action. The model can be live or videotaped.

**moderating variable** in statistics, a variable that alters the direction or strength of the relationship between an independent or predictor variable and a dependent or criterion variable. For example, the effects of an intervention might differ depending on the gender of the participants. In this case, gender would be a moderating variable. *See also* **mediating variable**.

**moment arm** the distance between an applied force and the fulcrum (pivot or axis) in a lever system.

**moment of force** the rotational 'turning effect' of a force. Calculated as the product of the force and the perpendicular (i.e. at 90°) distance between the point of application (and direction) of the force and the pivot; also known as *torque*. *net moment of force* the mathematical result of all the moments applied to an object or body, taking into account the size and direction of the moments. *See fig overleaf.*

**moment of inertia** a body or object's resistance to angular acceleration or deceleration. Depends on the mass of the object and the distribution of the mass in relation to the point of rotation. The summation of all the masses of the parts of the body multiplied by their distance squared from the axis of rotation ($I = \Sigma mr^2$) or the mass of the whole body multiplied by the radius of gyration squared.

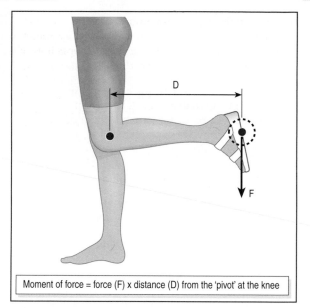

Moment of force = force (F) x distance (D) from the 'pivot' at the knee

Moment of force = force (F) × distance (D) from the 'pivot' at the knee.

**momentum** the 'quantity of motion' of a body or object. A **vector** quantity. *linear momentum* the product of mass and velocity. The change in linear momentum is equal to the linear impulse. *conservation of linear momentum* in the absence of external unbalanced forces, the total linear momentum of colliding bodies or objects will remain constant. Commonly applied to racquet/ball impacts. *angular momentum* the product of moment of inertia and angular velocity. *conservation of angular momentum* in the absence of an external moment (torque), the angular momentum of a rotating body will remain constant. Often applied to low-velocity flight (e.g. gymnastics) to explain how a body can increase or decrease angular velocity by manipulating moment of inertia (e.g. by 'tucking'). *trading of angular momentum* if, in the absence of an external moment (torque), an object or body is rotating about one axis (e.g. somersaulting) and rotation about another axis is introduced (e.g. tilt), the result will be a rotation about a third axis (e.g. twist) due to the vector nature of angular momentum. *transfer of angular momentum* can occur from one part of a body to another in the absence of an external moment (torque) (e.g. if one part of a body increases angular velocity, another part must decrease to conserve angular momentum).

**monocarboxylate transporters** transmembrane carrier molecules, co-transporting monocarboxylic acid anions (typically lactate) and protons ($H^+$) through cell membranes, notably those of skeletal and cardiac muscle fibres. Considered to be responsible for the major part of lactate transport at low concentrations but, as saturation of the carrier approaches, simple diffusion (which is primarily of the undissociated *lactic acid*) becomes more important. *See also* **lactate**, **lactic acid**.

**mood** a temporary but relatively enduring positive or negative affective state. Typically differentiated from emotion in that a mood is of longer duration and not necessarily evoked in response to a specific event. *moodstate* a person's current mood. *See also* **affect**, **emotion**.

**moral development** the development of a sense of right or wrong in children during the course of maturation through the influence of the social environment. Some developmentalists and educationalists claim that involvement in sport in childhood can assist in the process of moral development.

**Morton's metatarsalgia (Morton's neuroma)** *see* **metatarsalgia**.

**motion** change in position of an object or body. *linear motion* motion which takes place in straight lines (rectilinear) or curves (curvilinear), but note that this does not apply to rotation. *general motion* motion which includes translation and rotation. *See also* **Newton's laws of motion**.

**motivation** the internal and external drives and forces that energize, direct and regulate behaviour. Motivation is often conceptualized in terms of direction (the behavioural goal) and intensity (the level of motivation from low to high). *Extrinsic motivation* motivation directed towards the attainment of rewards that are separable from a behaviour or activity itself. For example, an athlete who engages in sport just to win medals would be extrinsically motivated. *intrinsic motivation* motivation driven by the pleasure and satisfaction inherent in engaging in a behaviour or activity. For example, an athlete who engages in sport purely for fun and enjoyment would be intrinsically motivated.

**motivational climate** the structure of the social environment with regard to the way that it influences individuals' motivation and motivational processes.

In achievement goal theories it is typically described in terms of the extent to which the environment is oriented towards promoting task mastery and learning goals or social comparison and performance goals.

**motivational hierarchy** *see* **need hierarchy theory**.

**motor control** the production and control of movement and the processes and mechanisms that underlie it. Also the study of such processes and mechanisms.

**motor endplate** term used variously to refer to the specialized region of skeletal muscle fibre membrane lying directly under the terminal of a motor nerve (the nerve's 'footprint' on the muscle, rich in receptors for acetylcholine, to which it responds by depolarization), or to the terminal arborization of the motor nerve. Now most frequently refers to both of these combined in the mammalian form of a **neuromuscular junction**. *See also* **motor unit**.

**motor learning** the internal processes that lead to an enduring change in a person's capacity for skilled movement. Also the study of such processes.

**motor nerve** general term for any nerve consisting of efferent nerve fibres en route to effectors (muscles, glands).

**motor neuron(e) (motoneuron(e))** a nerve cell and its axon which is part of a pathway for activation of muscle. An *upper motor neuron* has a cell body in the brain and its axon runs to a synapse with another at a relay station, or directly with a *lower motor neuron,* the final link to muscle. The cell bodies of the lower motor neurons are in the anterior horns of grey matter in the spinal cord or in nuclei of cranial nerves. *alpha motor neurons* serve the main (extrafusal) skeletal muscle fibres; *gamma motor neurons* serve the (intrafusal) fibres of **muscle spindles**. *See also* **gamma (motor) system**, **motor unit**; *appendix 1.1.*

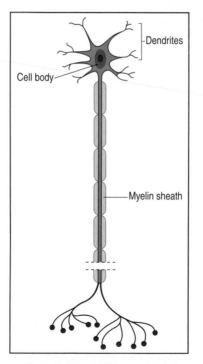

Alpha motor neuron from anterior horn cell to nerve terminals.

**motor pattern** a co-ordinated set of movements involving both voluntary and reflex actions, such as standing, sitting, etc. Typically the initiation and cessation of such acts are voluntary but once initiated, the movements continue without conscious control.

**motor point** small region of a skeletal muscle in which **motor endplates** are aggregated; the muscle is most sensitive to electrical stimulation at this point.

**motor programme** a prestructured set of commands stored in memory that, once initiated, organizes and controls a specific action or sequence of actions in an *open-loop* fashion without subsequent modification. *generalized motor programme* a motor programme for a class of similar actions that can be selected and modified according to the parameters (e.g. speed, direction) required for successful execution of a specific action from that class. For example, a generalized motor programme for jumping can be modified according to the distance, height, direction, etc. of a particular jump.

**motor skill** a co-ordinated pattern of movements acquired through practice involving the ability to execute movements effectively to achieve intended outcomes. *gross motor skill* movement involving the co-ordinated use of large muscle groups, such as when kicking a ball. *fine motor skill* movement involving the ability to manipulate small objects.

**motor unit** a single motor neuron and the skeletal muscle fibres that it innervates and so controls, all of which must respond, virtually simultaneously, to an action potential in the nerve axon. The number of muscle fibres

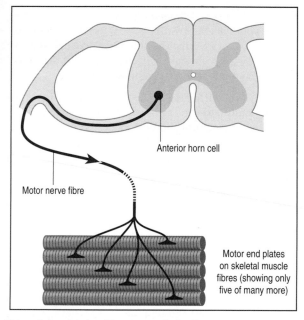

Motor unit, from spinal cord to neuromuscular junction.

in a single motor unit ranges from about 10 to 2000: fewest in small muscles where the control is finest (e.g. for eye and finger movements) and most in large muscles (e.g. quads) designed for force rather than precision. *See also* **muscle**, **neuromuscular junction**.

**mountain sickness** *see* **altitude**.

**murmur** *see* **heart murmur**.

**muscle** contractile soft tissue, responsible for all significant active movements and force-generations in an animal body. Divisible into three classes: (1) *skeletal* or *voluntary muscle* the class of muscle acting, in almost all body locations, to move one bone relative to another, the more superficial skeletal muscles being visible under the skin in all but the most obese subjects; (2) *cardiac muscle* the type unique to the heart; (3) *smooth muscle* composing the actively adjustable components of the walls of blood vessels and of the gastrointestinal, respiratory, urinary and reproductive tracts. Skeletal and cardiac are the *striated* muscles; cardiac and smooth share the property of being *involuntary*. *See also* **muscle fibres**, **muscle fibre types**, **myofibrils**; *figs appendix 1.2.*

**muscle conditioning** training of skeletal muscles to enhance strength and/or endurance; commonly abbreviated in the sport and exercise context to 'conditioning' but note the radically different meaning of this word in behavioural work, which may be relevant to sport in attempts to modify emotions or in certain forms of skill training.

**muscle contraction** the process of *force-generation* in the fibres of any class of muscle, by the interaction of **myosin** head-groups in the thick filaments with **actin** molecules in one of the immediately neighbouring thin filaments. This is set in train ('activated') by a rise in the concentration of calcium ions $[Ca^{2+}]$ in the muscle fibre cytoplasm in all types of muscle, but the mechanism for this rise differs in important respects between them. With reference to *skeletal muscle*, 'contraction', though literally implying shortening, is used to describe force-generation, whether it actually results in shortening (**concentric action**), tension without movement (**isometric action**) or even lengthening against the muscle's own resistance (**eccentric action**); the last is sometimes called an 'eccentric contraction' or, even worse, a 'lengthening contraction' – paradoxical usages better avoided. *See also* **excitation–contraction coupling**, **force–velocity relationship**, **myofibrils**.

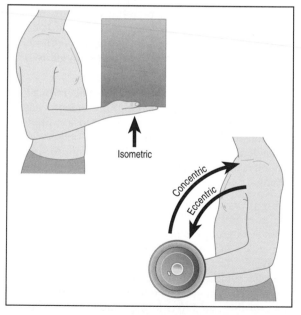

Isometric

Concentric

Eccentric

Types of skeletal muscle contraction.

**muscle enzymes** the table lists some of the most often-mentioned enzymes present in skeletal muscle, with their locations and functions. Apart from actomyosin and myosin ATPases which are associated with the contractile mechanism, they are by no means specific to muscle, being present and highly active also in other tissues. *See also* **Krebs cycle**, **muscle fibre types**.

## Muscle enzymes

| Name *Site* | Catalyses . . . |
|---|---|
| **Actomyosin ATPase (amATPase)** *myosin head groups* | hydrolysis (Mg-dependent and triggered by rise in $[Ca^{2+}]$) of terminal phosphate group of ATP when head-group is in interaction with actin, releasing energy that powers force-generation. (Compare myosin ATPase) |
| **Creatine kinase (CK)** *cytoplasm* | transfer of phosphate group from creatine phosphate to ADP, producing ATP and creatine. Isoenzymes can be distinguished in blood when either skeletal or cardiac muscle has been damaged. |
| **Hexokinase (HK)** *cytoplasm* | 'capture' of glucose after uptake from the blood, by conversion to the impermeant glucose 6-phosphate, in type 1 muscle fibres, which utilize glucose directly. |
| **Lactate dehydrogenase (LDH)** *cytoplasm* | reduction of pyruvate to lactate when oxygen tension is low, and the converse when it is high. Isoenzymes can be distinguished in blood when either skeletal or cardiac muscle has been damaged. |
| **Myosin ATPase (mATPase)** *myosin head groups* | hydrolysis ($Ca^{2+}$ dependent, $Mg^{2+}$ independent) of terminal phosphate group of ATP by head group alone, not interacting with actin (so not contraction-producing: *cf* actomyosin ATPase). Basic histochemical marker for fast vs. slow fibres. |
| **Phosphofructokinase (PFK)** *cytoplasm* | conversion of fructose 6-phosphate to fructose 1,6-diphosphate; rate-limiting for glycolysis, and sensitive to very many stimulatory and inhibitory influences. |
| **Phosphorylase (PPL)** *cytoplasm* | removal of hexose units, one at a time, from glycogen, to form glucose 1-phosphate: rate-limiting enzyme of, and histochemical marker for, glycogenolysis. |

*(Continued)*

## Muscle enzymes—Cont'd

| Name Site | Catalyses . . . |
|-----------|-----------------|
| Pyruvate dehydrogenase (PDH) *mitochondrial envelope* | oxidative decarboxylation of pyruvate (from cytoplasm) to form acetyl CoA, which thence feeds into tricarboxylic acid (Krebs) cycle |
| Sarcoplasmic reticulum ATPase (srATPase) *SR membrane* | pumping of $[Ca^{2+}]$ back into SR after its electrically stimulated release |
| Succinate dehydrogenase (SDH) *mitochondrial inner membrane* | oxidation of succinate to fumarate, in tricarboxylic acid (Krebs) cycle. Histochemical marker for aerobic capacity. |

**muscle fatigue** impairment of muscle force production or of shortening speed resulting from repeated and/or prolonged activity. Causes vary greatly according to the nature and duration of the effort. In all cases they appear to consist principally in disturbances of intramuscular biochemistry, differing substantially between circumstances. However, the possibility of contributory neural factors, resulting in reduced muscle activation, should never be overlooked. Note that cytoplasmic ATP concentrations never fall to less than about half resting levels in living muscle fibres (radical ATP depletion would lead to rigor, not weakness). *See also* **central fatigue, glycogen.**

**muscle fibres** the muscle cells. Usually refers to skeletal muscle, which has greatly elongated (fibre-like) cells, up to 15–20 cm in the largest muscles of the human body. Each skeletal muscle fibre has many nuclei (more than 2000 in the largest fibres), located, after initial development, just beneath the cell membrane. These nuclei cannot divide; skeletal muscle growth and repair depend on **satellite cells**. The term 'muscle fibre' may also be applied to the much smaller cells of smooth and cardiac muscle, which have one central nucleus. All types of muscle fibre have longitudinally oriented contractile filaments containing **actin** and **myosin**. Each skeletal muscle fibre receives its own branch of a motor nerve, but cardiac and smooth muscle fibres are innervated in looser groupings. *See also* **myofibrils**, **sarcoplasmic reticulum**; *appendix 1.2 fig 7*.

**muscle fibre types** categories of muscle fibre adapted for various modes of use. Normally taken to refer to skeletal muscle unless specified otherwise. The main types found in stable human skeletal muscles after infancy are shown in the table. Intermediate 'hybrid' forms also occur, commonly in non-stable states such as during intensive or recently changed training regimes, or in recovery from injury. Types termed 1, 2A and 2B, containing myosins similarly designated, have been recognized since about 1970; however, the separate existence in many mammals of type 2X (initially also known as 2D), distinguishable from 2B only by sophisticated techniques, was recognized during the 1990s and it is now accepted that most, if not all, human fibres formerly called 2B in fact have 2X myosin. The slower-contracting muscles have a majority of type 1 fibres (typically approaching 90% in the extreme instance, soleus), while the faster-contracting ones have rather more, and often rather larger, type 2. Only some small specialist muscles (e.g. extraocular) have 80–85% fast fibres; in large limb muscles above 60% fast is reported only for sprint athletes. *See also* **muscle enzymes**. *See table below.*

**Characteristics of the three main types of stable human skeletal muscle fibres**

| Fibre type and myosin type | 1 | 2A | 2X (formerly '2B') |
|---|---|---|---|
| Description | Slow (-twitch) red | Fast (-twitch) red | Fast (-twitch) white |
| Principal energy supply system | Oxidative | Oxidative and glycolytic | Glycolytic (anaerobic) |
| Abbreviated description | SO | FOG | FG |
| Mitochondrial density | High | Medium to very high | Low |
| Motor neuron size | Small | Medium | Large |
| Contraction speed | Slow | Fairly fast | Fast |
| Fatigue resistance | High | Medium to high | Low |
| Myosin ATPase activity after pH ~10.3 pre-treatment | Low | Fairly high | High |
| Ditto, after pH 4.6 pretreatment | High | Low | Medium |
| Ditto, after pH 4.3 pretreatment | High | Low | Low |

**muscle spasm** powerful involuntary muscle contraction, often of sudden onset and quite often painful, which interferes with voluntary movement; may be a consequence of neurological damage or disease. *See also* **cramp**, **spinal injury**.

**muscle spindles** specialized sensory structures within skeletal muscles, consisting of small *intrafusal muscle fibres* which do not contribute to load-bearing or power generation, but participate in control of the working (extrafusal) fibres. The intrafusal fibres are innervated

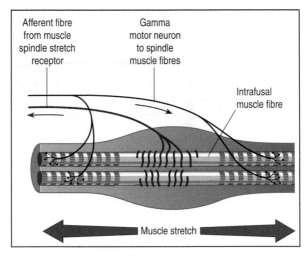

Simplified diagram of a muscle spindle.

towards their ends by gamma motor neurons, but are also invested more centrally by both primary and secondary sensory endings; these signal changes in length, and also rates of change in length of the muscle, to the central nervous system. The gamma motor neurons control the sensitivity of the sensory endings to stretching. They also compensate for the shortening of muscle spindles during extrafusal contraction by causing additional intrafusal contraction; this ensures that sensory feedback continues during muscle contractions. The overall system mediates both the **stretch reflex** and, in voluntary movement, appropriate adjustment of force-generation to load, provided the load is not varying too rapidly. *See also* **gamma motor system**, **tendon jerk reflex**.

**muscle tear** rupture of the tissue of a muscle. In sport, most commonly the result of a sudden movement beyond the normal range; may reflect poor muscle strength, flexibility or preparation.

**muscle tone** *syn tonus* (1) in skeletal muscle, a state of tension that is maintained continuously – minimally even when relaxed – and which increases in resistance to passive stretch. Pathologically, loss of tone (*flaccidity*) can be caused, e.g. by peripheral nerve damage, and exaggerated tone (*spasticity*) by overstimulation, e.g. when the activity of the relevant lower motor neurons is released from higher CNS control in spinal injury. The term is sometimes also used, incorrectly, to indicate general muscle strength. (2) In smooth muscle, steady tension maintained in the walls of hollow vessels; regulated mainly by autonomic innervation but influenced, e.g. in the walls of arterioles, by local variables: temperature, chemical factors or intravascular pressure, contributing to *autoregulation* of appropriate blood flow. *See also* **stretch reflex**.

**myalgia** (Greek *myos,* muscle; *algos,* pain) pain or ache in a muscle which may be the result of injury, inflammation, overuse or inappropriate activity. Normally settles with rest and anti-inflammatory medication. Also unexplained and persistent as part of the **chronic fatigue syndrome**.

**myalgic encephalomyelitis (ME)** *see* **chronic fatigue syndrome**.

**myocarditis** inflammation of the *myocardium,* the muscle of the heart, usually the result of viral infection (especially *Coxsackie*), sometimes during or after bacterial and other infections. Causes enlargement of the heart, impaired function and sometimes heart failure. It can present with chest pain, breathlessness, lethargy and fatigue and arrhythmias. Diagnosis is based on history, laboratory tests (to identify infective agent and inflammatory markers), ECG and echocardiography. A rare condition, but one of the causes of **sudden death** during exercise, especially if a sports participant returns to activity before the infection has resolved completely.

**myofibrils** longitudinally oriented cytoplasmic components of skeletal and cardiac **muscle fibres**, which are the loci of force-generation when the muscle is activated. Each myofibril extends the whole length of the fibre though it is typically only ~1 μm diameter; thus a fibre of 100 μm diameter has several thousand fibrils in its cross-section. In turn, each fibril is composed of numerous parallel filaments of *myofibrillar proteins*, chiefly **myosin** in *thick filaments* and chiefly **actin** in *thin filaments*, alternating and partially overlapping along the length of each myofibril, and so giving rise to the cross-banding pattern of the lengthwise repeating **sarcomeres**; these are aligned side by side across the fibre, giving it (under appropriate histological stains or optical imaging techniques) the striated appearance characteristic of these two classes of muscle. Interaction between the two proteins, myosin and actin, at the **cross-bridges** results in the generation of active force during **muscle contraction**. *See also* **sarcoplasmic reticulum**; *appendix 1.2 fig 1.*

**myoglobin (Mb)** iron-containing haem protein present at high density in the cytoplasm of oxidative muscle fibres (skeletal and cardiac) and substantially contributing to their redness. Related to haemoglobin (Hb), with which it shares affinity for oxygen. In diving mammals (whose tissues it makes almost black) Mb serves as a significant oxygen store but in terrestrial ones, including humans, its predominant function is considered to be facilitation of diffusion of oxygen from the blood through the cytoplasm, by the transfer of oxygen from Hb which has a lower oxygen affinity than Mb at the oxygen tension ($PO_2$) encountered in the muscle vascular bed. *See also* **muscle fibre types**.

**myosin** one of the two main *myofibrillar proteins* in the **myofibrils** of a **muscle fibre**. A dimeric molecule comprising two identical monomers. Each monomer consists of a long chain ('light meromyosin, LMM') which readily associates with the chains of other myosin molecules to form the *thick filaments*, and a more globular component ('heavy meromyosin, HMM'), itself further divisible into two subunits, S2 and S1. The latter are the *myosin head-groups*, embodying an ATPase and an actin-binding site; it is these that interact with **actin** in the thin filaments when the muscle is activated, to form the force-generating (*actin-myosin*) **cross-bridges.** This whole monomer constitutes one *myosin heavy chain (MHC)*. However, associated with the head-groups are two *myosin light chains (MLC)*, of uncertain function. (Since myosin is not the only constituent of thick filaments, the term 'myosin filament' is a misnomer and better avoided). *See also* **muscle contraction, sliding filament theory**.

**myosin ATPase** *see* **muscle enzymes**.

# N

**navicular bone** the boat-shaped tarsal bone on the medial side of the foot in front of the talus (ankle bone), with which its concave posterior surface articulates. Stress fractures of the navicular are seen in runners and should be considered if localized pain and discomfort fail to settle. *See also appendix 1.2.*

**neck injury** damage to the structure of the neck including soft tissue, bones, spinal column and nerves. In sport, most commonly injured by direct trauma with compression (rugby) or a fall from height (trampolining, horse riding). Appropriate first aid care is vital to prevent spinal cord damage and possible paralysis. It is essential to stabilize the neck and not to move the casualty until experienced help arrives, especially if the airway is compromised. Symptoms range from pain and stiffness to numbness, paraesthesia and paralysis, but the commonest neck injuries are muscle spasm and strains, which settle with rest and physiotherapy. *See also* **spinal injury**.

**need for achievement** *see* **achievement motivation**.

**need hierarchy theory** the theory proposed by American psychologist Abraham Maslow (1908–1970) that human needs are hierarchically ordered such that the gratification of a need lower in the hierarchy leads to the emergence of the next higher need in the hierarchy. From lower to higher, the needs are: basic physiological needs (food, water, etc.); security; love and belonging; esteem; and self-actualization (achieving one's true potential).

**negative reinforcement** *see* **reinforcement**.

**negative transfer** a degradation in performance because of practice or experience of another skill, typically where the new skill has similar characteristics and gaining familiarity with these interferes with prior learning of the similar but specific aspects of the prior skill. For example, some tennis players believe that practising other racquet sports such as badminton or squash degrades their tennis performance. *See also* **positive transfer**, **transfer of learning**.

**negative work** *see* **work**.

**nerve cell (neuron(e))** the structural unit of the nervous system. Each consists of a *cell body* with a great many fine short extensions from its surface (*dendrites*) and a long thin extension, the **nerve fibre** with an **axon** at its core. Other neurons which influence the activity of the cell (by excitation or inhibition) form **synapses** on the cell body or dendrites, and the axon terminates at a synapse on another neuron or on the effector which it innervates. *See also* **motor neuron**, **neurotransmitter**.

**nerve fibre** component of all nerves and their branches in the peripheral nervous system (PNS), and of the tracts in the central nervous system (CNS). The central **axon**

transmits nerve impulses (**action potentials**) to the nerve terminal in motor (**efferent**) nerves, or from a receptor to a nerve cell body in sensory (**afferent**) nerves. Also common to all nerve fibres are an outermost covering (*neurilemma*) and within that the

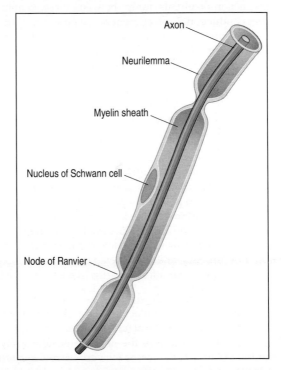

Part of a myelinated nerve fibre. Adapted from W.E. Le Gros Clark, 'The Tissues of the Body', 6th Ed. Oxford, Clarendon Press, 1971, p346.

*Schwann* **cells** which are crucial to the regeneration process if a fibre is damaged. In *myelinated nerve fibres* (including motor nerves to skeletal muscle) there is a fatty *myelin sheath* between the axon and the neurilemma, interrupted at intervals by the 'nodes of Ranvier'; action potentials 'jump' between these, enabling faster conduction. Each efferent nerve fibre runs from a nerve cell body to terminal branches at a nerve-to-nerve **synapse** or at an effector organ; each afferent fibre runs from a sensory receptor to a relay site in the CNS.

**neuralgia** pain in the distribution of a sensory nerve. Neuralgia is not an illness in itself but a symptom of injury or an underlying condition. In sport usually the result of pressure from equipment (e.g. helmet).

**neurohormone** a hormone that is formed in neuron cell bodies and passes down their axons to be stored in the axon terminals until secreted into the blood stream in response to **action potentials** generated in these neurons (compare **neurotransmitters**). Examples are the hormones which are formed in nerve cells in the **hypothalamus**, pass down their axons to their terminals in the **posterior pituitary**, and are secreted there into the blood when appropriate stimuli activate the hypothalamic cells.

**neuromuscular junction** the site where a motor nerve axon terminal makes close contact with the skeletal muscle fibre which it supplies. An action potential arriving at the terminal causes release of the neurotransmitter **acetylcholine (ACh)**, which crosses the very narrow *synaptic cleft* to binding sites on the muscle membrane and initiates its depolarization; this triggers an action potential

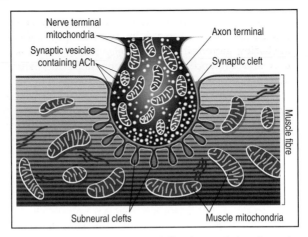

Nerve terminal mitochondria

Axon terminal

Synaptic vesicles containing ACh

Synaptic cleft

Muscle fibre

Subneural clefts

Muscle mitochondria

Axon terminal at its junction with a muscle fibre, from an electronmicrograph.

in the adjacent muscle fibre membrane and so sets in train the process of **excitation–contraction coupling**. In almost all mammalian/human extrafusal muscle fibres, the junction takes the form of a **motor endplate** but less extensive structures occur in some other locations.

**neuropathy** disease affecting peripheral nerves, causing neuralgia, paraesthesia and loss of sensory and/or motor function. Causes include trauma, diabetes, drugs, etc. Treatment is of the cause, but it is often irreversible.

**neuropeptides** peptides formed and released by groups of neurons within the central nervous system, that act on other neuron populations. Comparable to **neurotransmitters**, often made within the same cells, but acting via different types of specific receptors. Many have been recognized, of which better known examples are *enkephalins*, **serotonin** and *neuropeptide Y*. They have extensive influences, for example on mood and behaviour, pain and analgesia, appetite and the immune system. *See also* **endorphins**.

**neuroticism** one of the **big five** personality factors, characterized by a tendency to be tense, anxious and moody.

**neurotransmitter** a substance which is formed in a neuron cell body and passes down the axon to be stored in vesicles in the axon terminals. It is released in response to action potentials, to act at a synapse with another neuron or at an effector site: skeletal muscle, smooth muscle or gland. *See also* **acetylcholine, neuromuscular junction, noradrenaline**.

**Newton's laws of motion** three laws that relate the forces and motions of bodies or objects (from the viewpoint of a fixed observer), first proposed by Isaac Newton. (1) An object will remain at rest or continue with constant velocity unless acted on by an unbalanced force. (2) The rate of change of momentum (or acceleration for a body/ object of constant mass) is proportional to, and in the same direction as, the force applied to it (force = mass × acceleration). (3) When two objects are in contact, the force applied by one object on the other is equal and opposite to that of the second object on the first (for every action, there is an equal and opposite reaction).

**niacin** one of the vitamin B complex. *vitamin B$_3$* refers also to *nicotinic acid* and *nicotinamide*. *See also* **vitamins**; *appendix 4.2*.

**nitrogen balance** exists when nitrogen intake (in protein) equals nitrogen excretion. In *positive nitrogen balance* intake exceeds excretion, with the additional protein used to synthesize new tissues. This is required in growing children, during pregnancy, in recovery from illness and during resistance exercise training when overloading of muscle cells promotes protein synthesis. In *negative nitrogen balance* output is greater than intake, indicating that protein (primarily from skeletal muscle) is being used for energy. This occurs on starvation diets and those with low protein and carbohydrate intake; it reduces the lean tissue mass and is detrimental to exercise performance.

**nitrogen narcosis** a disturbance of mental function caused by an increase in the nitrogen dissolved in body fluids at high ambient pressure, e.g. diving at more than 2 atmospheres or 60 ft of water, if breathing air. Known as the *rapture of the deep.* Avoided by breathing mixtures containing oxygen and helium. *See also* **diving**.

**nomothetic** relating to the study of groups and generalizations rather than individuals and individual differences. *See also* **idiographic**.

**non-esterified fatty acids** *see* **fatty acids**.

**non-starch polysaccharides (NSP)** a form of carbohydrate, in foods such as wholegrain cereals, fruits and vegetables, which is not digested in the small intestine and so provides no source of calories; also known as *dietary fibre.* As well as providing 'bulk' and assisting weight maintenance or loss, fibre is important for the health of the colon (anti-cancer effect), reduces the risk of coronary heart disease (by combining with and preventing reabsorption of cholesterol from the gut) and assists blood sugar regulation in diabetes (by slowing the digestion of carbohydrates).

**non-steroidal anti-inflammatory drugs (NSAID)** a large group of drugs with varying degrees of anti-inflammatory, antipyretic and analgesic action. Related in their action to aspirin (**acetylsalicylic acid**), the earliest of the group to be in common use. They act by inhibiting enzymes needed for the synthesis of prostaglandins and thromboxanes. Used in sport as an anti-inflammatory agent to treat pain and reduce swelling. Commonest used is ibuprofen, which can be bought over the counter without a doctor's prescription. Sportsmen and women can be advised to take these drugs to facilitate healing, but not to continue with sport due to the risk of masking the signs of further, potentially serious, tissue damage. *See also appendix 6.*

**noradrenaline (*norepinephrine*)** the best known **neurotransmitter** at postganglionic sympathetic nerve endings (ATP and neuropeptide Y are also released). Also secreted into the blood stream from the adrenal medulla in response to activation of the **sympathetic nervous system**. Acts on all types of **adrenoceptors** but is less potent than **adrenaline** at the $\beta_2$ adrenoceptors that dilate skeletal muscle arteries and airways. Actions include vasoconstriction, relaxation of gut musculature, dilatation of the pupils. Both noradrenaline and adrenaline (to a much lesser extent) are neurotransmitters in the central nervous system.

**noradrenergic** *see* **adrenergic**.

**normal force** force acting at right angles to the surface of a body or object. *normal reaction* the force acting at right angles on the surface of a body or object due to opposition to another force, often coming from the ground or from another body or object.

**normoglycaemic** having the normal concentration of **blood glucose**.

**normothermia** the condition when **body temperature** is within the normal range. *normothermic adj. See also* **heat illness**, **hypothermia**.

**nutation** the result of the angular momentum and angular velocity vectors of a body or object being in different directions, leading to a rotation about a third axis.

**nutrient** a component of food that can be used to provide energy and/or in the synthesis of substances necessary for metabolism, growth and repair, and for all physiological functions (e.g. coenzymes, hormones, haemoglobin). *See also* **macronutrients**, **micronutrients**, **minerals**, **vitamins**; *appendix 4.1–4.4.*

**nutrition** the sum of the processes by which cellular organelles, cells, tissues, organs, systems and the body as a whole obtain necessary substances from foods and use them as sources of energy and to maintain structural and functional integrity.

**nutritional assessment** the assessment of an individual's nutritional status, used to identify those who are malnourished and those who are at risk of becoming malnourished. Factors included in the assessment are dietary intake, nutritional requirements, clinical condition, physical appearance, anthropometric and biochemical measurements. *See* also **anthropometry, dietary reference values, malnutrition**.

**obesity** a condition in which body fat stores are enlarged to an extent which impairs health. Develops when food intake is in excess of energy requirements. The most common nutritional disorder worldwide, and the incidence is increasing. Defined in terms of body mass index and circumference at the waist. *See also* **body composition, body weight, waist-to-hip ratio**.

**oestrogens (estrogens)** a group of steroid hormones produced mainly by the ovaries (predominantly in the first half of the menstrual cycle) and during pregnancy by the placenta; also in small amounts by the testes, and by the adrenal cortex in both sexes. Responsible for female secondary sexual characteristics and the development and function of the female reproductive system. Used in the combined oral contraceptive and in hormone replacement therapy. *See also* **hormones, menstrual cycle**.

**oligosaccharides** carbohydrates with 3–9 monosaccharide residues. The main dietary sources are vegetables, particularly seed legumes.

**omega-3 fatty acids** polyunsaturated fatty acids found in oil from oily fish and in certain plant/nut oils. The three major types contained in foods and used by the body are *alpha-linolenic acid (ALA), eicosapentaenoic acid (EPA)* and *docosahexaenoic acid (DHA)*. Fish oil contains EPA and DHA, while some nuts (English walnuts) and vegetable oils (canola, soybean, flaxseed/linseed and olive oil) contain ALA. Supplements are also widely available. Research indicates that omega-3 fatty acids reduce inflammation, improve plasma lipid profile and help to prevent certain chronic conditions such as **coronary artery disease** and arthritis; they are highly concentrated in the brain and have been reported to be important for cognitive and behavioural function.

**onset of blood lactate accumulation (OBLA)** *see* **metabolic and related thresholds**.

**open kinetic chain** exercise in which a distal body segment is free to move.

**open-loop control** in motor control, movement that is executed without regard to sensory feedback. Contrast **closed loop control**.

**openness to experience** one of the **big five** personality factors characterized by a tendency to be imaginative, curious, insightful and creative.

**opto-electronic motion analysis** equipment used to measure the motion of a body or object, using light (often infra-red) reflected from markers attached to its surface.

**oral rehydration fluids** *see* **hydration status**, **sports drinks**, **water balance**.

**origin** with reference to a skeletal muscle, the site of its attachment to bone which remains relatively fixed during its contraction compared to the site of its **insertion**. For example, in elbow extension, contraction of the triceps moves the forearm (site of insertion) while the upper arm and scapula (sites of origin) may remain still.

**orlistat** a drug which in conjunction with dieting has been proven to produce weight loss. It is a pancreatic lipase inhibitor which prevents fat breakdown in the intestine and therefore its absorption. About a third of ingested fat is passed through the bowel undigested when on a course of orlistat, reducing energy intake. Other beneficial effects include a lowering of serum cholesterol, reduction in blood pressure and better control of diabetes. Undesirable effects are abdominal discomfort, diarrhoea and anal leakage, and potential loss of fat-soluble vitamins. *See also* **lipolysis**.

**ornithine** dietary supplement which in combination with other amino acids arginine and lysine is claimed to increase muscle growth/lean body mass to a greater extent than strength training alone, but this has not been supported by properly designed trials. *See also* **ergogenic aids**; *appendix 4.4*.

**orthoses** from Greek *ortho*, to straighten. Custom-designed external devices used to control or counteract the effect of an actual or developing deformity. They include braces, splints, etc. In sport the term is most commonly used to describe foot-supporting insoles used to correct structural imbalance which may result in discomfort in the back, hips, knees or feet. Orthoses decrease the risk of further injury and make movement of the foot more efficient. *orthotics* the study and manufacture of orthoses.

**Osgood–Schlatter disease** osteochondritis/apophysitis of the tibial tubercle (tuberosity). Described by both Osgood and Schlatter (American and Swiss surgeons) in 1903. An 'overuse' injury, which produces pain (due to inflammation) at the attachment of the patellar tendon to the tibial tubercle at an age when this is not fully developed. Most common around puberty/adolescence (rapid skeletal growth), in boys more than girls, who take part in repeated or multiple sports, especially those with repetitive running (football, athletics) or with repeated knee bending and jumping (athletics, gymnastics). Some authors suggest up to 50% are precipitated by trauma. Symptoms include swelling, pain and tenderness on direct pressure, and pain (felt precisely on the tibial tubercle) during exercise and contraction of the quads. Heals spontaneously, with no individual treatment shown to be particularly helpful, except reduction in activity to levels where symptoms are acceptable. Rarely leads to problems in later life.

**osmolality** the concentration of osmotically active particles in a solution, expressed as the number of osmoles per kilogram ($Osm.kg^{-1}$) of solution. In blood plasma, osmolality (280–300 $mOsm.kg^{-1}$) is very slightly less than **osmolarity** (in $mOsm.L^{-1}$) because the presence of large molecules (e.g. lipids) adds to the volume that contains 1 kg of water (plasma is about 94% water). The two terms are often incorrectly used interchangeably; osmolality applies appropriately to body fluids. Measurement allows assessment of dehydration/overhydration.

**osmolarity** the concentration of osmotically active particles in a solution expressed in osmoles per litre

$(Osm.L^{-1})$ of the solution. Values for human body fluids (e.g. blood plasma) are usually expressed in milliosmoles per litre $(mOsm.L^{-1})$. Compare **osmolality.**

**osmole** the amount of a substance in a solution that forms one mole of osmotically active particles, irrespective of their size, e.g. a single sodium ion contributes as much to the osmolality as a large protein molecule; and 1 mole of glucose, which does not ionize, provides 1 osmole, while 1 mole of sodium chloride provides 2 osmoles – one of $Na^+$ and one of $Cl^-$.

**osmoreceptors** cells located in the hypothalamus, sensitive to a change in the **osmolality** of their surroundings, which will reflect any such change in the plasma and body fluids as a whole. A rise in osmolality (tending towards dehydration) triggers increased production and release of **antidiuretic hormone (ADH)** from the posterior pituitary (a neuroendocrine secretion), causing the kidneys to retain more water. Conversely, a decrease in body fluid osmolality (due to high water intake) reduces ADH release, leading to increased and less concentrated urine output (diuresis).

**osmotic pressure** the 'suction' exerted by a solution of higher, upon one of lower, osmolar concentration, which moves water by *osmosis* in the direction that will equalize concentrations if the solutions are separated by a semi-permeable membrane; this allows the passage of water but not of the solute particles. Applies to movements of water across cell membranes, maintaining *osmotic equilibrium* between extra- and intracellular fluids.

**osteoarthritis (OA)** a condition of the joints where articular cartilage becomes worn, exposing the underlying bone. More than just 'wear and tear', it is an evolving process with much research aimed at slowing its advance. Known aetiological factors include increasing age, female sex, manual occupations, obesity, malalignment and injury in sport. Genetic factors have been implicated, though not yet identified. There is little evidence that exercise *per se* produces OA. Clinically OA presents with pain, stiffness, limitation of movement and joint deformity. X-rays show joint space narrowing, osteophytes, subchondral sclerosis and bony deformity. Most commonly affects the weight-bearing joints (hips, knees, ankles and feet) and hands. Exercise is used in treatment to maintain mobility, flexibility and muscle strength. Analgesia and modification of activity are advised in mild to moderate OA, and osteotomy or joint replacement for severe disease in suitable joints.

**osteopathy** an established clinical discipline (now regulated by a statutory body) concerned with the interrelationship between structure and function of the body. Osteopaths have a holistic approach, treating the whole person in the prevention, diagnosis and treatment of illness, injury or disease. Osteopaths in sport mainly treat mechanical musculoskeletal problems.

**osteopenia** lower than normal bone mineral density.

**osteoporosis** reduction in bone mineral density with ageing, particularly in women; onset and progress are mitigated by regular exercise, particularly **weight-bearing exercise**. Increases the likelihood of fractures, often with relatively minor trauma. *See also* **bone scan, dual emission X-ray absorptiometry (DEXA)**.

**osteotomy** surgical division of a bone to achieve realignment. Used to encourage healing, e.g. in a poorly aligned healed fracture, or to reduce pain in osteoarthritis.

**outcome expectancy** in **social cognitive theory**, a person's expectations about the consequences of an action.

**outcome goal** a goal that specifies the outcome of a performance, usually involving a comparison with others such as winning a race. *See also* **performance goal, process goal**.

**ovary** the female **gonad**, the site of production of *ova*; one on each side, in the pelvic cavity, close to the open end of each Fallopian tube. An *ovum* is discharged into one of these tubes en route for the uterus at *ovulation* in each **menstrual cycle**. The ovaries are also endocrine glands (under the influence in turn of anterior pituitary *gonadotrophic* hormones), secreting the female hormones oestrogen and progestogen. These have actions both widely in the body and on the reproductive organs at specific times in the menstrual cycle and during pregnancy. *See also* **hormones**; *appendix 5*.

**overjustification effect** an explanation for the observation that if individuals are rewarded for engaging in an inherently enjoyable or satisfying activity, they are subsequently less likely to engage in the activity when given the opportunity to do so in the absence of a reward. It is proposed that the reward comes to justify engagement in the activity instead of the initial inherent enjoyment and when removed, there no longer remains a reason for taking part. For example, rewarding children for engaging in sport could undermine their inherent interest in sport.

**overlearning** the learning of a task or action beyond the point of mastery so that it becomes automated. Typically acquired through repetitive drills.

**overload principle** a term used less now than previously, indicating the need to place increased demand upon a tissue (e.g. connective), organ (e.g. muscle) or system (e.g. cardiovascular) if its performance is to improve. The demand concerned may be for strength, endurance or (less commonly) speed. Must be distinguished from 'overload' in engineering, which is a load greater than a structure can bear.

**overtraining** training exceeding the body's recovery capacity, indicated by excessive fatigue both physical and mental, and resulting in impaired performance. Also called *staleness*. Short-term overtraining is usually adequately countered by a period of reduced intensity or a few days' total rest but if extended, it leads to the *overtraining syndrome* – a set of symptoms and signs, probably of neuroendocrine origin. The psychological aspect of fatigue now usually predominates, while physical symptoms often include increased BMR, protracted elevation of pulse rate after exercise, and negative nitrogen balance leading to weight loss. Recovery may take months or never be fully achieved. Compare the unexplained **under performance syndrome (UPS)** which may apply in some instances previously classed as overtraining. *See also* **burnout**.

**overweight** *see* **body weight, body mass index, obesity.**

**oxidative phosphorylation** oxidation of products of carbohydrate, fat, protein and alcohol metabolism to carbon dioxide and water with formation of ATP from ADP and inorganic phosphate ($P_i$), associated with the transfer of electrons from substrate via coenzymes to oxygen, taking place in **mitochondria**. *See also* **adenosine mono-, di- and triphosphates (AMP, ADP, ATP).**

**oxidative stress** general term used to describe imbalance between **reactive oxygen species** and **antioxidants**. Oxidative stress can damage a specific molecule or the entire organism and is known to be implicated in the pathogenesis of a wide variety of disorders, including coronary heart disease, cerebrovascular disease, chronic obstructive lung disease, some forms of cancer, diabetes, skeletal muscular dystrophy and others. Oxidative stress-induced damage in muscle could be one of the factors that terminate muscular effort, but consecutive exercise bouts seem to induce antioxidant adaptations.

**oxygen consumption ($\dot{V}O_2$)** the rate of uptake of oxygen in the lungs, usually expressed in litres per minute. Measured in *indirect calorimetry* as an estimate of **metabolic rate**, taking the 'calorific value' of 1 litre of oxygen as 4.8 kcal (for an average ratio of carbohydrate to lipid oxidation), therefore $1\,L.min^{-1}$ as equivalent to $4.8\,kcal.min^{-1}$, $20\,kJ.min^{-1}$ or 333 watts.

**oxygen cost** the rate of oxygen usage for a particular task or work rate.

**oxygen debt** amount by which oxygen consumption during recovery from exercise exceeds resting level.

Consists of an initial rapid phase lasting ~1–2 min (formerly called the 'alactic' phase), in which muscle CrP and ATP stores are replenished, and a subsequent slow phase (~1 h) in which lactic acid is oxidized (hence the former term 'lactacid' phase), temperature falls toward resting level and blood hormonal concentrations are normalized. Also known as *elevated post-exercise oxygen consumption (EPOC)* or *recovery oxygen consumption*.

**oxygen deficit** shortfall of oxygen consumed during activity below that required to supply all necessary energy aerobically. Postexercise restoration of this deficit constitutes part, but not all, of the **oxygen debt.**

**oxygen delivery** the rate of supply of oxygen by the arterial blood to body organs and tissues, expressed as cardiac output (L.min$^{-1}$) × oxygen content of the blood (L.L$^{-1}$), e.g. typical resting value would be $5 \times 0.2 = 1$ L.min$^{-1}$. This is four times the typical oxygen usage at rest, since only a quarter of the oxygen in the arterial blood is removed by the tissues, reducing haemoglobin saturation from 100% to 75%. *See also* **oxyhaemoglobin dissociation curve**.

**oxygen plateau** the flattening out of oxygen consumption after the maximal value is attained in incremental exercise.

**oxygen poisoning** a hazard of exposure to high ambient pressure (typically in **diving**) when breathing high percentage oxygen. With 100% oxygen inspired oxygen pressure is ~100 kPa on the surface at 1 atmosphere, and increases by 100 kPa for every 10 m depth under water. Susceptibility varies between individuals and with the level of physical work, but limits typically advised are ~150–170 kPa, equivalent to breathing 100% oxygen at depths of 5–7 metres (or proportionately <100% mixed with nitrogen at greater depths). Toxic effects are mainly on the brain (causing epileptic fits) and on the lungs (cough, oedema, impairment of oxygen diffusion). Fits under water can be fatal and the more slowly developing pulmonary toxicity can be irreversible if severe. (Higher pressures than those advised above are safely used to treat **decompression illness** by 100% oxygen at rest.)

**oxygen transport** *see* **oxygen delivery, oxyhaemoglobin dissociation curve, partial pressure**.

**oxygen uptake** *see* **oxygen consumption**.

**oxyhaemoglobin dissociation curve** the graph which describes the relationship in the blood between partial pressure of oxygen ($PO_2$) and the percentage saturation of haemoglobin; it can also show the equivalent oxygen content of the blood when haemoglobin is in normal concentration. With normal lungs, saturation in arterial blood is determined by the $PO_2$ in the alveolar gas with which pulmonary capillary blood equilibrates. The S-shape of the curve has important physiological advantages, e.g. a relatively small decrease in $PO_2$ encountered where blood flows through tissues causes a 'steep' removal of oxygen from the blood; but there needs to be a relatively large decrease in $PO_2$ in the inspired air (and therefore in the alveoli, e.g. at **altitude** or in a confined space) before there is a serious decline in haemoglobin saturation. (*See fig overleaf.*)

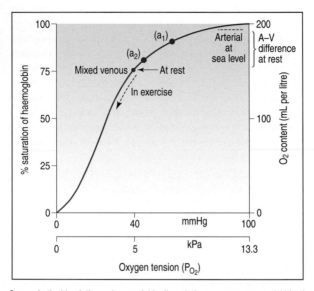

Oxygen in the blood: the oxyhaemoglobin dissociation curve. $a_1$, $a_2$: arterial blood at altitudes of ~2500m and ~5000m.

# P

**pacemaker** the region of the heart, normally the *sinoatrial node*, that rhythmically initiates the *cardiac action potential* and hence the whole electrical and mechanical **cardiac cycle**, varying the **heart rate** under the influence of the sympathetic and parasympathetic nerve supply. An *artificial pacemaker* may be implanted when normal rhythm generation is affected by heart disease.

**packed cell volume** *see* **haematocrit**.

**pain** the name that we give to the unpleasant and disturbing subjective experience that results from injury or other damage. Sensory receptors involved are known as *nociceptors* (from the *adj* noxious meaning harmful); thence afferent nerve impulses reach the central nervous system (CNS), where different influences can diminish or enhance them, acting where they are relayed and transmitted to the cerebral cortex and conscious perception. The pain pathways are separate from those serving other sensations, and even vigorous stimulation of other sensory receptors does not, by itself, cause pain. *pain management* involves a multdisciplinary approach, often by a specialist team. *See also* **endorphins, transcutaneous electromagnetic nerve stimulation (TENS)**.

**pain killer** *see* **analgesic**.

**palpation** examination of a body area by touch.

**palpitation** beating of the heart of which a person is strongly aware, as being rapid and/or forceful, or sometimes irregular. May be both unpleasant and worrying but most will experience palpitation on occasion. Physiological causes include exercise, excitement, caffeine intake, smoking and alcohol. May also be a symptom of underlying disease, e.g. anaemia, hyperthyroidism, cardiac disease (especially if linked with other symptoms such as faintness, sweating, chest pain). Investigations (ECG, ambulatory monitoring, echocardiography, exercise test) are used to identify the nature of the condition and possible underlying causes.

**panting** rapid shallow breathing; a mechanism in furry animals for losing heat. In humans, not a normal physiological pattern of breathing. *See also* **hyperventilation**, **tachypnoea**.

**paradigm** term introduced ca 1960 by the science-historian Kuhn; a widely followed way of approaching an area of research, deriving from a notable early achievement in the field and carrying forward both its experimental methodology and its theoretical outlook.

**paraesthesia** the sensations commonly known as *pins and needles*; may be due to pressure on, or damage to, a nerve or may have no evident cause.

**parallel axis theorem** mathematical method of relating the moment of inertia of a body or object around one axis to the moment of inertia of the same body or object around a parallel axis. Calculated as $I_2 = I_1 + md^2$ where $I_1$ and $I_2$ are the moments of inertia, m is the mass of the object and d is the distance between the two parallel axes.

**paralympics** the competitive events regularly held 'parallel to the Olympics' for disabled sportspeople. In the late 1940s Ludwig Guttmann, medical director of the Stoke Mandeville Spinal Injuries Unit, who had made wheelchair games a feature of rehabilitation, initiated competitive events in archery, netball and table tennis for his paraplegic patients. In 1952 he invited a small Dutch team to join in the local games, and this first international event led to his inauguration of the paralympics in Rome in 1960, with 400 wheelchair athletes. By 2004 successive occasions had extended the range of disabilities included, and there were 19 events for 4000 participants from 136 countries. *See also* **spinal injury**.

**paralysis** loss of muscle function, due to damage at any level in the pathway for neural activation, or to muscle disease or relaxant drugs. *See also* **spinal injury**.

**paraparesis** incomplete loss of motor function in the lower half of the body.

**paraplegia** paralysis of the lower part of the body, including both lower limbs. *paraplegic adj. See also* **spinal injury**.

**parasympathetic nervous system** one of the two components of the **autonomic nervous system**. Preganglionic nerve fibres come from the brain stem and from the sacral segments of the spinal cord ('craniosacral outflow'), i.e. from the central nervous system above and below the sympathetic outflow. These nerves relay in ganglia close to the organs where they act (including heart, lungs, gastrointestinal tract). Most of the cranial components travel in the **vagus nerves**. In general, parasympathetic nerves stimulate the functions of the alimentary and genitourinary systems, whereas effects on the cardiorespiratory system are appropriate to relative inactivity, e.g. slowing the heart rate. *See also* **acetylcholine, atropine, sympathetic nervous system**; *appendix 1.1 figs 5, 6.*

**parathyroid glands** small clumps of endocrine tissue (usually four) on the back of the thyroid gland which secrete *parathyroid homone (PTH)*. This acts to increase calcium ion concentration in the extracellular fluid, counterbalanced by calcitonin from the thyroid gland which has the opposite effects. Together they correct any changes in blood $[Ca^{2+}]$ by action on absorption of calcium from the gut, its deposition in bone and its excretion by the kidneys. *See also* **hormones**; *appendix 5.*

**partial pressure** the component of the total gas pressure accounted for by one gas in a mixture of gases, e.g. in air at 1 standard atmosphere (1 bar, $\sim$101 kPa, 760 mmHg or torr), 21% is oxygen and the partial pressure of oxygen ($PO_2$) is $\sim$21 kPa or 160 mmHg (torr). Partial pressure (*syn* **tension**) of a gas dissolved in a liquid is defined as the partial pressure of that gas in the gaseous phase with which the liquid is, has been or would be, in equilibrium. So, given near-perfect diffusion equilibrium across the alveolar-capillary membranes, blood leaves the lungs with virtually the same $PO_2$ and $PCO_2$ as in alveolar gas (normally close to 100 mmHg

$PO_2$ and 40 mmHg $PCO_2$). When blood reaches capillaries in active tissues, the lower $PO_2$ and higher $PCO_2$ in tissue fluids cause net molecular movement towards equilibrium, so that $O_2$ is removed from the blood and $CO_2$ taken up. *See also* **carbon dioxide, diffusing capacity, gas exchange, nitrogen, oxygen, oxyhaemoglobin dissociation curve**.

**participation motive** an individual's reason for engaging in activity. Often applied to reasons for engaging in exercise or sport, such as to manage weight, for enjoyment or for social reasons.

**patella** the knee cap. *patellar tendon syn patellar ligament* the strong flat fibrous band that runs from the lower margin of the patella to the tibial tubercle (tuberosity). The more superficial fibres are in fact continuous over the front of the patella with the quadriceps tendon, effectively providing insertion of the quadriceps onto the tibia. Injury is seen in jumping sports. *patellar tendonitis* inflammation of the patellar tendon. Causes include a change in training (intensity, frequency or type, e.g. more repetitive running on a hard surface), poor muscle strength and altered biomechanics at the knee. This results in pain and swelling over the tendon, especially after activity. Common in jumping sports such as basketball and athletics (*jumper's knee*).Treatment is as for any soft tissue injury. Rehabilitation includes changing technique, altering training load, biomechanical assessment and muscle strengthening. *See also* **knee joint**; *appendix 1.2 figs 1, 2*.

**Pavlovian conditioning** *see* **conditioning**.

**peak expiratory flow rate (PEFR)** the highest flow rate at the mouth during a rapid forced expiration, starting with the lungs at full capacity. Peak occurs almost immediately after the start of exhalation. Reduced in obstructive lung disease (asthma, bronchitis, emphysema). *See also* **lung volumes**.

**peak force** the greatest recorded instantaneous force on an object or body (e.g. during gait analysis).

**peak performance** a state in which the person performs to the maximum of their ability, characterized by subjective feelings of confidence, effortlessness and total concentration on the task.

**pectoral muscles** group of muscles on the front of the chest which link the trunk to the upper limb. *pectoralis major* the largest and most superficial, takes origin from the clavicle, sternum and ribs and crosses the front of the shoulder to insertions into the clavicle and humerus. *See appendix 1.2 fig 5A.*

**pedometer** device for counting the number of strides taken in a given period or event. Almost all modern pedometers also provide estimates of distance covered and average speed, based upon a user-entered mean value of stride length.

**peer group** a social group composed of people of a similar age or status.

**peer support** the social support provided by one's peer group.

**pelvis** (from Latin meaning 'basin') the bony framework of the lowest part of the trunk, where the *hip bones* together with the sacrum and coccyx enclose the pelvic cavity, which is continuous above with the abdominal cavity. Each hip bone has three fused components: the *ilium* with a flared upper rim, the *iliac crest*, and linked to the sacrum at the **sacroiliac joint**; the *ischium* with the socket for the head of the femur (the acetabulum) at the **hip joint**; and the *pubis* which is attached to its partner at the *pubic symphysis*, centre front. *See appendix 1.2 figs 1, 2.*

**perception** the act or process of becoming aware of internal or external sensory stimuli or events, involving the meaningful organization and interpretation of those stimuli. In psychology, perception also applies to evaluations of one's own and others' internal states and beliefs as well as sensory stimuli and a person's perceptions are not necessarily identical to the stimulus object or event being perceived. For example, a person's perceptions of their ability might not match their actual ability. Perception is to be distinguished from *sensation* which refers to the subjective experience that results from excitation of the sensory apparatus without any interpretation or imposition of meaning.

**perceptual motor skill** any skill involving the interaction and integration of perceptual processes and voluntary physical movement, such as the ability to perform a gymnastic routine.

**performance** the act of producing a co-ordinated sequence of behaviours. *See also* **ability**, **skill**.

**performance genes** the potential uses of genetic profiling and gene therapy within sport remain experimental and controversial. Suggested applications include (1) identification of potential athletes by the presence of the so-called performance genes, which may enable an athlete to perform at a higher level by their influence on muscle metabolism and endurance; (2) use as a 'screening' tool to identify athletes with particular body shape, e.g. tall athletes for basketball. This could result in discrimination and have implications for the funding for young athletes, should funding be withheld from those who 'fail' to have the ideal body habitus; (3) identification of those athletes who have a genetic predisposition to sports-related injury. Other moral dilemmas exist in this area. Should the limited funding for genetic research be used to enhance sports performance at the expense of research into disease prevention? Should we limit opportunities within sport and exercise because the young person does not have the ideal 'genetic makeup'? The **World Anti-Doping Agency (WADA)** and the **International Olympic Committee** have recently included the non-therapeutic use of genes, genetic elements and/or cells that have the capacity to enhance athletic performance in their list of proscribed substances and methods. They will continue to monitor the use of genetic testing and genetic information for identifying or selecting athletes, with a view to developing policies and guidelines for sports organizations and athletes. *See also* **human enhancement technologies (HET)**.

**performance goal** (1) a goal focused on gaining favourable judgements or avoiding unfavourable judgements by others; (2) a goal that specifies the achievement of an endproduct of performance that is relatively independent of the performance of other people, such as running a race in a certain time rather than beating others. *See also* **ego involvement**, **learning goal**, **process goal**, **outcome goal**.

**performance profiling** a method for helping athletes to identify their strengths and weaknesses in order to encourage them to be fully involved in decisions about developing appropriate training programmes to enhance their performance. It typically involves asking athletes to identify what they think are the major characteristics of an elite performer in their sport and then to rate themselves on those characteristics.

**perfusion** in physiology and pathology, refers to blood flow in a region, organ or tissue; *hypoperfusion* inadequate blood flow.

**peripheral nervous system (PNS)** all nerve cells and fibres that are outside the central nervous system (CNS, the brain and spinal cord) and which connect all parts of the body with the CNS. Includes the *somatic nervous system* – the nerves to skeletal muscles and from neural receptors in the musculoskeletal system and the skin, and the **autonomic nervous system** which controls the functions of the organs, the glands and the cardiovascular system via the outgoing nerves of its two divisions, the sympathetic nervous system and the parasympathetic nervous system; together with their associated *visceral afferents*. *See appendix 1.1 figs 3–5.*

**peripheral resistance** the sum total of resistance to blood flow in the systemic circulation, mostly located in the arterioles, dependent on the constriction/relaxation of the smooth muscle in their walls. The balance between cardiac output and total peripheral resistance determines the arterial blood pressure (BP), and physiological adjustments of either or both are the means of maintaining BP despite variations in local vasodilatation/vasoconstriction in different organs and tissues.

**personal construct theory** a theory of personality first described by American psychologist George Kelly in 1955 that views the person as actively constructing their view of reality and acting as an incipient scientist, constantly formulating and testing hypotheses about their world in order to bring sense and meaning to their lives.

**personality** the totality of behavioural, psychological and emotional characteristics that make a person an individual. *See also* **big five**, **trait**.

**Perthes' disease** avascular degeneration of the upper femoral epiphysis. Occurs in children aged 4–8, five times more commonly in boys, causing a limp, which may be painless. Revascularization occurs but residual deformity of the femoral head may subsequently lead to arthritic changes. Diagnosed on clinical suspicion with X-ray confirmation. Treatment aims to minimize the deformity and includes rest, traction, plaster cast or occasionally surgery (described in 1910 by German orthopaedic surgeon G. C. Perthes).

**pes cavus** high-arched or *claw foot*. An acquired or congenital condition, which results from plantarflexion of the forefoot relative to the rearfoot, with elevation of the longitudinal arch. Associated with clawing of the toes, depression of the first metatarsal and hindfoot varus. May be the result of underlying neuromuscular disease. Can present with pain, difficulty in getting suitable shoes or obvious foot deformity. In sport, good podiatry input and correctly fitted shoes will minimize secondary effects, which are seen primarily in weight-bearing sports.

**pes planus** *aka **flat foot*** an abnormally low longitudinal arch causes a greater contact area with the ground. Most do not cause problems but can result in loss of the gripping action of the toes, causing pain and discomfort during weight-bearing, especially when running. The foot becomes more rigid with age, with increased risk of later osteoarthritis. Common in children when the longitudinal arch has not yet developed.

**pH** the negative logarithm of the hydrogen ion concentration $[H^+]$, so a change by one pH unit means a tenfold change in $[H^+]$. pH 7 represents neutrality in water at $25°C$, when $[H^+] = 10^{-7}$ molar $= 100\,nmol.L^{-1}$. In the body, at $37°C$, 'neutral' would be $\sim$pH 6.8 but the *extracellular pH* of body fluids is more alkaline than this. Arterial blood pH (the most readily measured) varies in health within the range of 7.36–7.44 or $[H^+] = 40\,nmol.L^{-1} \pm$ about 12% – a tiny amount compared to other ions in the blood. *intracellular pH* is more acidic (e.g. 6.8–7.1 in skeletal muscle fibres), so there is a gradient promoting exit of metabolically generated $H^+$ from cells. Regulation, vital for normal metabolic processes, depends on this gradient, on intracellular buffers (predominantly proteins and phosphates) and on variations in $PCO_2$. The whole-body turnover of $H^+$ (by ingestion, metabolic production and excretion) is

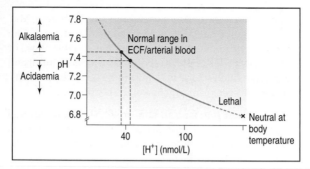

pH and hydrogen ion concentrations in extracellular fluids.

of vastly greater magnitude than the body fluid concentrations. *See also* **acid–base balance**.

**phenotype** an individual's characteristics, determined largely, but not entirely, by his/her genotype, as it can be influenced for example by environmental and maternal factors.

**phenylbutazone** a powerful anti-inflammatory drug first used in the 1940s in the treatment of arthritis. Limited by its potentially serious side effects (including fatalities), it is now rarely used in humans (ankylosing spondylitis is an exception) but interestingly is used in equestrian sports to treat soft tissue injuries in horses.

**phosphofructokinase (PFK)** the most important regulatory enzyme involved in the pathway of glycolysis, enabling the phosphorylation of fructose-6-phosphate to fructose 1,6-diphosphate. The activity level of PFK probably limits the rate of glycolysis during maximal exercise. *See also* **muscle enzymes**.

**phospholipids** *see* **lipids**.

**phosphorylase** *see* **glycogenolysis, muscle enzymes**.

**phosphorylation potential** the concentration ratio [ATP] / [ADP] [$P_i$] in the cytosol of a cell (where $P_i$ is the total of inorganic phosphate ions, $HPO_4^{2-}$ and $H_2PO_4^{-}$), proposed as an index of its energy status; this ratio is directly related to the free energy available from ATP. Also known as *cytoplasmic energy state*. *See also* **adenosine mono-, di- and triphosphates (AMP, ADP, ATP), energy charge**.

**physical activity level (PAL)** the ratio of daily energy expenditure to basal metabolic rate, reflecting the average activity at both work and leisure. PAL is estimated at 1.4 for inactive men and women, 1.6 for moderately active women and 1.7 for moderately active men. The PAL of athletes is of course much higher.

**physical self-concept** a person's perception or description of their physical self, including their physical appearance, typically not involving an evaluative component.

**physical self-esteem** a person's evaluation of their physical self, including evaluations of both physical appearance and physical competencies. Also known as *physical self-worth*.

**physical self-perception** a general term that denotes all aspects of a person's perceptions of their physical self, including evaluative and descriptive elements.

**physiological arousal** *see* **arousal**.

**physiology** the branch of biological science concerned with the normal bodily function of living organisms, hence *physiologist*. Also those functions themselves, as for example the physiology of digestion, of vision, of locomotion, etc. *adj physiological*.

**physiotherapy** a healthcare profession that provides treatment for physical problems due to accident, illness or disability, promoting normal function and mobility, using skills of **manipulation**, **electrotherapy** and/or appropriate exercise regimes. Physiotherapists are involved also in preventive healthcare as well as in rehabilitation and are key personnel in the provision of injury care and rehabilitation in sport.

**pituitary gland** endocrine gland at the base of the brain, attached by the *pituitary stalk* carrying blood vessels and nerve fibres from the hypothalamus. *See also* **anterior pituitary**, **posterior pituitary**.

**placebo** harmless inert substance given as medicine or supplement. In a randomized placebo-controlled trial, this is identical in appearance with the active material being tested. When neither the researcher nor the subjects know which is which, the trial is said to be 'double blind'. *placebo effect* a therapeutic effect or in the case of sport performance an enhancing effect observed after the administration of a placebo.

**planar analysis** motion analysis (may be *kinematic* or *kinetic*) which analyses movement in only one plane, i.e. is two-dimensional. If a body/object is moving three-dimensionally, planar analysis requires assumptions about out-of-plane movements. Kinematic planar motion analysis usually only requires one camera, so is simple.

**planes** for reference in the description of location and movements of parts of the body, three planes perpendicular to each other, passing through the middle of the body, are defined: *sagittal* vertical, front-to-back; *frontal* vertical, side-to-side; *transverse* horizontal. *See also* **principal axes**. *Fig overleaf.*

**plantar** pertaining to the sole of the foot.

**plantar fascia** the thick band of connective tissue on the sole of the foot, which runs from the calcaneum to the base of the toes; inflammation (*plantar fasciitis*) is one of the commonest causes of heel pain, usually at the attachment to the calcaneum. Pain is felt especially first thing in the morning (overnight rest with the foot in plantarflexion allows the fascia to contract) or on weight-bearing exercise: a dull pain felt along the sole of the foot. Associated with, but not caused by, a bony spur. More common in runners, gymnasts and dancers (who use repetitive maximal plantarflexion of the foot) and in those with flat feet. Management includes rest, anti-inflammatory medication, podiatry assessment, exercises to stretch the fascia, **orthoses** and, if severe, corticosteroid injection.

**plantarflexion** movement at the ankle joint that points the foot downwards away from the leg, or movement of the toes that curls them down towards the sole (compare **dorsiflexion**). *See appendix 1.2 fig 3.*

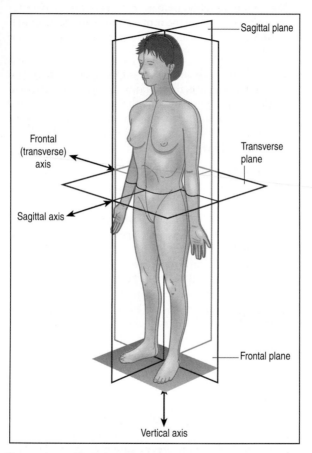

Sagittal plane

Frontal (transverse) axis

Transverse plane

Sagittal axis

Frontal plane

Vertical axis

Planes and axes of the body.

**plastic** describes a body, object or substance which after deformation does not return to its initial state. Contrast **elasticity**.

**platelets** *syn thrombocytes* cellular fragments in the blood, involved in **blood coagulation**. Platelets aggregate and adhere to form a temporary plug at the site of blood vessel damage.

**pleura** thin membrane in two layers in continuity, which cover the lung and line its compartment within the thorax on each side; the layers enclose between them the *pleural cavity*, a 'space' normally occupied only by a thin fluid film; this holds the lungs expanded against their *elastic recoil*, so that chest wall and lungs move together during the breathing cycle, but allows some sliding movement between them. The lung collapses if the layers become separated by entry of air (**pneumothorax**). *See appendix 1.3 fig 4.*

**plyometrics** type of exercise which utilizes the stretch-shortening cycle of musculotendinous tissue. Eccentric stretching is followed by concentric shortening of the same muscles. Often involves rebound activities.

**pneumotachograph** an instrument for recording respiratory airflow in terms of the pressure drop across a low resistance in its path (*flow head*). Flow can be electronically integrated with respect to time, to give a continuous record of volume breathed in or out, and hence the volume per minute (ventilation).

**pneumothorax** air in the pleural cavity, between the chest wall and the lungs, either by escape from damaged lungs or by entry from outside with a penetrating injury. Causes compression of lung tissue and potentially respiratory distress. Can occur spontaneously, especially in the young, as a complication of lung disease or in sport, most commonly as a result of direct trauma. May also occur by **barotrauma** in scuba diving and flying at altitude. Symptoms include sharp chest pain and shortness of breath. Diagnosis is clinical, confirmed by chest X-ray. If small, usually heals spontaneously but if larger and symptomatic may require the use of a chest drain to re-expand the lung. If recurrent, may require surgery.

**podiatry** the term that is now generally used to include *chiropody*, traditionally the practice of caring for the health, and treating disorders, of the feet. Now a paramedical profession responsible for the assessment, diagnosis and management of conditions of the feet and lower limbs. The input of podiatrists in sport is increasing with the greater understanding of the role of biomechanics of the lower limb in the prevention and treatment of injury. Biomechanical assessment may, for example, suggest the benefit of custom-made insoles to partially correct an abnormality. *See also* **orthoses**.

**polarity** in the context of rotation, one method of signifying the direction of rotational movements. Anticlockwise is usually positive, clockwise is negative.

**polycythaemia** greater than normal number of red blood cells (RBC) per unit volume of blood. A compensatory mechanism in **hypoxia** (arising either from lung disease or in healthy people at **altitude**) which leads to stimulation of RBC production in the bone marrow. Improves oxygen transport, but at the expense of increasing blood viscosity, adding to the resistance to blood flow in the circulation. *See also* **erythropoiesis**.

**polyunsaturated fatty acids** *see* **fatty acids**.

**position** the location of a body or object in space that may be specified by **co-ordinates** (e.g. Cartesian or polar).

**positive energy balance** *see* **energy balance**.

**positive transfer** an enhancement in performance because of practice or experience gained in practising another similar skill or the same skill under different conditions. For example, skill gained practising golf on a driving range should positively transfer to skill on the golf course. Similarly, practising overhand throwing of a ball should transfer positively to more complex skills such as the overhead serve in tennis. *See also* **negative transfer, transfer of learning**.

**posterior compartment syndrome** *see* **compartment syndrome**.

**posterior cruciate ligament** *see* **cruciate ligaments**.

**posterior pituitary** not itself the site of hormone synthesis, but the site of release of hormones formed in the **hypothalamus** by neurons whose axons form the hypophyseal-pituitary tract, store the hormones in their terminals, and release them into the blood stream in response to action potentials (**neurohormones**: compare adrenal medulla). *antidiuretic hormone* (*syn vasopressin*) regulates water loss in the kidneys, by increasing water retention; *oxytocin* stimulates uterine contractions and the ejection of milk from the breasts. *See also* **hormones**; *appendix 5*.

**postural hypotension** fall in arterial blood pressure on rising from lying or sitting to standing. Minimal and transient in healthy people, but exaggerated in people with inadequate autonomic response. Also known as *orthostatic hypotension*.

**postural muscles** those utilized predominantly in the maintenance of body posture against gravity, e.g. neck, back, knee and ankle extensors. They have a majority of slow (type 1, 'red') muscle fibres, e.g. the calf muscle *soleus* has close to 90% in most individuals and *erector spinae* has over 60%, although, as in all human muscles, there is substantial variation between individuals *See also* **muscle fibre types**.

**potassium** the major cation in intracellular fluid (ICF) accounting for over 90% of the body's potassium. Its many functions include a crucial role in the generation of the **membrane potential** and of an **action potential**. The level in the blood is regulated by the kidneys, under the influence of the hormone aldosterone. Intake in food and excretion (mainly in the urine) are typically balanced at about 60 mmol/day. *hypokalaemia* abnormally low, *hyperkalaemia* abnormally high, blood level of potassium. *See also* **minerals**; *appendix 4.3*.

**potential energy** the energy due to an object or body's position or form. May be elastic, gravitational or electrical.

**power** rate of doing work. In mechanics, over any period of constant applied force, power = force multiplied by displacement in the direction of that force, divided by the time for which it has operated, i.e. = force × velocity. In electricity, power = current × voltage.

**practice** in general, the repeated execution of an action in order to gain or improve a skill. *blocked practice* when executing a series of trials of one skill before moving on to practice another skill, typical of drills in which the same skill is repeated many times; *distributed practice* when there are periods of rest in between trials; *massed practice* when the order of executing different skills is randomized or mixed within a given session.

**prednisolone** *see* **glucocorticoids**.

**pre-event fuelling** *see* **carbohydrate loading**.

**pregnancy** the time from about 2 weeks after the last menstrual period (the time of ovulation) to parturition (labour/delivery), normally 40 weeks or 280 days. Most women feel and look better if they exercise while pregnant and it helps to alleviate backache and maintain posture, ease joint discomfort, allow better sleep and minimize excessive weight gain. Pregnancy confers physiological benefits to exercise and possibly performance during the first trimester (3 months), especially by virtue of changes in the cardiorespiratory systems. Modern thinking is that exercise is generally safe and should be encouraged, if comfortable, until well into the last trimester, provided that there are no complications of pregnancy (bleeding, hypertension, multiple pregnancy, placenta praevia, etc.). Walking, cycling, dance and water-based activity are popular with pregnant women. Exercise should be symptom-limited and should stop if the woman becomes dizzy or breathless. Contact sports such as boxing and those where a fall is likely, such as horse riding, climbing and trampolining, are not recommended in case of damage to the fetus.

**premenstrual syndrome (PMS)** group of physical and emotional symptoms defined as occurring in the 14 days prior to menstruation, relieved almost immediately by the onset of the period, and having at least a 7-day symptom-free break in each cycle. Athletes are encouraged to complete a menstrual diary to help confirm the diagnosis and rule out other gynaecological or psychological conditions. Symptoms include irritability, headache, poor concentration, mood swings, disrupted sleep pattern, headaches, breast tenderness and abdominal bloating and cramps. PMS occurs as a result of the hormonal changes, particularly the rise in progesterone, which occur at that phase of the cycle. The importance in sport is the potential effect on performance of some female athletes, though there is a huge variation among them and no attributable effect in the majority. Treatment can include lifestyle and training modification, with hormonal manipulation to alleviate the symptoms or to manipulate the cycle to avoid times of participation. *See also* **menstrual cycle**.

**pressor response** increase in arterial blood pressure in response to various internal or external conditions or to drugs, e.g. mental stress, sustained handgrip or other isometric exercise. A *cold pressor response* occurs on immersion of all or part of the body in cold water. *See also* **static exercise**.

**pressure** force divided by the area over which the force acts. Measured in pascals (Pa) or newtons per square metre ($N.m^{-2}$). *barometric pressure* the pressure due to the column of atmosphere above an object or body (measured also in millimetres of mercury or millibars).

**prime** *n*: a cue given to prompt, facilitate or inhibit a particular response in experimental studies; or *v*: the act of presenting a prime.

**principal axes** the axes of a body or object around which the moment of inertia (resistance to rotation) is greatest, least and intermediate. With reference to the human body in the standing position, the axis for maximum moment of inertia is the *sagittal axis* (front to back), for minimum is the *vertical axis* and intermediate is the *frontal (syn transverse) axis* (side to side), all axes passing through the midpoint of the body (where the frontal, sagittal and transverse **planes** intersect).

**process goal** a goal that specifies the processes a performer will engage in whilst performing. For example, a fielder in cricket might set a process goal to keep their eyes on the ball when making a catch. *See also* **performance goal**, **outcome goal**.

**progesterone** steroid hormone secreted from the ovaries in the second half of the menstrual cycle after ovulation, with actions that prepare the uterus for pregnancy; also by the ovaries in early pregnancy, and by the placenta during the later months, maintaining appropriate changes from conception onwards. Used in contraceptive pills, either alone or combined with oestrogens. *See also* **premenstrual syndrome (PMS)**.

**projectile** an object that moves through a resistive medium, usually the air above the surface of the earth. *projectile motion* motion above the surface of the earth, under the influence of gravity and also of air resistance and lift forces, including **Magnus forces**.

**prolapsed intervertebral disc** *syn slipped disc see* **intervertebral discs**.

**pronation** (1) of the foot: sequence during normal gait after the heel hits the ground, the ankle tends to angle inwards, the foot is supported briefly on its inner side, the arch tends to flatten whilst weight is transferred progressively forwards towards the toes. *overpronation* flattens the arch excessively; (2) of the forearm: twisting movement of the forearm which brings the palm of the hand to face downwards or backwards. Opposite of **supination**.

**prophylaxis** from the Greek, to guard or prevent beforehand. The attempt to prevent a condition or disease by, for example, immunization, antibiotics for dental work in certain cardiac conditions, low molecular weight heparin to prevent deep vein thrombosis.

**proprioceptive neuromuscular facilitation (PNF)** therapeutic technique, with questionable neurophysiological basis, in which maximal static stretch is first performed, with view to enhancement of subsequent range of movement.

**proprioceptors** sensory receptors in muscles, joint capsules and surrounding tissues, that signal information to the central nervous system about position and movement of body parts, for example the angle at a joint or the length of a muscle. *proprioception* the process of receiving this information, with or without conscious awareness. *See also* **Golgi tendon organ**, **joint receptors**, **muscle spindle**.

**propulsive force** force on a body or object used to accelerate it in a required direction (usually forward). *See also* **thrust**.

**protective equipment** equipment which has been developed and recommended for many different sports in order to help prevent and reduce the severity of injuries where research has identified a high risk of injury in a particular sport or recreational activity. Examples include shin guards, gum shields, helmets and knee pads.

**proteins** large polymers consisting of one or more sequences of **amino acid** subunits joined by peptide bonds: the major functional and structural components of body cells. The body of a 70 kg man contains about 11 kg protein. The protein mass can be influenced by nutritional status, physical activity and pathological factors. Proteins in the diet typically account for 10–15% of energy intake and the currently recommended *protein requirement* for sedentary individuals is 0.8 g per kilogram body mass per day. The optimal protein intake for strength athletes may be as high as 1.7–1.8 g and for endurance athletes 1.2–1.4 g per kilogram body mass per day. *See also* **nitrogen balance**.

**proximal (to)** in anatomy, nearer to some reference point.. For example, in a limb, nearer to the trunk – the forearm is proximal to the hand; in the gut, the small intestine is proximal to the large intestine. *proximally adj*. Opposite of **distal**.

**psych-up** to mentally prepare oneself for performance.

**psychological skills** *see* **mental skills**.

**psychometrics** the construction, validation and use of psychological tests and measurements. *psychometric* *properties* the reliability and validity of a psychometric measurement instrument.

**psychoneuromuscular theory** the theory that mental **imagery** of an action provokes subliminal stimulation of the muscles that are used in the actual movement patterns being imaged. Has been used to explain why mental practice can enhance performance.

**psychophysics** the study of the relationships between the subjectively perceived magnitude of sensations and their actual magnitude, particularly with regard to the ability to detect differences between stimuli of different magnitudes.

**psychotherapy** the treatment of emotional and psychological problems by psychological methods.

**pubic symphysis** the site where the two pubic bones are linked at the centre-front of the **pelvis** by a thick disc of fibrocartilage, allowing some flexibility, although there is no true joint cavity. Persistent pain in this area should suggest the symphysis as a possible cause but it is often misdiagnosed as arising from the groin or lower abdominal musculature. *osteitis pubis* is an inflammatory condition causing persistent discomfort especially in the midline with tenderness on pressure over the symphysis. Most common in kicking or running sports and in gymnastics and swimming (especially breast stroke). Treatment is often difficult and sometimes requires prolonged rest.

**pulmonary** pertaining to the lungs.

**pulmonary function tests** tests for assessment of the function of the lungs (*aka respiratory function tests*) to aid diagnosis of respiratory disease and assess effectiveness of treatment. Includes methods for measuring **lung volumes** and gas transfer. In sport, primarily used in the diagnosis and monitoring of treatment of **asthma,** especially exercise-induced asthma; **WADA** guidelines have now set criteria based on such tests, whereby an athlete may use certain inhaled medication. *See also* **blood gases**.

**pulmonary ventilation**  *see* **ventilation**.

**pulse** the transmitted heart beat felt, or recorded by a sensor, from pulsation of an artery, commonly the radial artery at the wrist. *pulse rate* the **heart rate** in beats per minute, counted by feeling the pulse.

**pulse oximeter** an instrument attached to a finger or ear for non-invasive measurement of the percentage saturation with oxygen of haemoglobin (Hb) in the blood. Based on the different light absorbance properties of saturated and desaturated Hb. Used to assess hypoxia in pathological conditions, and also to monitor oxygenation, e.g. in athletes/cyclists at high altitude or in any severely taxing exercise.

**pulse pressure** the difference between the highest (systolic) and lowest (diastolic) arterial **blood pressure** during each **cardiac cycle**.

**punishment** a stimulus that leads to a reduction in a behavioural response or, more generally, a stimulus that an organism seeks to avoid or escape. Often erroneously referred to as **negative reinforcement**. *See also* **conditioning**, **reinforcement**.

**pyramidal tracts** the nerve pathways from the motor cortex of the brain to the motor neurons in the spinal cord (some direct but the majority via relay stations) that activate voluntary movements. *See appendix 1.1 fig 3.*

**pyruvate dehydrogenase** *see* **muscle enzymes**.

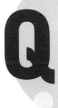

**Q**

**Q (quadriceps)-angle** the angle between the long axis of the femur (and thus the line of pull of the quadriceps) and the line of the patellar tendon (extended upwards); describes the extent to which the line of pull is not straight. In practice, it is measured as the angle between the line from the anterior iliac spine to the centre of the patella, and the line from there to the tibial tubercle. Normally less than 20° (14° in males, 17° in females) but often greater in some female runners who have a wider than average pelvis. Factors which increase the Q-angle include **genu valgum** (knock knees), patellar subluxation, weak quadriceps, tight hamstrings and overpronated feet. Relevant in the diagnosis of patello-femoral pain and used in treatment as an indication of relative quads strength, allowing appropriate strength work. *See fig overleaf.*

**quadriceps femoris** (commonly known as *quads*) muscle group on the front of the thigh comprising *lateral, intermediate* and *medial vasti* (all contributing to knee extension, with origin from the shaft of the femur) and *rectus femoris* (contributing also to hip flexion, by its origin from the ilium of the pelvis). Parts of the vasti are inserted into the top and sides of the patella, and

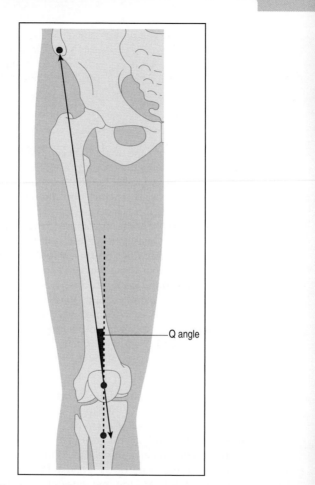

Q angle

The Q-angle.

contribute tendinous reinforcements to the joint capsule of the knee. The four muscles converge onto the single *quadriceps tendon* which spans the front of the knee to be inserted as the *patellar tendon (ligament)* into the tibial tubercle (tuberosity). *See also* **patella, Q(quadriceps)-angle**.

**quadriplegia** *syn* **tetraplegia** paralysis involving all four limbs. *quadriplegic adj. See also* **spinal injury**.

**quasi-isometric** term introduced 1997–1998 by Legg and Spurway, to indicate the condition in which muscles, though not strictly isometric, nonetheless remain for many tens of seconds under load sufficient to restrict blood flow substantially and thus produce metabolic and hence fatigue effects virtually indistinguishable from those experienced during strictly isometric contraction, sustained for similar time under equivalent load. Occurs for example in quadriceps of a dinghy sailor in a fresh breeze or of a jockey standing in stirrups.

**R**

**radiography** the use of electromagnetic radiation to create images of the body from which medical diagnoses can be made. Initially referred to 'plain' X-ray films but the general term has expanded to include other forms of diagnostic imaging such as ultrasound, CT and MRI scanning. Used in sports medicine to provide images of bone, soft tissue and internal organs to aid diagnosis and monitor the effects of treatment, e.g. the healing of a fracture or muscle tear. *See also* **X-rays**.

**radiology** the medical specialty covering the use and interpretation of X-ray images and, more recently, other imaging techniques.

**radius** the smaller of the two forearm bones. Articulates at the **elbow** with the humerus and at the **wrist** with the carpal bones. *adj* ***radial*** in descriptions of forearm structures, on or towards the side of the radius, i.e. the thumb side. *See appendix 1.2 fig 1*.

**range of movement (ROM)** how far a joint permits rotation of the moving parts about the axis of the joint. Usually measured in degrees or radians. Depends on the articulating surfaces, the length and elasticity of ligaments and the properties of muscle, tendon and other soft tissue surrounding the joint. Used as an index of flexibility and to assess progress in rehabilitation. For example, after repair of the anterior cruciate ligament, knee movement will be restricted and as rehabilitation progresses the ROM will increase back to normal. May be assessed by direct examination and measurement or using an isokinetic dynamometer.

**rating of perceived exertion (RPE)** a psychophysical measure of a person's subjective experience of the intensity of exercise based on the totality of physical sensations the person experiences during physical activity, including sensations of a racing heart, breathlessness and muscle fatigue. Often used to train people to regulate the intensity of their exercise to achieve optimal results without the need for technical equipment.

**reaction time** the time that elapses between the presentation of a stimulus and a response; also known as *response latency. choice reaction time* reaction time when two or more stimuli are presented and different responses are required, also known as *complex reaction time. discrimination reaction time* reaction time where a response is required to only one of two or more stimuli. *simple reaction time* reaction time when only one stimulus is presented and one response is required.

**reactive oxygen species (ROS)** any oxygen-containing compound that is particularly reactive. From both exogenous and endogenous sources, ROS are present in all aerobic organisms, which have evolved defences against their potentially damaging effects and also ways of utilizing them (e.g. for signalling between and within cells and in the immune system, for killing invading micro-organisms). Some but not all ROS are *free radicals* (e.g. the superoxide anion ($\cdot O_2^-$) and the hydroxyl radical (OH$\cdot$) where an atom has one or more unpaired electrons in its outer orbital, making it particularly reactive. All the better known free radicals in the body are oxygen-based (although other atoms can also exist in this form) and are generated as by-products of oxidative metabolism. They are formed by exposure to ionizing radiation, cigarette smoke and other environmental pollutants and increased by excessive alcohol consumption and in infections. Free radicals are believed to cause cellular damage by *lipid peroxidation* which incorporates oxygen into membrane lipids. Protein and DNA damage are also involved. They are implicated in ageing and disease, including atherosclerosis (hence coronary heart disease and stroke), cancers and obstructive lung disease. Antioxidant enzymes protect cell membranes by reacting with the free radicals and removing them (e.g. removal of $\cdot O_2^-$ by superoxide dismutase which produces hydrogen peroxide ($H_2O_2$), itself an ROS). In sport, ROS may be responsible for **delayed-onset muscle soreness (DOMS)**. *See also* **antioxidant enzymes**, **antioxidant nutrients**, **oxidative stress**, **lipids**, **vitamins**.

**receptor** (1) in the nervous system, the distal ending of an afferent nerve, or specialist structure served by such a nerve, which signals the incidence of a mechanical, chemical, thermal or other stimulus (termed *sensory receptor* if the signal can reach consciousness); (2) in the context of cell signalling, a molecular structure on the surface of a cell (*membrane receptor*) or in its nucleus, to which hormonal or other signalling molecules or drugs must bind to initiate their effect. *See also* **proprioceptor**.

**reciprocal inhibition** inhibition of spinal cord motor neurons innervating muscles whose contraction would oppose an initiated movement, e.g. when flexing the elbow to lift a weight, the elbow extensors are relaxed. Term introduced in the 1890s by Charles Sherrington (British neurophysiologist and Nobel prize winner) and later known as *Sherrington's law*.

**recommended daily allowance (RDA)** refers to standards for intake level of a particular nutrient for specific groups of people. In the UK it has offically been replaced by **dietary reference values (DRV)** and their subcategories, but is still widely quoted on packaging with reference to **vitamin** content. *See also appendix 4*.

**recovery position** urgent first aid position to protect the airway of an unconscious or semi-conscious person, whatever the cause (e.g. victims of drowning or poisoning) until further medical assistance arrives. This position prevents the tongue falling back in the mouth, obstructing the airway, or the possible aspiration of blood or vomit into the lungs. The casualty is laid on one side with the underneath leg straight while the other leg is fully flexed at the hip, with the knee bent and resting on the ground, altering the centre of gravity to prevent rolling onto the back. The head is supported by the arm, maintaining the desired position with the face tilted towards the ground. It is important not to move the casualty if a spinal injury is suspected, unless for resuscitation. Also known as *coma position*.

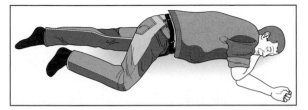

The recovery position.

**recruitment** activation of additional cells in response to increased stimulus strength. In skeletal muscle contraction, activation by the central nervous system of progressively more motor units, hence of more muscle fibres, as the strength of contraction increases.

**rectus abdominis** *see* **abdominal muscles**.

**rectus femoris** *see* **quadriceps femoris**; *appendix 1.2 fig 6A.*

**red blood cells (RBC)** *see* **erythrocytes.**

**red muscle** *see* **muscle fibre types**.

**reference nutrient intake (RNI)** *see* **dietary reference values (DRV)**; *appendix 4.*

**reflex** rapid innate response by an effector (muscle or gland) to a stimulus detected by neural receptors and signalled by afferent nerves to neurons in the central nervous system whose efferent nerves activate the effector. *reflex arc* this neural pathway, including one or more synaptic connections. *See also* **stretch reflex, tendon reflex (tendon jerk)**.

**reframing** a technique for altering negative or self-defeating thought patterns by deliberately replacing them with positive, constructive **self-talk**. For example, athletes might reframe negative self-talk following failure in a competition by telling themselves that it was a useful learning experience. Frequently included in mental training programmes. Also known as *cognitive restructuring*.

**rehabilitation** planned, supervised and progressive programme to return an individual to their maximum degree of physical and psychological independence. In sports medicine, this usually refers to the process, commencing at the time of injury or operation, which aims to return the athlete to both training and competition at their previous level, as soon as possible.

**reinforcement** in psychological terms: (1) in operant conditioning, a stimulus that, when presented following a response, leads to an increase in the frequency of emission of the response in the future. Also known as a *reinforcer* and more colloquially as a *reward*; (2) the process of strengthening the frequency of a response through presenting a reinforcement. *reinforce vt. negative reinforcement* the strengthening of the frequency of a response by removing an aversive stimulus. *See also* **conditioning**, **punishment**.

**relaxation techniques** methods for reducing physiological arousal or cognitive anxiety. *progressive muscular relaxation* a relaxation technique that involves successively tensing and relaxing different skeletal muscle groups in the body. Also known as *Jacobson's progressive relaxation*.

**renal** pertaining to the **kidneys**.

**renal function**  *see* **kidneys**.

**repertory grid test** an **idiographic** psychological test developed by American psychologist George Kelly (1905–1966) derived from his **personal construct theory** that elicits the ways in which an individual views their world by presenting them with a number of sets of three familiar elements (for example, people that they know) and asking them to identify in what way any two are similar to each other but different from the third. In this way a series of **bipolar constructs** are elicited (e.g. friendly versus unfriendly) that are said to describe how the person construes their world.

**repetitions** repeats (*'reps'*) of training actions at short or minimal intervals; contrast '**sets**'.

**residual volume (RV)** the volume of gas remaining in the lungs after a full expiratory effort. *See also* **lung volumes**.

**resistance training**  *see* **strength training**.

**respiration** used generally to mean breathing; hence *respiratory system* the lungs and the air passages leading to them; *respiratory rate* number of breaths per minute. In animal physiology *external respiration* refers to breathing and pulmonary gas exchange and *internal respiration* to oxygen uptake and carbon dioxide release in the tissues, serving energy production.

**respiratory acidosis**  *see* **acidosis**.

**respiratory alkalosis**  *see* **alkalosis**.

**respiratory centres** complex of neurons in the brain stem where the breathing rhythm is generated, and where various neural inputs influence the neural output to the respiratory muscles which in turn determines the depth and frequency of breathing. *See also* **chemoreceptors**.

**respiratory exchange ratio (RER or R)** the ratio of carbon dioxide released to oxygen taken in, by exchange between the body and the atmosphere, over a period of measurement by analysis of expired gases. Used in the estimation of **oxygen consumption ($\dot{V}O_2$)** and from that the equivalent **energy expenditure** to allow calculation of the 'true' difference between inspired and expired oxygen percentage when the RER is other than 1:1. In a steady state (when carbon dioxide is neither being stored nor over-excreted by hyperventilation) RER is equal to the **respiratory quotient** which reflects the proportion of the different nutrients being used for energy production.

**respiratory frequency (f)** number of breaths per minute; *aka* **breathing frequency** or *respiratory rate*.

**respiratory function tests** *see* **lung volumes**, **pulmonary function tests**.

**respiratory quotient (RQ)** the ratio of carbon dioxide produced to oxygen used by the whole body, or by any of its tissues, over the period of measurement. Differs according to the metabolic substrate, ranging from 0.7 for fat alone to 1 for carbohydrate alone. Overall whole-body RQ on a typical mixed diet is about 0.8. Compare **respiratory exchange ratio**.

**response latency** *see* **reaction time**.

**rest re-injury cycle** a pattern that occurs when an athlete returns to activity after an injury and aggravates that injury due to inadequate recovery.

**resting metabolic rate** *see* **metabolic rate**.

**revolution** one complete rotation of a body or object about an axis. Measured as $360°$ or $2\pi$ radians.

**RICE (rest, ice, compression, elevation)** used in the management of acute injuries to minimize inflammatory processes and to accelerate the recovery process by minimizing swelling; basic, efficient and key first aid treatment in sports injuries, especially soft tissue injuries.

**right hand rule** (1) used to relate direction of rotation of an object to its vector representation: if the right hand is 'wrapped' from palm to tips of fingers in the direction of rotation, the vector lies in the direction of the outstretched thumb of the right hand (e.g. vector representation of angular momentum); (2) the organization of a three-dimensional cartesian co-ordinate system. X direction can be considered as acting along the outstretched first finger of the right hand, Y direction is along the outstretched second (middle) finger of the right hand (at right angles to the first finger) and Z is along the outstretched thumb (at right angles to the other two) of the right hand.

**rigid-body mechanics** analysis of bodies or objects that do not deform due to the forces upon them. The bones of the human skeleton are often assumed to be rigid links.

**ringworm** generic term used to describe contagious fungal infections (*tinea*) of the skin, characterized by circular scaly patches. Treated with topical antifungal cream or, if severe, oral antifungal tablets. *See also* **athlete's foot**.

**rotation** movement of a body or object about an axis. The axis may be external (e.g. gymnastic high bar) or within the body (e.g. at a joint). May be combined with **translation** to give general motion.

**rotator cuff** four muscles (supraspinatus, subscapularis, infraspinatus and teres minor), which act in synergy at the **shoulder joint** to facilitate movement and provide stability by maintaining the head of the humerus in the glenoid cavity. In sport, most commonly injured in throwing, swimming and racquet sports with tears, tendonitis or (in young athletes) **impingement**.

**runner's haematuria** *see* **march haemoglobinuria**.

**runner's knee** a non-specific term used to describe pain felt in or around the knee in runners. Includes conditions such as patellofemoral pain and iliotibial band syndrome. *See also* **chondromalacia patellae**, **iliotibial band**.

**runner's nipples** term used in sports medicine to describe the irritation of the nipples due to friction caused by the runner's shirt rubbing over them; relieved by the use of lubricating jelly.

**runner's toe** painful, black discoloration at the base of the toe nail, usually the result of inappropriate footwear (too small or too wide) or direct trauma. A significant amount of blood gathering under the toenail may form a *subungual haematoma* which may require immediate release from its pressurized space by a sterile, heated needle.

**running economy** defined as the volume of oxygen required per km, relative to body mass, to run at a submaximal speed, so expressed in $mL.kg^{-1}.km^{-1}$. Most commonly reported, however, in terms of the rate of oxygen usage relative to body mass, in $mL.kg^{-1}.min^{-1}$, in a run at a standard speed of 16 km per hour: note the lower the value, the greater the 'economy'.

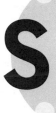

# S

**saccade** a rapid movement of the eyes as they move from one fixation point to another or track a moving object.

**sacroiliac (SI) joint** the joint between the sacrum and the ilium of the pelvis. A synovial plane joint with very limited movement. The SI joint facilitates the torsional or twisting movement of the pelvis as the lower limbs move. Often involved in inflammatory arthritis, seen in sport in athletes with lower limb biomechanical problems. *See appendix 1.2 figs 1, 2.*

**salbutamol** short-acting beta-agonist drug, used to relieve the bronchoconstriction of **asthma**. Use in sport is restricted due to its anabolic (and thus potentially performance-enhancing) effects. New **WADA** guidelines require the degree of bronchoconstriction to be measured by formal lung function testing, with the use of salbutamol allowed only if specific criteria are reached. Requires a *Therapeutic Use Exemption (TUE)* form for use in sport.

**salt** there has been controversy in the past about the potentially harmful effects of excessive salt intake (specifically the sodium component). A statement from the Faculty of Public Health of the Royal College of

Physicians UK has endorsed evidence that intake above the recommended maximum of 6 g per day for adults (less for children, proportional to age group) is strongly linked to the development of hypertension, and is therefore in turn a risk factor for coronary artery disease and stroke, whereas the average intake over the population is closer to 9 g per day. More than 6 g per day is, however, likely to be appropriate for athletes whose training or competition involves excessive **sweating**. Salt in the diet (apart from added table salt and that used in cooking) is derived mostly from processed food and there are also other minor sources of sodium. *See also* **sodium**, **minerals**, **water balance**; *appendix 4.3.*

**sarcolemma**  cell membrane of skeletal **muscle fibre**, plus an extracellular layer of carbohydrate and collagenous macromolecules which imparts some mechanical strength and is contiguous at fibre ends with tendons or aponeuroses of origin and insertion.

**sarcomere**  length-wise repeating unit of striated muscle, from one *Z line* to the next; length about $2.5 \times 10^{-6}$ m in fully extended muscle, less in shortened. *See also* **myofibrils**.

**sarcoplasmic reticulum (SR)**  membrane-bounded system within the cytoplasm of all muscle cells (particularly prominent in large, skeletal fibres), which on excitation releases calcium ions (thereby activating force-generation). In skeletal muscle this occurs when an **action potential (AP)** invades abutting t-tubes. If the AP, and thus the release process, is not repeated within a few tens of msec, the active reabsorption of $Ca^{2+}$ into the SR

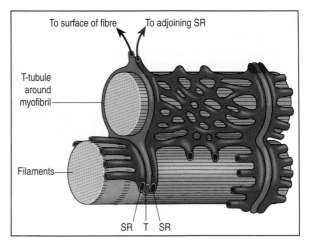

Two adjoining myofibrils of skeletal muscle, with sarcoplasmic reticulum (SR) and t-tubules (T).

by the **calcium (Ca) pump** leads to relaxation. *See also* **muscle fibre**; *appendix 1.2 fig 7.*

**sarcoplasmic reticulum ATPase** *see* **muscle enzymes**.

**Sargent jump test** an elementary test of lower limb impulsive power, consisting of comparison between a subject's upward reach when standing and the height attained in a standing vertical jump; most simply performed against a blackboard, against which chalk is pressed by the subject's hand.

**satellite cell** small cell, a nucleus surrounded by minimal cytoplasm, lying outside but as close as possible to the membrane of a skeletal **muscle fibre**, and within the

**sarcolemma**. When fibre enlargement (**hypertrophy**) or repair is required, satellite cells divide, one daughter becoming active in developing new muscle cytoplasm and the other being retained as a further-generation satellite cell.

**satiety** with reference to food, the converse of hunger – the sensation of satisfaction or fullness. Mediated by the **hypothalamus** and influenced by many complex factors, including hormone secretions from the gut in response to a full meal, vagal afferent stimulation by stomach distension, insulin/glucagon secretion and blood glucose concentration.

**scalar** describes a variable, quantity or measurement that has only magnitude (size), i.e. no directional component. Can be added arithmetically. Examples are area, speed, temperature.

**scaphoid bone** a (tarsal) bone in the foot and a (carpal) bone in the wrist. Latter is commonly damaged by compression, causing *scaphoid fracture*, when there is a fall onto the outstretched hand in hyperextension. If the fracture involves the proximal third of the scaphoid, there is a high risk of non-union and threat of avascular necrosis, due to the poor blood supply.

**schema** in psychology, an abstract mental representation or set of rules for organizing one's experience or an aspect of one's world that is based on experience and stored in memory. It is accessed either consciously or subconsciously in response to relevant environmental cues and facilitates and guides the person's perception and interpretation of events. *schemata pl. schema* *theory* a theory of motor learning, positing that as individuals practise a motor skill, they acquire a schema for the actions involved, which generalizes and guides the execution of similar actions in the future.

**sciatica** pain felt from the lower back to the buttock, and down the back of the leg to the outside of the foot, due to compression of the spinal nerve roots that form the sciatic nerve, aggravated by bending forwards – the 'slump test'. May cause detectable sensory loss and occasionally foot-drop. *See also* **intervertebral disc**.

**segment angle** the angle of a segment of the human body (e.g. limb or trunk) to a fixed reference line (e.g. the horizontal).

**selenium** functions as an **antioxidant** by serving as cofactor for the enzyme glutathione peroxidase. A few studies have suggested a benefit of selenium supplementation in improving antioxidant capacity and diminishing cancer occurrence. Selenium may possibly be effective in athletes who are ingesting insufficient amounts, but it is not known if marginally insufficient intake compromises efficiency of training. Excessive amounts of selenium could have toxic effects. *See also* **minerals**; *appendix 4.3*.

**self-concept** the totality of a person's perceptions or description of their self, typically not involving an evaluative component. *See also* **self-esteem**.

**self-confidence** a generalized tendency to believe that one is capable of being successful within or across behavioural domains. *See also* **self-efficacy**.

**self-determination theory** a theory of human personality and motivation predicated on the assumption that people have an innate tendency toward personal growth and development which is facilitated when their psychological needs to feel competent, autonomous and socially related are supported. Widely employed in the study of motivation in sport and exercise.

**self-efficacy** in social cognitive theory, a person's belief in their ability to execute the behaviours necessary to achieve desired outcomes. In contrast to self-confidence, self-efficacy refers to beliefs about specific behaviours in specific situations. *self-efficacy level* the individual's beliefs about their expected level of performance attainment, ranging from easy to difficult, such as a tennis player's beliefs about the percentage of first serves they could successfully make in a match. *self-efficacy strength* the degree of certainty with which an individual expects to successfully execute a behaviour. *See also* **outcome expectancy**.

**self-esteem** the totality of a person's evaluation of their worth as an individual. Also known as *self-evaluation* and *self-worth*.

**self-handicapping** the imposition of an impediment to successful performance by a person so that they can subsequently either attribute failure to the impediment rather than to lack of ability or effort, or gain increased credit for success. For example, an athlete might avoid training for a race in order to self-handicap.

**self-serving bias** the tendency to attribute successes to internal factors such as ability and effort and failures to external factors such as bad luck. *See also* **attributions**.

**self-talk** a person's internal dialogue, which can be positive and motivational or negative and demotivating.

**semantic differential** a method for measuring affective responses or attitudes to objects or events by asking people to rate the object or event along a bipolar scale, for example ranging from good to bad.

**semilunar cartilage** *see* **meniscus**.

**sensation seeking** a personality trait associated with a preference for high levels of sensory stimulation, often achieved by engaging in risk-taking behaviours and adopting non-conventional lifestyles.

**sensory** strictly, applies only to the reception and processing by the nervous system of information from the outside world such that it reaches consciousness as a subjective experience (*sensation*); often used loosely in relation to any **afferent** nerve pathway or process, including those serving only reflex function.

**series-fibre muscle** skeletal muscle in which fibres do not extend from one end to the other, but are a fraction of muscle length and overlap their lengthwise neighbours only enough to convey force from one to another via molecular linkages between their sarcolemmae. Chief benefit is in co-ordination of contraction: in, say, sartorius, which may be 50 cm long, muscle action potential (AP) conduction over the whole length could not initiate contraction at the ends before relaxation had started under the motor endplate; 'series' construction allows motor nerve APs, propagating 10–20 times faster, to trigger contractions almost simultaneously throughout the muscle. *aka short-fibre muscle*.

**serotonin** a monoamine (*5-hydroxytryptamine, 5-HT*) formed from the essential amino acid tryptophan. Its widespread actions include vasoconstriction, inhibition of gastric secretion and stimulation of smooth muscle. It is also an important neurotransmitter in the central nervous system; as such it is involved in pain transmission and perception, and can influence a variety of behaviours, including tiredness, sleep, mood and mental fatigue. It is suggested that an increased level of serotonin makes it mentally harder to maintain a steady pace of exercise, as in running or cycling (**'central fatigue'**). Administration of branched-chain amino acids has been claimed to reduce uptake of tryptophan by the brain and therefore to diminish serotonin production. *See also* **ergogenic aids**; *appendix 4.4.*

**serum** the fluid that separates when a sample of blood coagulates after withdrawal from the body. Has the contents that were present in plasma, except for those that have taken part in the clotting process. Used for many biochemical investigations, and in the preparation of specific immunoglobulins for short-term prevention or urgent treatment of some infections in those who are not themselves immune. *See also* **immunity**.

**sets** groups of 'reps', separated by substantial recovery intervals. *See also* **repetitions**.

**shear force** force acting parallel to the surface of a material so as to tend to deform it, usually through a *shear angle*, the angle between a deformed body and its original position.

**shoulder girdle** the parts of the musculoskeletal system that link the upper limbs to the sternum in front and to the vertebral column behind, including sternoclavicular joint, clavicle, acromioclavicular joint, scapula and attached muscles.

**shoulder joint** *syn glenohumeral joint* synovial 'ball- and-socket' joint, the 'ball' of the head of the humerus articulating with the 'socket' of the shallow glenoid cavity of the scapula, which allows the shoulder to move around multiple axes – the greatest range of movement of any joint in the body, providing flexion, extension, abduction, adduction, circumduction and rotation. This flexibility sacrifices stability, which has to be maintained by the surrounding muscles and ligaments, notably the muscles of the **rotator cuff**; also the socket of the joint is deepened by the *glenoid labrum*, a ring of cartilage attached to the rim of the glenoid cavity to which the joint capsule, ligaments and tendons are partly attached. *labral tears* are not uncommon in throwing athletes, including *superior labrum anterior-posterior (SLAP)* lesions which can be visualized on MRI scan and require arthroscopic surgical repair. *See also* **Bankart's lesion**, **dislocation**; *appendix 1.2 figs 1–5. See fig overleaf.*

**shuttle test** test of aerobic power requiring minimal apparatus, introduced by Leger and colleagues in 1982 and *aka Leger shuttle run, multi-stage fitness test* or, informally, *bleep test.* Starting at $8 \, km.h^{-1}$, subjects run to and fro over 20 m at a pace increased every minute until exhaustion.

**sit-up** exercise of abdominal muscles, in which the subject lying on the floor raises the upper body towards vertical before lowering again; importantly, for safety, should

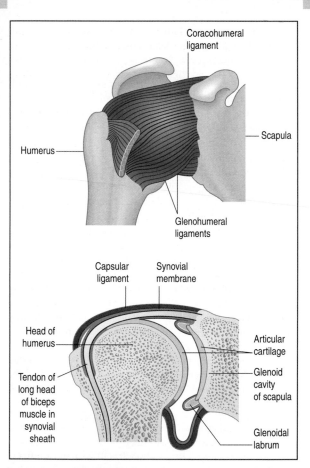

Right shoulder joint from the front.

be performed with knees bent to approximate right angle, when the target becomes touching of elbows to knees. *aka trunk curl* although this term is sometimes reserved for the particular case where chin is pressed against chest during the upper-body elevation.

**skeletal muscle** *see* **muscle, muscle contraction, muscle fibre, neuromuscular junction**; *figs appendix 1.2.*

**skier's thumb** a colloquial expression used in sports medicine to describe instability of the metacarpophalangeal joint caused by forced abduction whilst the thumb is extended (e.g. holding the ski stick in a fall); this stretches or ruptures the ulnar collateral ligament which normally limits movement of the thumb away from the hand. Also known as *gamekeeper's thumb* since similar damage was caused by breaking the neck of birds or rabbits held between finger and thumb.

**skill** the learned ability to competently and consistently coordinate a complex pattern of behaviours in order to accomplish a task with minimum effort and maximum effect. *closed skill* a skill executed in an environment that is stable and predictable, such as a floor routine in gymnastics. *open skill* a skill executed in an environment that is variable and unpredictable, such as dribbling the ball past an opponent in soccer. *See also* **ability, performance**.

**skin** human skin serves the functions of sensation, protection and insulation and has a major role in regulation of **body temperature**, by variations in heat loss or conservation (increasing loss by vasodilatation and **sweating**, decreasing it by vasoconstriction), under the control of the **autonomic nervous system**. Sensory nerve endings

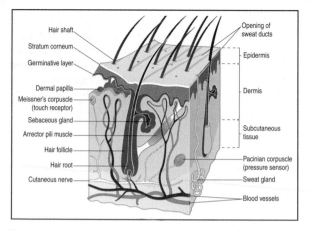

The skin. Meissner's corpuscles serve touch sensation (named after the 19th-century anatomists who described them). Pacinian corpuscles serve pressure and vibration sensation (named after the 19th-century anatomists who described them).

and receptors include those that mediate the sensations of touch, pain and pressure.

**skinfold thickness** measurement of subcutaneous skinfold thickness as a technique for the determination of body fat. A fold of skin and subcutaneous fat is grasped between the thumb and forefinger and pulled away from the underlying muscle. The thickness of this double layer is then read, using a caliper. The five sites most frequently measured are the upper arm, below the scapula, above the hip bone, the abdomen and the thigh. The values are used in an equation that estimates body fat. *See also* **anthropometry**, **body composition**.

**sliding filament mechanism** the process by which striated muscles change length, the overlap of thin and thick filaments increasing as the muscle shortens and decreasing as it lengthens. Describes the manner in which these length changes occur, but is not an explanation of the mechanism of active shortening. *See also* **cross-bridge (XB)**, **muscle fibre**, **myofibrils**; *appendix 1.2 fig 7.*

**slow-twitch fibre** *see* **muscle fibre types**.

**smooth muscle** *see* **muscle**.

**social cognitive theory** a general theory or class of theories of human behaviour based on the assumption that thoughts, beliefs and expectations influence behaviour and that these are shaped by the person's social environment. Also known as *social learning theory*.

**social facilitation** the effects of the presence of an audience on a person's or team's performance. The term is a misnomer because the effects are not always facilitative and it has therefore been replaced with *audience effects* when the audience observes the activity but is not actively involved and *coaction effects* when the audience is concurrently engaged in the same activity.

**social learning theory** *see* **social cognitive theory**.

**social loafing** a tendency for individuals to exert less effort on a task when working in groups than when they work on the same task alone.

**social physique anxiety** anxiety that individuals experience in response to a perception that others will negatively evaluate their physique.

**sodium** the main cation in the extracellular body fluids (ECF). The concentration of ECF sodium, [Na$^+$], is regulated by variations in its reabsorption/excretion in the kidneys, dependent in turn upon mechanisms within the kidneys themselves, and on the adrenal cortical hormone **aldosterone** (promoting renal Na$^+$ reabsorption), and *atrial natruretic hormone* (promoting Na$^+$ excretion). Variations in ECF [Na$^+$] and its renal and hormonal control are closely linked to control of blood volume and ECF fluid volume as a whole. *See also* **hormones**, **salt**; *appendix 4.3.*

**sodium-potassium (Na-K) pump** one of many similar molecular complexes embodying ion-binding sites and an ATPase, found in surface (plasma) membrane of all cells, which actively transports sodium ions (Na$^+$) out of the cytoplasm and potassium ions (K$^+$) into it (usually in the ratio 3Na$^+$ out to 2K$^+$ in), using energy derived from hydrolysis of ATP by the action of *sodium-potassium (Na-K) ATPase.* All cells have at least a minimum density of these pumps but nerve and muscle cells have greater numbers to cope with the greater ion fluxes in these cells. The high intracellular [K$^+$] and low intracellular [Na$^+$] in cells (in contrast to their concentrations in extracellular fluid) are due to these pumps; the maintenance of the **membrane potential** and of cell volume results from this ion distribution. Formerly, on the basis of inadequate understanding, termed simply 'sodium pump'. *See also* **cell**.

**somatic** *adj* from *soma* *n*, derived from the Greek for 'body'; used to refer to (1) the body as distinct from the mind (e.g. as in 'psychosomatic', ascribing physical symptoms to mental causes); (2) the substance of the body, excluding the internal organs, i.e. as distinct from **visceral.** Hence *somatic nerves*, the components of the peripheral nervous system both sensory and motor, that serve the skin and musculoskeletal structures.

**somatic anxiety** *see* **anxiety**.

**somatostatin** hormone secreted at several sites, with widespread inhibitory effects on other secretions: from the hypothalamus, as *growth hormone-inhibiting hormone (GH-IH)* acting in the anterior pituitary; in the pancreas, inhibits other pancreatic secretions; from the intestinal wall, inhibits many hormonal and enzyme secretions in the gut.

**specific gravity** the relative density of one body or object compared to another. If compared to water, an object will float if its specific gravity is less than 1.0 (assuming water has a density of $1.0 \, kg.m^{-3}$).

**speed** the change of distance with respect to time. A scalar quantity (i.e. having no directional component). *linear speed* is usually measured in metres per second $(m.s^{-1})$, kilometres per hour $(km.h^{-1})$ or miles per hour (mph), and *angular speed* in degrees per second $(°.s^{-1})$ or radians per second $(rad.s^{-1})$ *See also* **velocity**.

**spinal column (spine)** *see* **vertebral column**.

**spinal cord** the part of the **central nervous system** that extends, in continuity with the brain, from the base of the skull down the vertebral (spinal) canal as far as the top of the second lumbar vertebra. Surrounded by the membranous tube of the meninges (in continuity

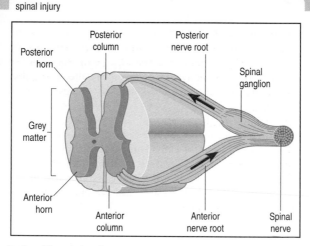

Section of the spinal cord.

with the coverings of the brain) and bathed within this by *cerebrospinal fluid*. Consists of nerve cells (grey matter) and nerve tracts (white matter). Anterior (efferent) and posterior (afferent) *spinal nerve roots* leave and enter through the intervertebral foramina, linking it to the **peripheral nervous system**. *See also* **vertebral column**; *appendix 1.1 figs 2–5.*

**spinal injury** injury to the vertebral column (fracture-dislocation) which may or may not involve *spinal cord injury* and/or injury of the nerve roots within the vertebral (spinal) canal. Cord injury can occur in the cervical, thoracic and upper lumbar regions, ranging from minor damage to complete transection. *Cauda equina injury* occurs with damage below the first lumbar vertebra, where the 'horse's tail' of lumbar and sacral nerve roots descend to their exits from the vertebral (spinal) canal. Cord and nerve root injuries cause complete or partial paralysis of voluntary movement and sensory loss in the regions served by the nerve tracts or roots affected. *See also* **back injury**, **cervical spine**, **neck injury**, **paraplegia**, **quadriplegia**, **whiplash injury**.

**spirometer** apparatus for measuring movement of air in and out of the lungs. *See also* **lung volumes**, **pulmonary function tests**.

**sport cohesion** a sport team's tendency to stick together in its pursuit of common objectives.

**sport competition anxiety** *see* **anxiety**.

**sport psychology** the application of psychological science to the study and understanding of human behaviour and mind in sport, and to the enhancement of performance in sport. Includes the areas of **motor learning**, sport skill acquisition, **motivation** and psychological skills training.

**sports drinks** commercially available drinks, designed for optimal delivery of water and carbohydrate during and after exercise. Water is often equally effective for hydration, but the taste of sports drinks makes them more likely to be taken in adequate quantities. The composition of commercial sports drinks is generally based on studies which have defined the content of carbohydrate (to supplement energy supply) and of electrolytes (mainly sodium salts) to promote fluid retention during and after prolonged exercise and to avoid

**hyponatraemia**. There has, however, been some controversy about the standard recommendations, as some experts have disputed their adequacy in avoiding hyponatraemia, exemplified recently in studies of its occurrence in endurance athletes. **Osmolality** of these drinks varies according to the concentration of carbohydrate, most often in the form of glucose polymers. *isotonic sports drinks* contain glucose in a concentration of 6–8% and are best for events such as middle- and long-distance running and team sports, rapidly replacing fluid lost by sweating as well as supplying an energy source. *hypotonic sports drinks* are suitable, for example, for jockeys, gymnasts and dancers, who need fluid but have less need for a carbohydrate top-up. *hypertonic sports drinks* have the most carbohydrate and are taken after exercise to supplement daily intake in the replacement of muscle glycogen stores; also used during very long-distance events when high levels of energy are required. *See also* **hydration status**.

**stability** the property of an object or body that determines how difficult it is to displace it to another position.

**stance** way of standing or the phase of gait (walking or running) in which the body is supported, usually by one or both feet being on the ground (although can include other methods of support such as crutches).

**state anxiety** *see* **anxiety**.

**static exercise** *see* **isometric contraction**.

**static stretching** technique in which an extreme stretched position is slowly reached, then held for some time (typically 20–30 s), with view to increasing the range of movement; by contrast with rapid ('ballistic') stretching, static stretching is considered not to elicit the **stretch reflex**, which would counteract the attempted muscle lengthening.

**statics** the study (or analysis) of systems (of bodies or objects) that are at rest or moving with constant velocity (i.e. not accelerating). Such systems are considered to be in equilibrium.

**step length** the distance between the position (e.g. heel contact) of one foot and the next similar position of the opposite foot in gait (walking or running). May also include other support devices such as crutches. May be different for each foot. May also be positive, negative ('dragging' one foot so that it never reaches the other) or zero (when one foot is advanced only to the position beside the other foot). Usually measured in metres.

**step test** test of aerobic fitness involving stepping up and down with alternate legs for a predetermined period followed by a series of measurements of postexercise heart rate, to determine its rate of return to resting level. Variants in current use include those prescribed by the YMCA and the Association College of Sports Medicine. The original *Harvard step test*, devised in the 1940s, used a higher step and longer exercise period (up and down 20 inches, every 2 s, for up to 5 min) than in most recent specifications.

**steroid hormones** those secreted by the adrenal cortex, the testis and the ovary, all made from cholesterol as precursor. A variety of synthetic steroids is used in treatment mainly of rheumatic conditions or of relevant hormonal disorders; others are marketed for body-building. *See also* **aldosterone**, **anabolic steroids**, **androgens**, **glucocorticoids**, **hormones**.

**steroids** organic compounds based on a nucleus of four 5-carbon rings. Those in the body include cholesterol, bile acids, sex hormones and adrenal cortical hormones. *See also* **aldosterone**, **anabolic steroids**, **androgens**, **corticosteroids**, **glucocorticoids**.

**stitch** a sharp, stabbing pain or spasm felt in the ribcage or abdomen, particularly on the right during exertion. The exact cause is unknown though insufficient blood flow and thus oxygen supply to the intercostal muscles or diaphragm has been implicated. While inconvenient and painful, a stitch has no medical significance.

**stomach** the part of the alimentary tract just below the diaphragm. Colloquially: abdomen, belly. *See also* **alimentary**, **digestion**.

**strain** the extent to which a body or object is deformed when an external force is applied to it. Often measured as a percentage change in the object's dimensions (e.g. length) or in its position (e.g. angle moved).

**strength training** training achieved by working dynamically against high loads or statically against fixed resistances. In both cases the forces involved must be such that relatively few repetitions are possible without a substantial rest period. A sustained strength-training programme will progressively increase the loads and number of lifts over a period of months, the exercises being performed in several sets, each embodying a specified number of repetitions. In the first 2–3 months the main improvement in strength is attributable to increased recruitment of motor units within the pre-existing muscle mass (the 'neural phase' of strength training); thereafter, increase of muscle fibre diameters is the major factor ('hypertrophic phase'). *aka resistance training*. *See also* **weight training**.

**stress** (1) in mechanics, the force per unit area applied to a body or object. Measured in newtons per square metre ($N.m^{-2}$) or pascals (Pa); (2) the psychological and/or physiological response of an organism to any demand made upon it by agents threatening its physical or emotional well-being. *stressor* any factor that causes a stress response. *stress management* any of a range of methods used to reduce or manage the negative effects of stress, such as relaxation techniques and biofeedback. *See also* **anxiety**.

**stretch reflex**  contraction of skeletal muscles in response to an applied stretch. Accounts for *muscle tone* including the continually adjusted background contraction in the postural muscles (mainly the extensors of the trunk and limbs), and for the resistance which an observer can feel in response to stretching any muscle by passive movement. Mediated by afferent impulses from the stretched intrafusal fibres in **muscle spindles** relayed via mono- and polysynaptic connections in the spinal cord (and also via long-loop supraspinal pathways) to the alpha motor neurons that supply the extrafusal fibres of the same muscle. *See also* **tendon jerk reflex**.

**striated muscle**  *see* **muscle**, **muscle fibre**, **myofibrils**.

**stride** in gait (usually walking or running): the interval between an event of one foot (e.g. heel-strike or toe-strike) and the next occurrence of the same event of the same foot. *stride length* the distance between the position (e.g. heel contact) of one foot and the subsequent position of the same foot. May also include other support devices such as crutches. Should be the same for each foot as long as movement is in a straight line (i.e. not in a curve). Usually measured in metres. *stride rate* the number of strides per minute.

**stroke volume** the output from each of the ventricles of the heart during a single beat (systole). Typically ~70 mL at rest, and rises during exercise as the venous return increases, raising the ventricular filling pressure, so that a greater volume of blood enters the relaxed ventricles during diastole, to be ejected during systole. The resting stroke volume may be doubled in exercise, exceptionally even more, but the increase is limited by the decreasing duration of diastole as heart rate rises. *See also* **cardiac output**, **heart rate**, **venous return**.

**Stroop effect** a phenomenon in which individuals take longer to name the colour of words printed in a non-matching colour, such as the word blue printed in red ink, than when the words are printed in the same colour as the word designates, such as the word blue printed in blue ink. *Stroop test* a test for this effect in which individuals are presented with lists of colour words in matching and non-matching colours and the time they take to read the different words, or the number of errors they make, is recorded. Often used as a stressor in experimental studies. (Described by American psychologist J R Stroop in 1935.)

**subjective norm** in the theory of reasoned action/planned behaviour, the person's perceived social pressure to engage or not engage in a behaviour.

**succinate dehydrogenase** *see* **muscle enzymes**.

**sucrose** a disaccharide that is hydrolysed into glucose and fructose during digestion. Occurs naturally in sugar and is added to many manufactured foods. Over-consumption of sucrose with inadequate dental hygiene can cause dental problems.

**sudden death** in sport, refers to sudden cardiovascular death, defined under the IOC Lausanne recommendations as death occurring without prior symptoms, or within 1 h of symptoms, in a person without a previously recognized cardiovascular condition. This specifically excludes cerebrovascular, respiratory, traumatic and drug-related causes. Ninety percent of non-traumatic sudden death in athletes is related to a pre-existing cardiac abnormality. *See also* **aortic valve stenosis, electrocardiography (ECG), heart attack, heart murmur, hypertrophic obstructive cardiomyopathy (HOCM), medical screening, myocarditis, Wolff–Parkinson–White (WPW) syndrome**.

**sugar** the colloquial term for sucrose. Commercial table sugar comes from either sugar cane or sugar beet. Chemically, the term *sugars* includes sucrose and other disaccharides (maltose, lactose) and also the simple sugars, the monosaccharides (pentoses, hexoses).

**supination** (1) of the foot: during normal gait immediately before 'take-off' from the toes, the ankle tends to angle outwards and the foot is supported briefly on its outer side. *oversupination* can cause the ankle to roll over towards the outer side, with possible ligament damage; (2) of the forearm: twisting movement which brings the palm of the hand to face upwards or forwards. *See also* **pronation.**

**supine** as applied to the whole body: lying on the back. Opposite of **prone.**

**supplements** *see* appendix 4.4.

**support** situation when an object or body has a force applied to resist the force of gravity. Often used to refer to the phase of gait when one or more feet are on the ground. *See also* **stance.**

**supramaximal exercise** *see* **anaerobic exercise**.

**sweating** secretion from the sweat glands in the skin: a major factor in the control of body temperature. Sweating is stimulated by the sympathetic nervous system and that in turn by the hypothalamus, in response to a rise in blood temperature. Corrective heat loss by evaporation of sweat is effective except in excessively humid conditions. Both salt (typically about $2.6\,g.L^{-1}$) and water are lost in the sweat, but at a moderate sweating rate water loss is proportionately greater because sodium is reabsorbed in passage through the sweat ducts. Sweat loss can be as much as 4 litres per hour in heavy exercise in the heat, and more sodium per litre escapes reabsorption at higher flow rates: hence the need to replace both water and salt. *See also* **electrolyte balance**, **hydration status**, **sodium**, **sports drinks**.

**swing** the phase of gait when one leg is being moved, to support the body when it is next placed upon the ground. Also known as *swing phase*.

**sympathetic nervous system** one of the two divisions of the **autonomic nervous system (ANS)**. Efferent fibres from nerve cells in the thoracolumbar segments of the spinal cord relay in a chain of *sympathetic ganglia* on each side of the spine in the thorax and abdomen; thence sympathetic *postganglionic nerves* reach all parts of the body except the central nervous system. They supply the heart, smooth muscle and many secretory glands. The main neurotransmitter is **noradrenaline** which has different actions depending on the type of receptors on the effector cells. This system is at all times active in the regulation of **cardiac output**, arterial **blood pressure** and regional **blood flow** (all contributing to adjustments in exercise), as well as priming the body for emergency 'fight or flight', when sympathetic nerves stimulate release of **adrenaline** from the adrenal medulla. The outflow from the spinal cord is influenced by inputs from the hypothalamus related to **body temperature** control, from the cardiovascular control centres in the brain stem, and by afferents from the alimentary tract and other organs. Dual sympathetic and parasympathetic innervation provides for synergistic interaction, although the effects are often opposite; most vascular smooth muscle is an exception, having only a sympathetic nerve supply. *See appendix 1.1 figs 5, 6.*

**synapse** the name given by Charles Sherrington in 1897 to the site of transmission of information from one neuron to another or (in current usage) to individual cells of a muscle or gland. The majority are *chemical synapses* involving release of a neurotransmitter from the presynaptic nerve ending which binds to receptors on the postsynaptic cell, opening ion channels and leading to local depolarization. At the very many fewer *electrical synapses (gap junctions)* the abutting cells are in tight contact and there is faster, direct electrical coupling, e.g. between neurons within the brain. *See also* **action potential**, **neuromuscular junction**.

**synergist** commonly refers to a muscle which acts together with another muscle (*adv* *synergistically*) to produce a greater effect; may also be applied to any pair or group of biological agents of the same kind, e.g. hormones.

**synovial** describes joints that have a cavity lined by *synovial membrane* which secretes *synovial fluid.*

**systematic desensitization** *see* **desensitization**.

**systemic** (1) relating to a system as a whole, e.g. with reference to pathological conditions, affecting the whole body, as opposed to being localized; (2) with reference to the **circulation of the blood**, the route from the left side of the heart through the vessels supplying the whole body except the lungs, and returning to the right side of the heart.

**systole** the phase in each heart beat when the ventricles are contracting and ejecting blood. *See also* **cardiac cycle**, **electrocardiogram**, **venous return**.

**T**

**tachycardia** rapid heart rate.

**tachypnoea** rapid breathing. In most situations when ventilation increases, there is normally an increase in both depth and frequency of breathing. Increase in frequency alone may occur in response to sudden immersion in cold water, and also can accompany anxiety. Tachypnoea with shallow breathing may increase only the **dead space** ventilation (as in **panting**) and so may not affect gas exchange.

**taping** the use of tape to prevent or treat injury. Taping is used to limit movements which would exacerbate the injury, whilst not inhibiting function. There is a lack of scientific evidence on its use to prevent injury, but it is widely used in the treatment of conditions such as ankle sprains and patellofemoral pain.

**target heart rate** heart rate (HR) range aspired to during aerobic training, with view to enhancing cardiovascular fitness. Always best set in relation to the individual's measured maximal heart rate ($HR_{max}$) or heart rate reserve (HRR), rather than general population figures. In exercise for health, 60–85% $HR_{max}$ or 55–80% HRR may typically be prescribed.

**tarsal tunnel syndrome** common, painful foot condition, caused by compression of the posterior tibial nerve as it passes through the tarsal tunnel on the inner side of the ankle to the foot. Results in pain, numbness, burning and tingling along the sole of the foot towards the first three toes. Often the result of excessive pronation. Treatment aims to reverse the cause but surgery may be required.

**tarsus** the back half of the **foot**, containing the seven *tarsal bones*.

**task involvement** a state in which the individual's goal is to demonstrate mastery of a task or personal improvement relative to self-referenced criteria, such as improving on their previous personal best. *adj **task-involved**. See also* **ego involvement, learning goal**.

**task orientation** a dispositional tendency to feel most successful in an activity when one demonstrates ability relative to one's self and personal improvement rather than in comparison to the performance of others. *See also* **ego orientation, goal orientation**.

**team cohesion** *see* **group cohesion**.

**telemetry** literally 'measurement at a distance'. Achieved by portable radio transmitter sending data measured from the subject to the observer's receiver. In exercise physiology, these data invariably include heart rate (HR); more sophisticated (but bulkier) equipment will also report other values, e.g. oxygen consumption.

**tendon** a band of white fibrous connective tissue that joins muscle to bone. Tendons consist of parallel bundles of collagen with little elastic tissue. This results in excellent mechanical strength but little elasticity. Tendons focus the strength of muscle contraction on a relatively small area of bone, maximizing pull and facilitating movement of the bone. *paratendon* the fibrous sheath around a tendon, with a thin synovial lining.

**tendon jerk reflex** rapid reflex contraction of a muscle in response to a sudden stretch, elicited by tapping its tendon, and involving direct (monosynaptic) excitation of **alpha motor neurons** in the spinal cord by afferent fibres from primary sensory endings in **muscle spindles**. The best known is the **knee jerk**: when the patellar tendon is tapped, the quadriceps is caused to contract. Similar rapid *monosynaptic reflexes* operate, e.g. when the tendon of the biceps is tapped at the elbow or the Achilles tendon at the ankle. Also known as a *phasic stretch reflex*. *See also* **stretch reflex**.

**tendonitis** inflammation of a tendon. Usually the result of repetitive overuse movements, especially at high intensity. This causes micro-tears in the collagen matrix with inflammation, swelling, tenderness and pain, especially on specific movements. More common in older athletes. Treatment aims to identify and reverse the cause, together with local anti-inflammatory measures such as **RICE**, anti-inflammatory medication, **electrotherapy** and occasionally corticosteroid injection (into the paratendon to avoid tendon rupture). *See also* **tenosynovitis**.

**tennis elbow** *see* **epicondyles**.

**tenosynovitis** inflammation of the thin synovial lining of a tendon sheath, as distinct from its outer fibrous sheath.

It may be caused by mechanical irritation or by bacterial infection.

**tension** force with which a body or object resists extension. Also known as *tension load*.

**testis** the male *gonad*, the site of *spermatogenesis*, whence sperm are discharged via the vas deferens into the urethra at ejaculation. This and also testicular endocrine function (secretion of *testosterone* and related hormones) are under the control of gonadotrophic hormones from the anterior pituitary, and in turn of the hypothalamus.

**testosterone** *see* **anabolic steroids, testis**.

**tetanus** disease caused by the bacterium *Clostridium tetani*, an anaerobic spore-forming micro-organism present in the intestines of domestic animals and humans and commonly found in soil, dust and manure. Potentially the most serious of all sports-related infections due to the presence of the spores in many sports fields. Important in sports where the athlete comes into contact with soil (e.g. grass pitches); cuts and grazes can not only allow entry of the bacteria but also facilitate their growth and neurotoxin production. Active immunization with tetanus toxoid (TT) is available as part of routine programmes, as regular booster doses and when risk is increased.

**tetany** condition of muscular hyperexcitability in which mild stimuli produce cramps and muscle spasms in the hands and feet (carpopedal spasm). It is due to a reduction in ionized calcium levels in the blood, for example as a result of hypoparathyroidism, or in healthy people as a result of alkalosis from alkali ingestion or **hyperventilation** (which may be seen in sport).

**theory of planned behaviour** an extension to the **theory of reasoned action** which incorporates the construct of perceived behavioural control, these being a person's beliefs about whether or not they possess the necessary skills and resources to overcome any difficulties in engaging in the behaviour.

**theory of reasoned action** a social cognitive theory of the relationships between attitudes and volitional behaviour which holds that intention is the immediate determinant of behaviour and that intentions are determined jointly by attitudes towards the behaviour and perceived social pressures to engage in the behaviour.

**thiamine (vitamin B₁)** *see* **vitamins**; *appendix 4.2.*

**thick filaments** *see* **myofibrils, myosin**.

**thin filaments** *see* **actin, myofibrils**.

**thirst** sensation arising when there is body fluid depletion, in response to increase in local **osmolality** in the hypothalamus and to neural and hormonal signals related to decreased blood volume and/or blood pressure; accompanied by production by cells in the **hypothalamus** of the water-retaining **antidiuretic hormone (ADH)** and its release from the **posterior pituitary**.

**thoracic breathing** inhalation by expanding the thorax, using the intercostal muscles to elevate the ribs, as compared to abdominal breathing using the **diaphragm**.

**thorax** the chest. *thoracic cage* the framework (ribs, costal cartilages, sternum and thoracic vertebrae) which protects the internal thoracic structures (especially lungs and heart) and provides attachment for muscles. Traumatic damage in sport can range from local discomfort to fractured ribs and potential damage to the lungs and, rarely, the heart. The liver and spleen, although not in the thorax, are also protected by the lower ribs and can be damaged by their injury. *See also* **pneumothorax;** *appendix 1.3 fig 4.*

**thought stopping** a technique of cognitive behaviour therapy in which individuals are trained to stop intrusive negative thoughts when they occur, either by the self-administration of a painful stimulus, such as snapping an elastic band worn around the wrist, or by bringing to mind a vivid mental image such as a stop sign. Typically, individuals are also trained to reframe the negative thoughts or replace them with positive self-talk. Sometimes known as *thought stoppage*.

**thresholds** *see* **metabolic and related thresholds**.

**thrust** force that propels a body or object in the required direction of motion. *See also* **propulsive force**.

**thyroid gland** the gland in the front of the neck which secretes the iodine-containing hormones *thyroxine (T4)* and *triiodothyronine (T3)* necessary for normal growth in childhood, and crucial in the control throughout life of energy metabolism. The hormones target most body cells (except in the CNS) where they modify enzyme synthesis, thereby controlling the rate of aerobic metabolism and heat production. Thus overactivity (*hyperthyroidism*) causes increase in BMR and body temperature with weight loss, and deficiency (*hypothyroidism*) the reverse. Regulated by thyrotrophic hormone from the anterior pituitary, and in turn by the hypothalamus. Also secretes *calcitonin* which acts to decrease blood [$Ca^{2+}$]. *See also* **hormones**, **parathyroid glands**; *appendix 5*.

**tibia** the *shin bone*, the larger of the two bones of the lower leg; articulates above with the femur in the **knee joint**, below with the talus in the **ankle joint**, and at the outer side of its upper and lower ends with the **fibula**. *See appendix 1.2 figs 1–3*.

**tibialis muscles** occupy the anterior and posterior compartments of the lower leg with tendons extending into the foot: *tibialis anterior* (dorsiflexion) and *posterior* (plantarflexion and inversion). Acute inflammation, usually the result of overuse, results in the so-called *tibialis syndrome* where swelling in the tight compartment causes pain and tenderness on specific movements. Treatment is of the inflammation and of any identified cause such as overpronation. *See also* **compartment syndrome**.

**tidal volume** *see* **lung volumes**, **ventilation**.

**time-to-event paradigm** in sport psychology, a research paradigm for manipulating the components of **anxiety** or examining their relationships with other variables based on the reliable observation that cognitive and somatic anxiety tend to dissociate during the period leading up to a competitive event. Cognitive anxiety tends to be high and stable during the days leading up to an event and then falls when the event begins, whereas somatic anxiety remains low and stable during the days leading up to an event, rises just before the start of the event, and falls once the event begins.

**tone** *see* **muscle tone**.

**torque** *see* **moment of force**.

**torque–angular velocity relation** obtained from a series of measurements of the two parameters on an **isokinetic** dynamometer; the nearest approximation to a muscle **force–velocity relationship** which can be obtained from an intact limb but falling short of exact fit, both inevitably, because no anatomical joint retains constant geometry throughout its range of movement, and also often for neurophysiological reasons, as voluntary muscle activation varies with shortening velocity, a feature which is particularly marked in knee extension. *See also* **moment of force**, **momentum**.

**torsion** force applied to a body or object that deforms (or tends to deform) it in a 'twisting' manner. Also known as *torsion load*.

**total lung capacity (TLC)** *see* **lung volumes**.

**trait** an enduring individual behavioural characteristic or aspect of personality that is exhibited in a wide range of contexts.

**trait anxiety** *see* **anxiety**.

**trajectory** the plotted path of an object through space.

**transcutaneous electrical nerve stimulation (TENS)** a method of non-invasive pain control using pads placed either side of the spine to apply a mild electric current from a battery-operated device, which can be controlled by the patient for pain relief. Used for the control of both acute and chronic pain. Suggested to work through either blocking 'pain' nerves by stimulating other nerve channels or by **endorphin** release. Useful in sports injuries as an adjunct to other treatments, especially if drug treatment options are limited by doping regulations.

**transfer of learning** the extent to which practice or learning of one skill influences the learning or performance of a different skill, or the same skill in a different context. Also known as *generalizability of learning*. *See also* **negative transfer**, **positive transfer**.

**translation** movement from one position to another along a straight or curved line (rectilinear or curvilinear motion). *translational adj.*

**transverse plane** a plane perpendicular to the long axis of a body or object dividing it (e.g. the human body) into upper and lower parts. *See also* **planes**.

**trapezius** large, triangular, superficial muscle on each side of the upper back, its origin extending in the midline from the base of the skull down to the spine of the lowest thoracic vertebra. From there its fibres converge towards the shoulder, and partly over it, round the side of the lower neck, to be inserted in a continuous line into the outer end of the clavicle and the spine of the scapula. The tone of the two muscles keeps the shoulders braced and they act with the scapular spine as a lever when lifting the arms at the shoulder. *See appendix 1.2 fig 5.*

**traveller's diarrhoea** infectious illness common where hygiene conditions are poor and caused by a variety of infectious agents. Seen in sport where teams travel to countries where food and water hygiene and sanitation are poor. Can be passed from one member to another quickly, limiting numbers available to compete.

**Trendelenburg sign** test of hip stability, especially of hip abductors that maintain the horizontal position of the pelvis. Normally when one leg is raised in a standing position, the pelvis tilts upwards on that side, but downwards if the abductors on the opposite side are weak. Used in sport in biomechanical assessment of lower limb conditions.

**triacylglycerol (TG)** the officially approved term to replace the older but still widely used *triglyceride*. A hydrophobic compound made from the combination of glycerol and three fatty acids, which is the major energy store of the body and main component of dietary fat. Present in the body in adipose tissue, in the circulating blood and as *intramuscular triacylglycerol (IMTG)*. *See also* **lipoproteins**, **medium-chain triglycerides**.

**tricarboxylic cycle** *see* **Krebs cycle**.

**triceps** the major extensor muscle of the elbow, and the only muscle on the back of the upper arm. Arises partly from the scapula below the shoulder joint but the main bulk from the back of the humerus. Forms a broad tendon which passes behind the elbow joint (separated from it by a small bursa) to be inserted on the back of the olecranon process of the ulna. *See appendix 1.2 fig 5B.*

**trigger finger** a condition in which the finger can be actively bent but cannot be straightened without help; usually due to tenosynovitis of the flexor tendon sheath resulting in thickening or nodules which prevent free gliding. Seen particularly in gripping sports such as climbing. Treatment is by local corticosteroid injection or surgical release.

**trigger point** a localized hypersensitive band of tissue which, when irritated, refers pain to another part of the body. For example, shoulder trigger point resulting in headache.

**triglyceride (TG)** *see* **triacylglycerol (TG)**.

**trochanteric bursitis** pain over the greater trochanter – the bony prominence on the femur on either side of the thigh. Caused by inflammation of the bursa between the bone and the overlying muscle. Occurs as a result of repeated friction due to poor running gait or technique, altered biomechanics or poor muscle co-ordination. Management is as for bursitis elsewhere, including analgesia and identification of the underlying cause.

**troponin and tropomysin** the *control proteins*, components of the thin filaments in striated muscle, that work in partnership. Troponin has high affinity for calcium ions, which are released into the cytoplasm from the sarcoplasmic reticulum in response to excitation. When ionized calcium ($Ca^{2+}$) binds to it, the troponin molecule changes shape and in so doing, is thought to move the associated tropomyosin molecule around the thin filament, making previously masked binding sites on a number of actin molecules accessible to the head-groups of myosin. The resultant myosin/actin inter-action then develops force. *See also* **myofibrils**.

**tryptophan** *see* **amino acids, serotonin**.

**t-tubes (t-tubules)** in full *transverse tubules*. Tubules continuous with the surface membrane of a striated muscle fibre, which contain extracellular fluid yet penetrate in a network pattern the whole cellular cross-section, encircling every myofibril. The tubules are separated from the **sarcoplasmic reticulum (SR)** only by closely adjoining membranes, and are the route of excitation as an action potential spreads inward from the surface of the fibre to instigate $Ca^{2+}$ release from the SR.

**turbulent flow** the flow of a medium (e.g. air or water) in which the molecules are moving in a random, non-ordered manner. Can be an effect of an object or body travelling through the medium.

**ulna** larger of the two forearm bones, articulating at the elbow with the humerus and at the wrist with the carpal bones. *ulnar adj* in descriptions of forearm structures: on or towards the side of the ulna, i.e. the fifth finger side. *See appendix 1.2 fig 1.*

**ultrasound** sound frequencies above the limit of human hearing (20 kHz). *ultrasonography* imaging technique for body structures by reflection of ultrasound waves (up to 20 MHz). Used in sports medicine as a diagnostic tool in both cardiovascular and musculoskeletal assessment, e.g. cardiac screening, muscle tears. Ultrasound equipment is portable and accessible, costs less than MRI scanning but requires a skilled operator. It also allows dynamic imaging, e.g. of rotator cuff during shoulder movement. *ultrasound treatment (ultrasonics)* (1–3 MHz) is used especially for soft tissue injuries, to reduce swelling and inflammation and to encourage the healing process. The vibratory effect has been suggested to increase local blood supply, relieve pain, produce local heat and reduce sensory stimulation. One of the key treatments for sports injuries. *See also* **echocardiography**.

**unconditioned response** in classical conditioning, a response to an unconditioned stimulus that is naturally evoked by that stimulus. For example, in Pavlov's experiments with dogs, salivation at the presentation of food is the unconditioned response. *See also* **conditioning**.

**unconditioned stimulus** in classical conditioning, a stimulus that automatically evokes a particular reflexive response. For example, in Pavlov's experiments with dogs, the presentation of food is the unconditioned stimulus that automatically evokes the salivatory response. *See also* **conditioning**.

**underperformance syndrome (UPS)** an enduring deficit in performance which persists despite a period of rest or reduced training load and is not explained by any major diagnosed pathology. Characterized by a wide range of symptoms including fatigue, frequent minor infections and disturbed mood. It differs from **chronic fatigue syndrome** in that the symptoms do not have to last at least 6 months. *See also* **overtraining**.

**underwater weighing** an accurate method for the measurement of body density from which the percentages of body fat and lean body mass can be determined using standard equations. Weight in air is compared with weight in water during brief immersion, holding the breath after full expiration (at residual lung volume which is separately measured). Density is calculated from the volume of water displaced according to the Archimedes principle, which states that an object submerged in water is buoyed up by the weight of water displaced. *syn* *hydrostatic weighing*. *See* also **body composition**.

**V**

**vaccination** administration of antigenic material (*vaccine*) to induce active artificial immunity to specific infections. Important to prevent disease in sporting groups, especially with widespread foreign travel. *See also* **immunity**.

**vagus nerves** the tenth pair of cranial nerves, originating from the brain stem and descending through the neck, thorax and abdomen, giving off branches with both afferent and efferent components to many organs and tissues. The efferent fibres are mainly part of the **parasympathetic nervous system**, including those that slow the heart and those that innervate smooth muscle and glands in the respiratory and gastrointestinal tracts. The main afferent fibres are *visceral afferents* from thoracic and abdominal organs.

**valgum, valgus** angled inwards – deviation away from the midline of the body, of a part distal to a joint, e.g. **genu valgum** where the tibia is deviated laterally in relation to the femur, resulting in a 'knock-kneed' appearance in adults, often due to osteoarthritis of the knee joint. Opposite of **varum, varus**. *See also* **hallux**.

**valine** *see* **amino acids**.

**value–expectancy theory** *see* **expectancy–value theory**.

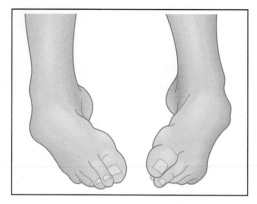

Talipes varus.

**varum, varus** angled outwards – deviation towards the midline of the body, of a part distal to a joint, e.g. **genu varum** where the tibia is deviated medially in relation to the femur, resulting in a 'bow-legged' appearance in adults. *talipes varus* inward tilt of the distal part of the foot at the talonavicular joint resulting in a *club foot*. Opposite of **valgum, valgus**.

**vasoconstriction** narrowing of the lumen of a blood vessel, due to contraction of the smooth muscle in its wall, mediated by neural (autonomic) control, local or blood-borne chemical factors, or fall in temperature. Part of the rationale for the use of ice in acute injury to minimize blood flow (and therefore swelling) in the damaged tissue.

**vasodilatation** widening of the lumen of a blood vessel, due to relaxation of the smooth muscle in its wall, mediated by neural (autonomic) control, local or blood-borne chemical factors, or rise in temperature. *Syn vasodilation*.

**vasopressin** *syn* **antidiuretic hormone (ADH)** *see* **hormones, hypothalamus, osmoreceptors, posterior pituitary, thirst**.

**vector** a variable, quantity or measurement that has both size and directional components. Cannot be added arithmetically due to directional component.

**vegan diet** consists totally of vegetables, vegetable oils and seeds, excluding all foods of animal origin – meat, fish and dairy foods, and also honey. Vegans need to make sure that they are getting enough protein and micronutrients such as iron and vitamin $B_{12}$.

**vegetarian diet** excludes any meat, fish, seafood or animal-body by-products such as gelatine, but usually allows milk, cheese and eggs; *lactovegetarian diet* excludes all animal-body foods and eggs but does allow milk and milk products; *lacto-ovo-vegetarian diet,* the most liberal, excludes all animal-body foods, but includes milk, milk products and eggs.

**velocity** rate of change of position with respect to time. A vector quantity so has both magnitude (speed) and direction; *linear velocity* the linear displacement per unit time; *angular velocity* the angular displacement per unit time, i.e. speed of rotation in a particular direction (e.g. clockwise or anticlockwise); *instantaneous velocity* velocity of a body or object measured over a very short (infinitesimal) period of time: effectively a continuous measurement of velocity; *tangential velocity* the velocity of an object or body acting at a tangent to its direction of motion (often when it is moving in a circle or around a curve). *See also* **displacement**.

**venous return** the flow of blood from the whole body (except the lungs) via the great veins to the right side of the heart. Apart from minor beat-by-beat variations, this is equal at any one time to the cardiac output (from each of the ventricles), as the whole circulation, with the systemic and pulmonary components in series, is a closed loop. When heart rate increases and muscle supply vessels dilate in exercise, stroke volume is maintained (so that cardiac output is increased) by an increase in venous return, assisted by constriction of peripheral veins, reduction in the blood flow to the abdominal organs, and by the 'pumping' effects of increased depth of breathing (promoting flow into the thorax), and of the contracting muscles, which 'milk' blood along their local veins towards the heart.

**ventilation** in physiology and medicine, refers to *pulmonary ventilation*, the movement of air in and out of the lungs, whether during normal breathing, or by artificial means. *total ventilation* or *minute volume* $\dot{V}_E$ (or $\dot{V}_I$) is the volume breathed out (or in) in litres per minute: the tidal volume multiplied by the number of breaths per minute. May be measured, e.g. by collecting the expired gas over a known time (**Douglas bag method**), or by integrating inspired or expired airflow with respect to time (by **pneumotachograph**). The effective component, *alveolar ventilation* $\dot{V}_A$, refers to that which reaches the regions of the lungs where gas exchange occurs, and is equal to the total ventilation minus *dead space ventilation* $\dot{V}_D$. Normally, at rest, $\dot{V}_A : \dot{V}_D = 2:1$ or typically, $\dot{V}_E - \dot{V}_D = \dot{V}_A$, $6 - 2 = 4\,L.min^{-1}$. When ventilation increases in exercise, the dead space is unchanged, so $\dot{V}_D$ rises only in proportion to the rise in frequency of breaths, but $\dot{V}_E$ rises relatively more as tidal volume also increases. *See also* **artificial ventilation**, **dead space, lung volumes and capacities**.

**ventilatory equivalent** describes the ratio of ventilation (minute volume) to oxygen intake, or to carbon dioxide output. For oxygen, the volume of gas breathed out (and in) in litres per minute (ventilation, $\dot{V}_E$) divided by the oxygen consumption in litres per minute ($\dot{V}O_2$) over the same period: an index of the efficiency of oxygen uptake in the lungs. When there is significant anaerobic metabolism, decrease in blood pH is countered by stimulation of ventilation to increase $CO_2$ excretion, such that $\dot{V}_E$ increases at a higher rate than $\dot{V}O_2$, raising the ventilatory equivalent (for $CO_2$ the ventilatory equivalent, $\dot{V}_E / \dot{V}CO_2$, increases in this instance less than that for $O_2$ because as $CO_2$ in the blood and lungs decreases, the same output is achieved by a smaller expired volume).

**ventilatory threshold** *see* **metabolic and related thresholds**.

**ventral** at or towards the front of the body; applies to the front of the hands and arms in the **anatomical position** when the palms face forwards. Opposite of **dorsal**.

**ventricles** the paired major chambers and muscular pumps of the **heart**. The *left ventricle* receives oxygenated blood from the lungs via the left atrium, and in an average-sized person at rest ejects a *stroke volume* of around 70 mL at each beat (contraction, systole) into the aorta, increasing during exercise by virtue of greater filling and stretching during each relaxation (diastole); the *right ventricle* receives venous blood from the rest of the body via the right atrium, and ejects the same volume as the left ventricle, in synchrony with it. The heart beat can normally be felt over the apex of the left ventricle. *See appendix 1.3 fig 1.*

**vertebral column** *syn back bone, spinal column* the dorsal axis of the body in all vertebrates. A bony and ligamentous structure extending from the uppermost (atlas) vertebra which articulates with the base of the skull, and ending above and behind the anus. Consists of 24 separate vertebrae linked by joints and by the intervertebral discs (seven cervical, 12 thoracic, which give attachment to the ribs, and five lumbar), plus five fused to form the *sacrum* (articulating with the ilium of the pelvic bones) and four rudimentary 'tail' vertebrae fused in the *coccyx*. Allows a limited amount of movement of the trunk and provides a protected tunnel, the *vertebral (spinal) canal*, for the spinal cord and the paired anterior and posterior spinal nerve roots, which leave through openings (intervertebral foramina) at the sides of the column, each being numbered according to that of the vertebra above the foramen. *See also* **cervical spine**, **intervertebral discs**, **spinal injury**; *appendix 1.2 figs 1, 2.*

**vestibular apparatus** sensory organs of the inner ear: the *otolith organs* and the *semicircular canals*. They detect tilt of the head with respect to the ground, and the direction and rate of any acceleration of the head in space. This input interacts with sensory information from muscles and joints, eyes and ears to co-ordinate reflex postural adjustments.

**vicarious experience** knowledge or information about a skill or behaviour derived from seeing the performance of others.

**video analysis** the use of video cameras and equipment to analyse motion, often for kinematic analysis.

**viruses** microscopic particles that can replicate only within a living animal or plant cell, so widely considered not to be themselves truly 'living', and not possible to destroy directly without also destroying the host cells. For those that cause human diseases, antiviral drug treatment is limited (antibiotics have no effect) but **vaccination** can provide immunity and in the second half of the 20th century this eradicated smallpox worldwide and much reduced the incidence of poliomyelitis. Viral conditions include colds, influenza, chickenpox, measles, hepatitis and herpes of different types (e.g. cold sores, shingles). *See also* **human immunodeficiency virus (HIV)**.

**visceral** pertaining to the *viscera* or internal organs. Hence *visceral afferents* the components of the peripheral nervous system that carry information from the organs. The outgoing nerves to the viscera are the sympathetic and parasympathetic nerves of the **autonomic nervous system** but are not usually known as visceral efferents.

**viscosity** the property of a fluid medium that provides resistance to motion of the fluid itself or of an object moving through it. Also can be considered to be friction within fluids.

**visual imagery** *see* **imagery**.

**visualization** *see* **imagery**.

**vital capacity** the volume of air that can be inspired with maximal effort after forcefully emptying the lungs, or expired from full lung volume. *See also* **lung volumes**.

**vitamins** organic substances that are necessary in the diet, in very small quantities, for normal growth and health: the **recommended daily allowance (RDA)** for any vitamin, widely quoted on food and drink labels, is less than 200 mg. Originally identified by alleviation of conditions caused by their deficiency (e.g. of scurvy in ships' crews in the 1750s by providing citrus fruit, the vital component being found later to be ascorbic acid, vitamin C). Nowadays *hypovitaminosis* due to lack of one or more vitamins is rare on a well-balanced diet, although occasionally an athlete may suffer from a deficiency, e.g. if dieting for weight loss or eliminating particular foods or food groups from the diet. *hypervitaminosis* can occur with excessive intake of one or more vitamins. The International Olympic Committee states that no vitamin supplements should be required if the diet is well balanced but athletes do often take them, especially vitamins C, B-complex and E, with a possible danger to their health by overconsumption. For sources, functions and deficiency effects, *see appendix 4.2*.

**volitional behaviour** in the **theory of reasoned action**, behaviour that a person intentionally enacts and that has no barriers or obstacles that would impede its enactment.

**volume** the amount of space taken up by an object or fluid. Expressed as cubic metres ($m^3$). The more commonly used litre (L or l) and it subdivisions are not SI units, but accepted for use with them: $1\,L = 1$ cubic decimetre $(1\,dm^3) = 10^{-3} m^3$.

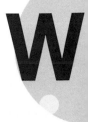

**waist–hip ratio (WHR)** circumference at the waist divided by that at the hips; an index of body fat distribution, said to be ideally not >0.8 in women and not >0.9 in men, i.e. a low ratio ('pear-shape') is healthier than a high ratio ('apple shape'). Some large-scale studies have found evidence that WHR is a better predictor than **body mass index** for coronary heart disease.

**warm-down** period of progressively less intense dynamic activity and stretching, undertaken promptly after a competition or bout of high-intensity training with a view to preventing blood pooling (leg exercise), better clearing of lactate and other waste products and minimizing subsequent stiffness. Also known as *cool-down*.

**warm-up** period of dynamic activity and stretching, initially gentle and loose but increasing in intensity and focus over 5–10 min, which gradually elevates heart rate and oxygen uptake as well as raising the tem1perature of muscle and other soft tissues. Undertaken shortly before competition or bout of high-intensity training (which itself may be dynamic or static), with a view to enhancing performance and reducing the likelihood of soft tissue injury or cardiovascular incident.

**water balance** the state when the amount of water consumed in food and drink plus that generated by metabolism equals the amount of water excreted. Intake is regulated by behavioural mechanisms, including thirst and salt cravings. While almost a litre of water per 24 hours is unavoidably lost via the skin, lungs and faeces, the kidneys are the site of regulated excretion of water in the urine. In a moderate climatic environment, to achieve water balance a sedentary individual should consume ~2 litres of water daily; in hot dry environments up to 4 litres may be needed. Athletes require additional intake to match the loss due to a high sweating rate, depending in turn on the type and severity of exercise, on the temperature and humidity, and on **heat acclimatization**. *See also* **hydration status**, **posterior pituitary**, **sports drinks**, **thirst**. *Fig facing.*

**weight** the force due to the effect of gravity on the mass of a body or object. Can be calculated by multiplying the mass by the acceleration due to gravity. Correctly, expressed in newtons. Commonly (usually, in the public context) but incorrectly referred to in units of mass (e.g. kg).

**weight-bearing exercise** exercise in which the legs support the body weight.

**weight-lifting** sport consisting of lifting maximum possible free weights through a variety of previously stipulated body positions.

**weight training** strength ('resistance') training using either free weights or those providing the loads in exercise machines. *See also* **strength training**.

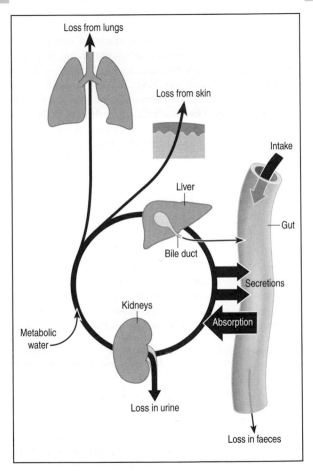

Water balance. Size of the arrows represents relative volumes of water moving in and out of the body, and exchanged internally with the gut, over a typical 24-hour period, with moderate activity in temperate conditions. The circle represents the circulating blood and other extracellular fluids

**whiplash injury** damage to the structures of the neck, particularly the cervical vertebrae, muscles, tendons and ligaments and, most importantly, the spinal cord and nerve roots. Term describes the mechanism of injury rather than a precise diagnosis. Usually caused by the sudden, uncontrolled movement of the neck forwards and backwards, like the crack of a whip. Seen in road traffic accidents when a vehicle comes to a sudden stop at speed. In sport, most common in rugby and American football when a player is tackled. *See also* **spinal injury**.

**white blood cells** *see* **leucocytes**.

**white muscle** *see* **muscle fibre types**.

**Wingate test** test of **anaerobic power** production, originating in the Wingate Institute, Israel, in 1974. Consists of flat-out pedalling on a **cycle ergometer** for 30 s against a resistance chosen to suit the subject's body weight (BW), sex and fitness, and the design of the ergometer, e.g. 7.5% BW for a normally healthy young adult male on the widely used Monark ergometer. Both peak power output and the extent to which output is maintained over the 30 s are usually reported.

**Wolff–Parkinson–White (WPW) syndrome** a cardiac arrhythmia (usually supraventricular tachycardia) resulting from an abnormal conduction pathway between the atria and ventricles. The characteristic ECG pattern has a wide QRS complex with a 'delta wave' and a short PR interval. A recent study of routine ECGs in over 130 000 adults over a wide age range detected the syndrome in about 1 in 1000, with the highest incidence in the 20–40 age group, equally in men and women. Usually asymptomatic but requires further investigation (by echocardiography and exercise testing) if discovered opportunistically or by cardiac screening. *See also* **sudden death**.

**work** the magnitude of a force applied to a body or object multiplied by the distance through which it is moved (linearly) in the direction of that force. Also the moment applied to a rotating body or object multiplied by the angular displacement through which it is moved (angularly). If there is no motion of the object there is no mechanical work done on it. A scalar quantity. Measured in joules (J). *external work* work done on an external body or object (e.g. by the human body); *internal work* work by forces inside a body or object (e.g. the human body); *negative work* the usually accepted convention for the situation of an object having work done on it by an external force, e.g. a muscle being extended by an external load during eccentric action. *positive work* the usually accepted convention for work done by an agent on surroundings, e.g. when a net muscle moment acts in the same direction as the direction of motion that it induces in the object.

**work–energy theorem** states that the change in the energy of a body or object is equal to the work performed.

**workload** in general usage, the amount of any type of work to be done, or being done, by a person or group. Used often, but inappropriately, in describing the level of various types of exercise and should be avoided since it has no precise definition or specific units, whereas each type may be properly quantified, e.g. as power output in cycling or treadmill exercise, or as force or tension during isometric contraction. The term 'intensity' has been recommended as preferable when referring to the level of activity during any exercise; it does not imply any particular units of measurement and so can be used with respect to the magnitude of force (in N), of power (in W), of speed (in $km.h^{-1}$) or to any of these as percentage of maximal.

**workrate** term used in exercise physiology for the power produced by a living body. May be expressed directly in units of power (joules per second ($J.s^{-1}$) or watts (W)) or indirectly in terms of oxygen consumed per unit time.

**World Anti-Doping Agency (WADA)** *see* **banned substance**.

**wrist** refers to the two rows of *carpal bones* between the metacarpal bones of the hand and the **wrist joint.** *Syn carpus. Fig facing.*

**wrist joint** links the forearm bones to the proximal row of the **carpal bones,** allowing movement of the hand forward (palmar flexion), backward (dorsiflexion) and side-to-side (and combinations of these) by the action of muscles that have their origins in the forearm and around the elbow, and tendons that span the wrist to be inserted beyond it. *wrist injury* is most common in sports where a strong grip is required, especially with twisting, such as gymnastics, golf and tennis, or in throwing sports (causing soft tissue injuries), contact sports or where falls are likely such as boxing or horse riding (causing fractures). *See also* **scaphoid bone**.

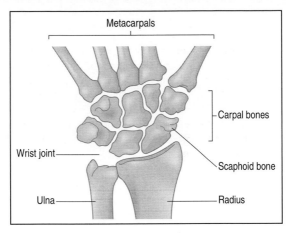

Bones of the right wrist from the front.

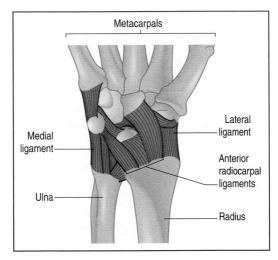

Right wrist and radioulnar joints, from the front.

**X-rays** short-wavelength electromagnetic ionizing radiation, which can penetrate the body structures to varying degrees. Discovered in 1895 by Wilmhelm Röntgen, a German physicist (the very first X-ray photograph showed the bones of his wife's hand, with her wedding ring). Used in general, and in sport, to produce photographic images of body structures, notably bones (to detect fractures), also heart and lungs. *See also* **radiography**, **radiology**.

**Y**

**Yerkes–Dodson law** *see* **inverted-U hypothesis**.

**yips** a movement disorder that can affect sports performers, seen particularly in golfers but also in cricketers and darts players, involving uncontrollable movements of the hand or wrist or an inability to release the ball or dart, making effective performance impossible. Its causes are unknown but both neurological deficits due to long-term overuse and psychological factors such as performance anxiety have been implicated.

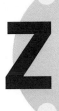

**zinc** *see* **minerals**; *appendix 4.3.*

**zone of optimal functioning (ZOF)** in sport psychology, a model of optimal performance, proposed in 1980 by Russian psychologist Yuri L Hanin, that hypothesizes a bandwidth of arousal within which an athlete will perform at their optimal level. This bandwidth is held to be different for different individuals with some performing better within higher bandwidths and others within lower bandwidths. In acknowledgement of these individual differences, the model was later renamed the *individual zone of optimal functioning model (IZOF)*. The more recent conceptualization also extends the model to include optimal patterns of positive and negative affect, taking account of particular emotions that might influence different performers differently and the optimal intensity of those emotions.

# Appendices

**Appendix 1** Human anatomy     411

1.1 Nervous system     411
1.2 Bones, joints and muscles     418
1.3 Heart, lungs, circulation     429
1.4 Alimentary system     433

**Appendix 2** SI units and the metric system     435

**Appendix 3** Normal values     443

**Appendix 4** Nutrients     445

4.1 Macronutrients     446
4.2 Micronutrients: vitamins     447
4.3 Micronutrients: minerals     451
4.4 Ergogenic aids     455

**Appendix 5** Hormones     459

**Appendix 6** Drugs     463

**Appendix 7** Abbreviations and acronyms     471

**Appendix 8** Useful addresses, including websites     479

**Appendix 9** References and further reading     481

# Human anatomy

## 1.1 Nervous system

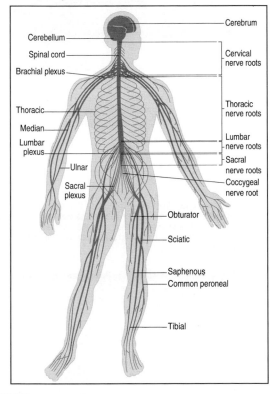

Fig 1.1.1 The nervous system.

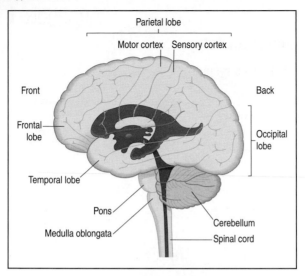

Fig 1.1.2 The brain viewed from the left showing the lobes of the cerebral hemisphere, the cerebellum and the lower parts of the brain stem in continuity with the spinal cord. Coloured area: the position of the ventricles, lying deep in the brain, containing cerebrospinal fluid and continuous with the central canal of the spinal cord.

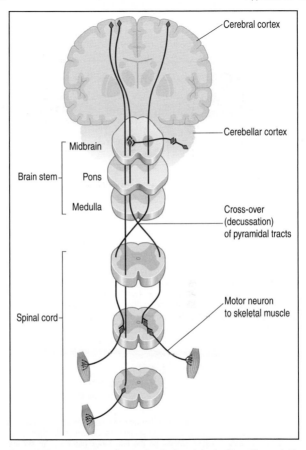

Fig 1.1.3 The sites of the main nerve centres and descending pathways in the brain and spinal cord that control voluntary movement, represented in diagrammatic sections.

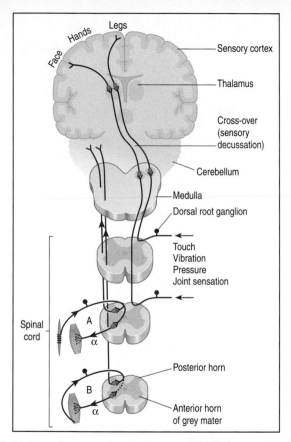

Fig 1.1.4 Ascending nerve pathways and proprioceptive reflex arcs, represented in diagrammatic sections of the brain and spinal cord. Shown on the right: those serving the sensations listed. Shown on the left: reflex pathways for skeletal muscle control. (A) From a muscle spindle, to a synapse with an alpha motor neuron, and a branch to the brain. (B) From a tendon organ, inhibitory branch (*broken line*) to an alpha motor neuron, and a branch to the brain.

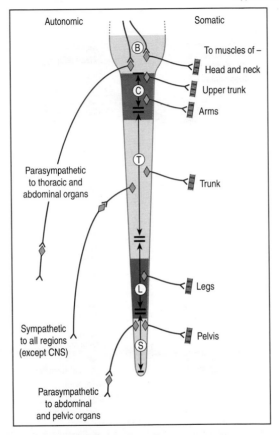

Fig 1.1.5 Efferent nerve pathways from the brainstem and spinal cord. Shown on the right: somatic, to skeletal muscles. Shown on the left: autonomic. B brain stem, C cervical, T thoracic, L lumbar, S sacral segments of the spinal cord. (Red shaded regions are those with no autonomic outflow.)

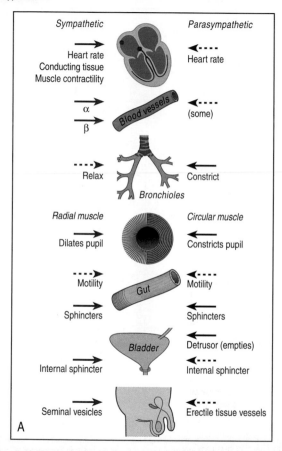

Sympathetic

Parasympathetic

→ Heart rate
Conducting tissue
Muscle contractility

◀···· Heart rate

α →
β →
Blood vessels

◀···· (some)

···▶ Relax

← Constrict

*Bronchioles*

*Radial muscle*

*Circular muscle*

→ Dilates pupil

→ Constricts pupil

···▶ Motility

◀···· Motility

→ Sphincters
*Gut*

← Sphincters

*Bladder*

← Detrusor (empties)

→ Internal sphincter

◀···· Internal sphincter

→ Seminal vesicles

◀···· Erectile tissue vessels

**A**

Fig 1.1.6A The autonomic nervous system. Actions on the heart and on smooth muscle. *Sympathetic* actions on the left and *parasympathetic* actions on the right. *Solid arrows*: stimulation (contraction or secretion); *broken arrows*: inhibition.

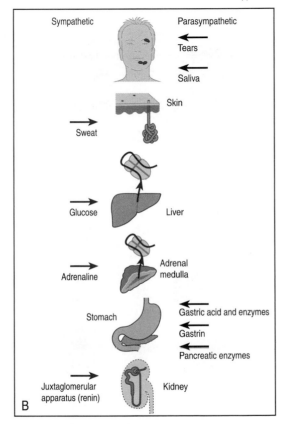

Fig 1.1.6B The autonomic nervous system. Actions on secretory functions (heart diagrams indicate release into the circulation). *Sympathetic* actions on the left and *parasympathetic* actions on the right. *Solid arrows*: stimulation (contraction or secretion); *broken arrows*: inhibition.

# 1.2 Bones, joints and muscles

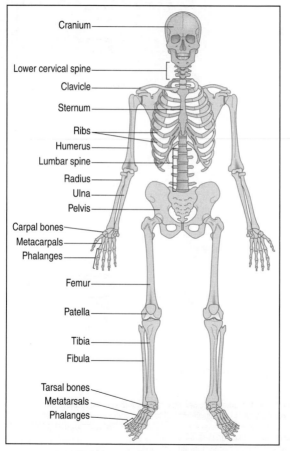

Fig 1.2.1 Front view of the skeleton.

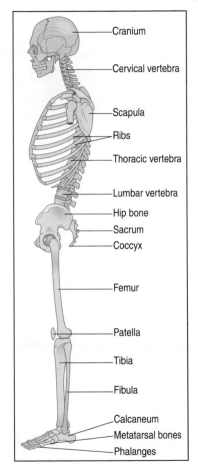

Fig 1.2.2 The skeleton from the left.

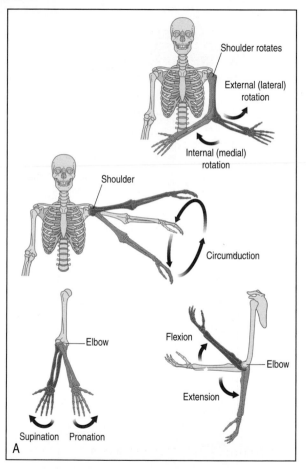

Fig 1.2.3A Movements at the joints. Upper limb.

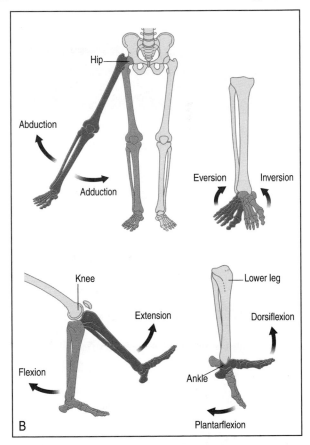

Fig 1.2.3B Movements at the joints. Lower limb.

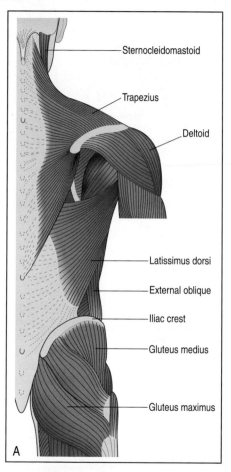

Fig 1.2.4A Muscles of the back.

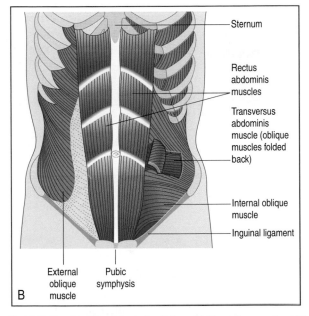

Fig 1.2.4B Muscles of the abdominal wall. Superficial layer shown on the right side of the body, deeper layer on the left.

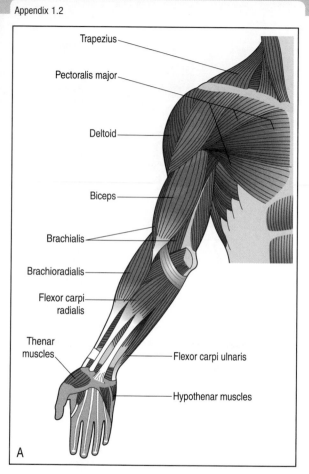

Fig 1.2.5A Muscles of the shoulder girdle and upper limb. Right arm from the front.

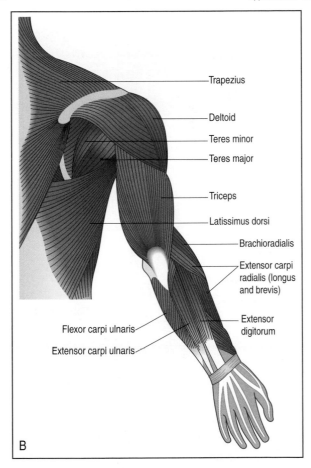

Fig 1.2.5B Muscles of the shoulder girdle and upper limb. Right arm from the back.

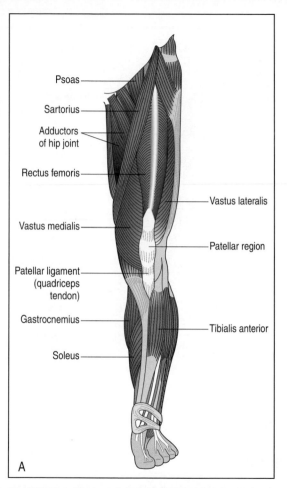

Psoas

Sartorius

Adductors
of hip joint

Rectus femoris

Vastus lateralis

Vastus medialis

Patellar region

Patellar ligament
(quadriceps
tendon)

Gastrocnemius

Tibialis anterior

Soleus

A

Fig 1.2.6A Muscles of the lower limb. Left leg from the front.

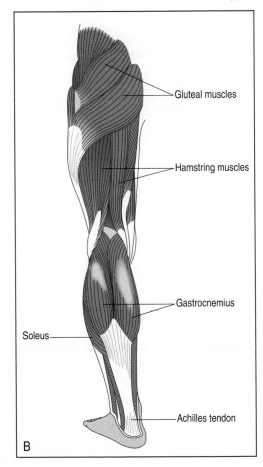

Fig 1.2.6B Muscles of the lower limb. Left leg from the back.

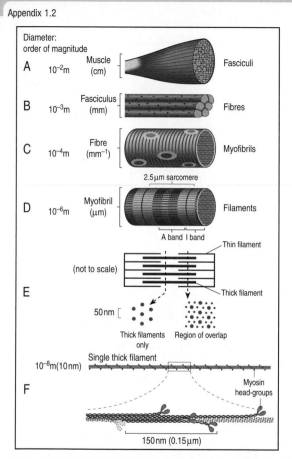

Fig 1.2.7 Structure of skeletal muscle at progressively higher magnification, from whole muscle to contractile proteins (A–D, F). E represents the 'sliding filaments' diagrammatically.

# 1.3 Heart, lungs, and circulation

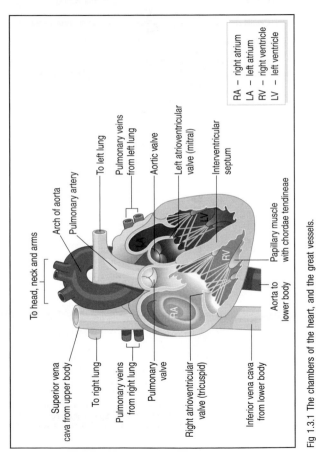

RA – right atrium
LA – left atrium
RV – right ventricle
LV – left ventricle

To left lung

Pulmonary veins from left lung

Aortic valve

Left atrioventricular valve (mitral)

Interventricular septum

Arch of aorta

Pulmonary artery

Papillary muscle with chordae tendineae

To head, neck and arms

Aorta to lower body

Superior vena cava from upper body

To right lung

Pulmonary veins from right lung

Pulmonary valve

Right atrioventricular valve (tricuspid)

Inferior vena cava from lower body

Fig 1.3.1 The chambers of the heart, and the great vessels.

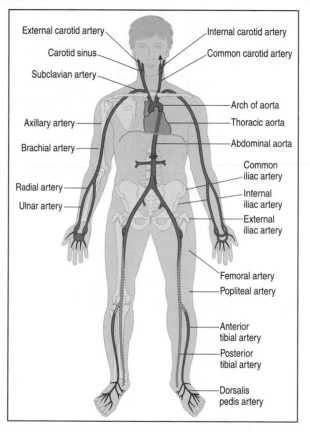

Fig 1.3.2 The aorta and the main arteries that supply the head and limbs. (*Broken outlines:* vessels deep in the thigh, or in the back of the leg.)

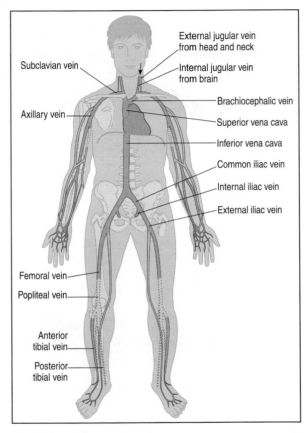

Fig 1.3.3 The main veins returning blood to the heart from the head and the limbs. (*Broken outlines:* vessels deep in the thigh, or in the back of the leg.)

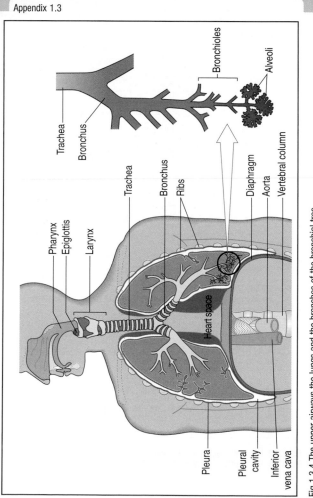

Fig 1.3.4 The upper airways the lungs and the branches of the bronchial tree.

# 1.4 Alimentary system

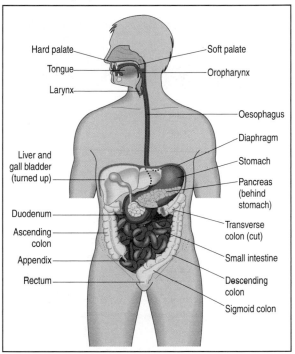

Fig 1.4.1 The alimentary tract. The small intestine (pink) opens into the large intestine (grey) at the caecum.

# SI units and the metric system

## Système International (SI) units

At an international convention in 1960, the General Conference of Weights and Measures agreed to an International System of Units: SI or Système International, the name for the current version of the metric system, first introduced in France at the end of the 18th century.

In any system of measurement, the magnitude of some physical quantities must be arbitrarily selected and declared to have unit value. These magnitudes form a set of standards and are called **base units**. All other units are **derived units**.

The SI measurement system is used for medical, scientific and technical purposes in most countries and comprises seven base units with several derived units. Each unit has its own symbol and is expressed as a decimal multiple or submultiple of the base unit by use of the appropriate prefix; for example, a millimetre is one thousandth of a metre.

### SI base units

| Name of unit | Symbol | Quantity |
|---|---|---|
| Metre | m | Length |
| Kilogram | kg | Mass |
| Second | s | Time |
| Mole | mol | Amount of substance |
| Ampere | A | Electric current |
| Kelvin | °K | Thermodynamic temperature |
| Candela | cd | Luminous intensity |

**SI derived units (obtained by dividing or multiplying two or more base units)**

| Name | Symbol | Quantity |
|------|--------|----------|
| Joule | J | Work, energy, heat |
| Pascal | Pa | Pressure |
| Newton | N | Force |
| Watt | W | Power |
| Volt | V | Electrical potential, potential difference, electromotive force |
| Hertz | Hz | Frequency |
| **Other values expressed in terms of base units** | | |
| Square metre | $m^2$ | Area |
| Cubic metre | $m^3$ | Volume |
| Metres per seond | m/s m.s$^{-1}$ | Speed, velocity |
| Metres per second per second | m/s$^2$ m.s$^{-2}$ | Acceleration |
| Kilogram per cubic metre | kg/m$^3$ kg.m$^{-3}$ | Density |
| Mole per cubic metre | mol/m$^3$ mol.m$^{-3}$ | Concentration |

# Decimal multiples and submultiples

The metric system uses multiples of 10 to express number. Multiples and submultiples of the base unit are expressed as decimals, with appropriate prefix to the name of the unit. The most widely used prefixes are kilo, milli and micro: e.g. $0.000\ 001\ g = 10^{-6}g = 1$ microgram.

# Rules for using units and numbers

- The symbol for a unit is unaltered in the plural and should not be followed by a full stop except at the end of a sentence: 5 cm *not* 5 cm. or 5 cms.
- The decimal point between digits is indicated by a full stop. Commas are not used to divide large numbers into groups of three: a space is left after every third digit. If the numerical value of the number is

**Multiples and submultiples of units**

| Multiplication factor | | Prefix | Symbol |
|---|---|---|---|
| 1 000 000 000 000 | $10^{12}$ | tera | T |
| 1 000 000 000 | $10^{9}$ | giga | G |
| 1 000 000 | $10^{6}$ | mega | M |
| 1000 | $10^{3}$ | kilo | k |
| 100 | $10^{2}$ | hecto | h |
| 10 | $10^{1}$ | deca | da |
| 0.1 | $10^{-1}$ | deci | d |
| 0.01 | $10^{-2}$ | centi | c |
| 0.001 | $10^{-3}$ | milli | m |
| 0.000 001 | $10^{-6}$ | micro | μ |
| 0.000 000 001 | $10^{-9}$ | nano | n |
| 0.000 000 000 001 | $10^{-12}$ | pico | p |
| 0.000 000 000 000 001 | $10^{-15}$ | femto | f |
| 0.000 000 000 000 000 001 | $10^{-18}$ | atto | a |

less than 1, a zero should precede the decimal point: 0.123 456 *not* .123,456.

- The SI symbol for 'day' (i.e. 24 hours) is 'd' but excretion of substances, fluid intake or output, for example, should preferably be expressed as amount or mass or volume 'per 24 hours'.
- 'Squared' and 'cubed' are expressed as numerical powers and not by abbreviation: square centimetre is $cm^2$ *not* sq cm.

# Units used for common measurements

**Temperature** The SI base unit is the kelvin but temperature is normally expressed in degrees Celsius (°C).

1° Celsius = 1° Centigrade

**Energy** The SI unit **joule** replaces the **calorie**.

1 calorie = 4.2 J

1 kilocalorie (calorie) = 4.2 kilojoules

Energy requirement, expenditure and content of food are expressed in kilojoules (kJ), but the kilocalorie (kcal) remains in common use.

**Amount** of substance in SI units is expressed in moles (mol), and concentration (amount per unit volume) in moles per litre (mol/L) or millimoles per litre (mmol/L). This replaces milliequivalents per litre (mEq/L). There are some exceptions: grams per litre (g/L), e.g. for haemoglobin and plasma proteins; international units (IU, U or iu) for enzyme activity.

**Pressure** The SI unit is the pascal (Pa); the kilopascal (kPa) replaces millimetres of mercury pressure (mmHg) for arterial blood pressure and partial pressure (or tension) of oxygen and carbon dioxide ($PO_2$ and $PCO_2$) in gas or in blood.

1 mmHg = 133.32 Pa

1 kPa = 7.5006 mmHg

Arterial blood pressure is, however, still widely measured in mmHg, cerebrospinal fluid pressure in $mmH_2O$ and central venous pressure in $cmH_2O$.

**Volume** is calculated as length × width × depth. The metre(m) is the SI unit for length but a cubic metre is not a practical unit of volume for most purposes. The litre (L or l – the volume of a 10 cm cube) and the millilitre (mL, ml) are therefore used ($1\,L = 10^{-3}m^3 = 1\,dm^3$).

# Weights and measures

## Linear measure

| | |
|---|---|
| 1 kilometre (km) | = 1000 metres (m) |
| 1 metre (m) | = 100 centimetres (cm) or 1000 millmetres (mm) |

| 1 centimetre (cm) | = 10 millimetres (mm) |
| 1 millimetre (mm) | = 1000 micrometres (μm) |
| 1 micrometre (μm) | = 1000 nanometres (nm) |

*Conversions*

| Metric | Imperial |
|---|---|
| 1 metre (m) | = 39.370 inches (in) |
| 1 centimetre (cm) | = 0.3937 inches (in) |
| 30.48 centimetres (cm) | = 1 foot (ft) |
| 2.54 centimetres (cm) | = 1 inch (in) |

## Volume

| 1 litre (L) | = 1000 millilitres (mL) |
| 1 millilitre (mL) | = 1000 microlitres (μL) |

*Conversions*

| Metric | Imperial |
|---|---|
| 1 litre (L) | = 1.76 pints (pt) |
| 568.25 millilitres (mL) | = 1 pint (pt) |
| 28.4 millilitres (mL) | = 1 fluid ounce (fl oz) |

## Mass

| 1 kilogram (kg) | = 1000 grams (g) |
| 1 gram (g) | = 1000 milligrams (mg) |
| 1 milligram (mg) | = 1000 micrograms (μg) |
| 1 microgram (μg) | = 1000 nanograms (ng) |

*Conversions*

| Metric | Imperial |
|---|---|
| 1 kilogram (kg) | = 2.204 pounds (lb) |
| 1 gram (g) | = 0.0353 ounce (oz) |
| 453.59 grams (g) | = 1 pound (lb) |
| 28.34 grams (g) | = 1 ounce (oz) |

# Temperature

### *Conversions*

- Fahrenheit $(9/5 \times x°C) + 32$
- Centigrade $= °Celsius = (x°F − 32) \times 5/9$

where $x$ is the temperature to be converted.

## Conversion scales

*Fig 2.1 facing.*

For Body Temperature: *Fig 2.2 over leaf.*

Conversion scales

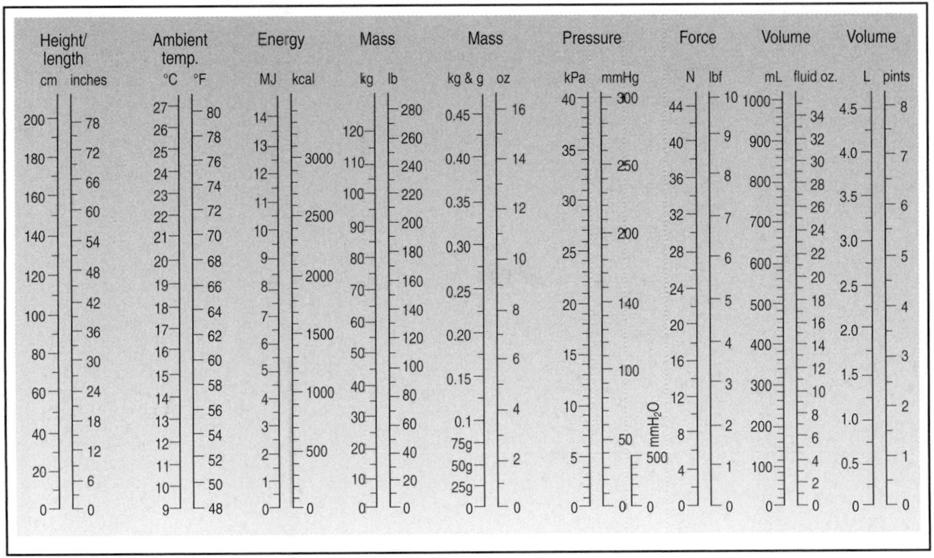

Fig 2.1

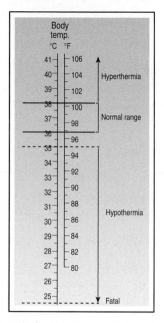

Fig 2.2 Conversion scale for body temperature showing the normal and abnormal ranges.

# Normal values

## Cardiac output

**Resting** 4–6 L.min$^{-1}$ depending on body size. Typically **stroke volume** 70 mL × heart rate 70 per min = 4.9 L.min$^{-1}$ (SV higher, HR lower after athletic training).

**Working/exercising**

|          | HR    | SV       | CO             |
|----------|-------|----------|----------------|
| Moderate | ∼120  | ∼ 80 mL  | ∼10 L.min$^{-1}$ |
| Strenuous| ∼150  | ∼100 mL  | ∼15 L.min$^{-1}$ |
| Maximal  | ∼180  | ∼140 mL  | ∼25 L.min$^{-1}$ |

Maximal CO can be higher after endurance training

## Metabolic rate and oxygen consumption

**Resting** typically  ∼4.2 kJ per kg body mass per hour
∼3.5 mL O$_2$ per kg of body mass per minute
4000–7000 kJ per 24 hours depending on body mass

**Working/exercising** (average for 70 kg man)

|          | Oxygen consumption | Energy expenditure |
|----------|--------------------|--------------------|
| Moderate | 1 L.min$^{-1}$     | ∼20 kJ.min$^{-1}$  |
| Strenuous| 2 L.min$^{-1}$     | ∼40 kJ.min$^{-1}$  |
| Maximal  | 4 L.min$^{-1}$     | ∼80 kJ.min$^{-1}$  |

# Blood gases (arterial)

| | |
|---|---|
| Haemoglobin oxygen saturation | 97–100% |
| Oxygen tension $PO_2$ | 12.0–13.3 kPa |
| | (90–100 mmHg) |
| Carbon dioxide tension $PCO_2$ | 5–5.6 kPa (38–42 mmHg) |

# Blood pH (arterial)                7.36–7.44

# Blood: biochemistry

| | |
|---|---|
| Bicarbonate (arterial blood) | 22–28 mmol.$L^{-1}$ |
| Calcium | 2.1–2.6 mmol.$L^{-1}$ |
| Chloride | 97–106 mmol.$L^{-1}$ |
| Cholesterol (total) | $< 5.2$ mmol.$L^{-1}$ (ideal) |
| HDL-cholesterol | 0.5–1.9 mmol.$L^{-1}$ |
| Triglycerides | 0.45–2.0 mmol.$L^{-1}$ |
| Protein (total) | 60–80 g.$L^{-1}$ |
| Glucose (venous, fasting) | 3.6–5.8 mmol.$L^{-1}$ |
| Potassium (plasma) | 3.3–4.7 mmol.$L^{-1}$ |
| Sodium | 135–143 mmol.$L^{-1}$ |

# Blood: haematology

| | |
|---|---|
| Haemoglobin | |
| Female | 115–165 g.$L^{-1}$ |
| Male | 130–180 g.$L^{-1}$ |
| Red cell count | |
| Female | $3.8–5.3 \times 10^{12}$ per litre |
| Male | $4.5–6.5 \times 10^{12}$ per litre |
| White cell count | |
| Total | $4.0–11.0 \times 10^9$ per litre |

# Appendix 4

## Nutrients

4.1 Macronutrients                          446

4.2 Micronutrients: vitamins                447

4.3 Micronutrients: minerals                451

4.4 Ergogenic aids                          455

**Table 4.1. Macronutrients**

| Energy value | Reference nutrient intake (RNI) | Sources | Functions | Deficiency | Excess | Notes |
|---|---|---|---|---|---|---|
| **Carbohydrate** 1 g yields 16 kJ (3.75 kcal) | Minimum of 47% of total daily energy intake; not >10% should be provided by added sugars. RNI for non-starch polysaccharide: 18 g/d | Sugar, potatoes, rice, pasta, noodles, bread, breakfast cereals | Provides energy for metabolism | Weight loss, ketosis | Obesity, elevated blood triglyceride | Diets high in carbohydrate tend to be low in fat |
| **Protein** 1 g yields 17 kJ (4 kcal) | About 15% of total daily energy intake: e.g. Women 45 g/d Men 55 g/d | Meat, fish, eggs, nuts, pulses, dairy products, tofu, Quorn | Component of all body tissues; energy source in some situations | Retarded growth; weight loss and muscle wasting; poor wound healing; impaired immune system; fat deposition in the liver | Possible link with loss of minerals from bone and age-related deterioration in renal function | Protein content of Western diets is usually higher than the RNI |
| **Fat** 1 g yields 37 kJ (9 kcal) | Should not exceed 35% of total daily energy intake. Of this no more than 10% should be saturated fatty acids | Butter and other full-fat dairy products, margarine; cooking oils and fried food; pastry, cakes, biscuits; meat, oily fish, seeds, nuts, chocolate, crisps | Provides energy for metabolism; energy stores and insulation in body fat; synthesis of steroid hormones; constituent of cell membranes, and of nerve fibres | Weight loss; deficiency of essential fatty acids can lead to neurological damage | Obesity, with increased risk e.g. of cardiovascular disease and some cancers | Normal development of the nervous system depends on the essential fatty acids, linoleic and alpha linolenic |

**Table 4.2. Micronutrients: vitamins**

| Vitamin | RNI (DoH 1991) | Sources | Action/functions | Deficiency | Excess | Special points |
|---------|----------------|---------|------------------|------------|--------|----------------|
| **Vitamin B group** | | | | | | |
| | | | Water soluble | | | |
| $B_1$ Thiamin(e) | 0.4 mg/1000 kcal | Fortified breakfast cereals, yeast extract, veget-ables, fruit, whole-grain cereals, milk, liver, eggs, pork | Coenzyme for carbohydrate metabolism | Encephalopathy can occur with alcohol excess and low food in-take. Beri-beri where polished rice is staple | Headache, insomnia, irritability, contact dermatitis | Requirement related to carbohydrate intake |
| $B_2$ Riboflavin | Female 1.1 mg/d Male 1.3 mg/d | Milk, milk prod-ucts, offal, yeast extract, fortified breakfast cereals | Coenzyme for the metabolism of carbohydrate, fat and protein | Fissures at corners of mouth; tongue inflammation; corneal vascularization | No toxic effects, since large quantities are not absorbed | Destroyed by sunlight |
| $B_3$ Niacin (nicotinic acid and nicotinamide) | 6.6 mg/1000 kcal as nicotinic acid equivalents | Meat, fish, yeast extract, pulses, wholegrains, fortified breakfast cereals | Energy metabol-ism, as part of co-enzymes NAD and NADP involved in oxidation and re-duction reactions | Pellagra: dermatitis, diarrhoea and dementia | Liver damage, skin irritation | Also synthesized from the amino acid tryptophan |
| $B_5$ Pantothenic acid | None set | Widespread in food, e.g. liver, eggs, yeast, vegetables, pulses, cereals | Protein, fat, carbohydrate and alcohol metabolism | Vomiting, insomnia | Not reported | |

*(Continued)*

**Table 4.2. Micronutrients: vitamins—Cont'd**

| Vitamin | RNI (DoH 1991) | Sources | Action/functions | Deficiency | Excess | Special points |
|---------|----------------|---------|------------------|------------|--------|----------------|
| $B_6$ Pyridoxine | Female 1.2 mg/d Male 1.4 mg/d | Meat, fish, eggs, some vegetables, wholegrains | Production of haemoglobin and of coenzymes involved in many metabolic processes | Rare. Metabolic and nervous system disorders | Peripheral nerve damage | Requirement is related to protein intake |
| Biotin | None set | Widely distributed in many foods, e.g. offal, egg yolk, legumes, etc. Can be synthesized by intestinal bacteria | Essential in fat metabolism | Rare; dermatitis, hair loss, nausea, fatigue and anorexia | None known | |
| $B_{12}$ Cobalamins | 15 μg/g of protein | Animal products, meat, eggs, fish, dairy products, yeast extract | Essential for red blood cell formation and nerve myelination. Needed for use of folate | Anaemia; irreversible spinal cord damage | Not reported | Absorption requires 'intrinsic factor' produced by the stomach. Only in foods of animal origin, so strict vegetarians and vegans require supplements |
| Folates (folic acid) | 200 μg/d | Green leaf vegetables, bread, fortified breakfast cereals, yeast extract, liver | Red blood cell production; DNA synthesis | Anaemia; growth retardation. May contribute to Alzheimer's. Fetal defects | Can mask the effects of $B_{12}$ deficiency | Supplements before and during pregnancy reduce the incidence of spinal cord defects |

| Vitamin | Amount | Function / Sources | Deficiency | Toxicity | Notes |
|---|---|---|---|---|---|
| Vitamin C ascorbic acid | 40 mg/d | Citrus fruits, kiwi fruit, blackcurrants, strawberries; green peppers; green leaf vegetables, potatoes, tomatoes. Content decreases with storage. Collagen synthesis, formation of bones, connective tissue, teeth. Iron absorption for red blood cell production. Acts as an antioxidant | Sore mouth and gums; capillary bleeding; scurvy; delayed wound healing, scar break down | Diarrhoea; oxalate stones in kidneys | Destroyed by cooking in the presence of air and by plant enzymes released when cutting and grating raw food |

### Fat soluble

| Vitamin | Amount | Function / Sources | Deficiency | Toxicity | Notes |
|---|---|---|---|---|---|
| Vitamin A retinol | Female 600 µg/d Male 700 µg/d | As retinol in liver, kidney, oily fish, egg yolk, full-fat dairy produce. As the provitamin carotenes in green, yellow, orange and red fruit and vegetables, e.g. broccoli, carrots, apricots, mangoes, sweet potatoes and tomatoes. Visual pigments in retina, aids night vision. Normal growth and development of tissues; essential for healthy skin and mucosae. Acts as an antioxidant | Poor growth; rough dry skin and mucosae; xerophthalmia and eventual blindness; increased risk of infection; poor night vision | In pregnancy, high doses can cause fetal malformations | Synthesized in the body from carotenes present in the diet |

(Continued)

**Table 4.2. Micronutrients: vitamins — Cont'd**

| Vitamin | RNI (DoH 1991) | Sources | Action/functions | Deficiency | Excess | Special points |
|---------|----------------|---------|------------------|------------|--------|----------------|
| Vitamin D cholecalciferol ergosterol | 10 μg/d if housebound | Oily fish, egg yolk, butter, fortified margarine; action of ultraviolet rays (sunlight) | Calcium and phosphorus homeostasis | Rickets (children); osteomalacia (adults) | Rare; weight loss and diarrhoea | Produced in the body by action of sunlight on a provitamin in the skin: deficiency develops in those who are not exposed to sun |
| Vitamin E tocopherols tocotrienes | None set | Wheat germ, vegetable oils, nuts, seeds, egg yolk, cereals, dark green vegetables | Antioxidant. Protects against cell membrane damage | Neurological abnormalities; anaemia: rare, from malnutrition or malabsorption | Muscle weakness, gastrointestinal disorders | Requirement is increased with increased intake of polyunsaturated fatty acids |
| Vitamin K phylloquinones menaquinones | None set | Green leafy vegetables, fruit and dairy products | Needed for the production of prothrombin and other coagulation factors | Impaired clotting; liver damage | Not so far observed from naturally occurring vitamin | Synthesized by intestinal bacteria so deficiency unusual |

Table 4.3. Micronutrients: minerals

| Name and chemical symbol | Reference nutrient intake (adults, per day) | Sources | Functions | Deficiency | Excess |
|---|---|---|---|---|---|
| Calcium Ca | 700 mg | Milk and milk products, green vegetables, soya beans, white bread, hard water | Crucial role in all cellular function, in neural transmission, muscle contraction, blood coagulation. As phosphate in bones and teeth | Dietary deficiency not uncommon. Rickets, osteomalacia from failure of Ca absorption in Vit D deficiency. Low blood [$Ca^{2+}$] causes tetany | Calcium deposits in soft tissue can occur, but probably not related to high intake |
| Chlorine Cl | 3.4 g (as chloride) | Salt-containing foods | Major anion in ECF. Role in maintaining electrical gradient across cell membranes | Unlikely with normal diet | As NaCl, risk factor for high blood pressure |
| Chromium Cr | 25 μg | Vegetables, cereals, meats, vegetable oils, whole grains | Co-factor for some enzymes involved in glucose and energy metabolism | Rare. Impaired glucose metabolism | Inhibition of enzymes. Occupational exposures can cause skin and kidney damage |

(Continued)

Table 4.3. Micronutrients: minerals—Cont'd

| Name and chemical symbol | Reference nutrient intake (adults, per day) | Sources | Functions | Deficiency | Excess |
|---|---|---|---|---|---|
| Copper Cu | 900 μg | Meat, drinking water | Co-factor for some enzymes; intermediate in electron transfer during oxidative phosphorylation | Low activity of antioxidant enzymes | Very high intake can cause liver damage |
| Iodine I | 140 μg | Seafood, iodized salt, milk and milk products, meat and eggs | Synthesis of thyroid hormones | Thyroid swelling (goitre) with hypothyroidism: low BMR, lethargy | Rarely any effect; may exacerbate some skin diseases |
| Iron Fe | Women 14.8 mg Men 8.7 mg | Liver, kidney, red meat, egg yolk, wholegrains, pulses, dark green vegetables, dried fruit, treacle, cocoa, molasses | Component of haemoglobin, myoglobin and many enzymes | Iron deficiency anaemia not uncommon. In childhood, poor growth; impaired intellectual development | Can be toxic if very excessive. (from blood transfusions rather than from diet); gastrointestinal upset; may promote vascular disease |

| | | | |
|---|---|---|---|
| Fluoride F | 3-4 mg | May be important in maintenance of bone structure | Increased risk of tooth decay | Unlikely from dietary sources |
| Magnesium Mg | Women 270 mg Men 300 mg | Cereals, milk, nuts, seeds, and green vegetables | Co-factor for enzymes essential in metabolism; role in calcium homeo-stasis; skeletal development; neuromuscular function | Uncommon; can occur with malabsorption or in chronic renal failure, when it accompanies hypocalcaemia | Unlikely from dietary sources |
| Phosphorus-P | 550 mg (as phosphate) | Milk, cheese, yogurt, meat, poultry, grains, fish | Adenosine phos-phate compounds vital in energy metabolism. With Ca in bones and teeth | Only in severe malnutrition; muscle weakness, bone pain, rickets, anorexia, anaemia | In treatment of osteoporosis or bone cancer with biphosphonates |
| Potassium K | 3.5 g | Fruit, vegetables, meat, wholegrains | Major intracellular cation; muscle contraction and nerve excitability. Linked to acid–base regulation | Poor dietary intake rare. Can occur with prolonged use of diuretics and purgatives. Muscular weakness; depression; confusion; cardiac arrhythmia | High ECF [$K^+$] (hyperkalaemia) causes cardiac arrest |

(Continued)

**Table 4.3. Micronutrients: minerals—Cont'd**

| Name and chemical symbol | Reference nutrient intake (adults, per day) | Sources | Functions | Deficiency | Excess |
|---|---|---|---|---|---|
| Selenium Se | Women 50 µg Men 70 µg | Seafood, meat, grains, wheat flour | Key component in the endogenous antioxidant, glutathione peroxidase | Health implications of low intake in UK currently under DoH review. May cause abnormality of heart muscle | Excessive supplements: hair loss, skin rash, neurological disorder |
| Sodium Na | 1.6 g | Mainly as salt: table salt, and in milk, meat, vegetables, sauces, pickles, processed foods, snacks, cheese | Major extracellular cation; linked to ECF volume, hence to blood volume and blood pressure. Component of bone mineral | Loss in sweat and diarrhoea; dilution in body fluids due to excess water intake. Weakness, cramp; faintness, confusion | Oedema, hypertension |
| Zinc Zn | Women 7.0 mg Men 9.5 mg | Red meat, dairy products, eggs, wholegrains, peas, beans, nuts, lentils | Co-factor for many enzymes. Synthesis of some proteins. Wound healing; immune system; physical and sexual development | Retarded skeletal growth; sexual immaturity. Anorexia, fatigue | Nausea, vomiting, or anaemia with chronic excess. Also decreases iron and copper bioavailability |

**Table 4.4. Ergogenic aids: supplements used by athletes**

| Substance | Description | Claimed ergogenic effect | Supporting evidence |
|---|---|---|---|
| | | **With clear scientific evidence** | |
| Caffeine | Stimulant in coffee and tea | Benefits performance by improving alertness, concentration, reaction time. Increases fat oxidation during endurance exercise. | Improves performance in most events, except very short high-intensity exercise; increases cognitive functioning during exercise. |
| Creatine | Carrier of high-energy phosphates in muscle | Increases the energy reserve, improves strength, reduces fatigue, and increases protein synthesis | Increases intramuscular Cr and PCr; improves performance in repeated sprint bouts (and reported to do so after even a single bout); improves recovery between bouts (but response varies between individuals). Anabolic properties unclear. |
| Sodium bicarbonate Sodium citrate | Buffers | Improves high-intensity exercise performance by limiting decrease in pH in ECF as a whole and indirectly in muscle ICF | Large doses can improve performance |

(Continued)

**Table 4.4. Ergogenic aids: supplements used by athletes—Cont'd**

| Substance | Description | Claimed ergogenic effect | Supporting evidence |
|---|---|---|---|
| | | **With mixed scientific evidence** | |
| Antioxidant nutrients | Vitamins, especially C and E | Provides protection against muscle damage by reducing oxidative stress | Benefits established at cellular level; no detectable aid to performance |
| Arginine | Amino acid in normal diet | Stimulates release of growth hormone, promoting gain in muscle mass and strength | Some evidence of GH promotion when combined with other amino acids (ornithine, lysine, BCAA); no conclusive evidence of effect when taken alone |
| Branched-chain amino acids (BCAA) | Leucine, isoleucine and valine | Retards the development of central fatigue and so improves performance. Improves efficiency of training | No good evidence of improved endurance performance. Evidence of accelerated recovery from muscle fatigue when given with other amino acids during eccentric exercise training |
| Glutamine | Amide of amino acid glutamate | Maintains a healthy immune system during training and improves muscle glycogen resynthesis | Does not affect immune function; possibly affects muscle glycogen re-synthesis |
| Glycerol | Component of triacylglycerol molecule | Induces hyperhydration, decreases heat stress, and improves performance | Does have the first two actions, but effects on performance are unclear |

## Lacking scientific support

| | | |
|---|---|---|
| Androstenedione | Synthetic product | Increases testosterone and thus muscle mass and strength, and improves recovery | Does not increase testosterone secretion; has no effect on strength |
| Hydroxy-methyl butyrate (HMB) | Metabolite of the amino acid leucine | Enhances gain in body mass and strength associated with resistance training, and improves recovery | Possible small effects only on lean body mass and strength |
| Boron | Micronutrient present in vegetables and non-citrus fruits | Increases testosterone levels, to improve bone density, muscle mass, and strength | Improves bone mineral density in postmenopausal women; no effect on bone density, muscle mass or strength in men |
| Carnitine | Substance important for fatty acid transport into mitochondria | Improves fat oxidation, helps weight loss | No supporting evidence |
| Choline | Precursor of acetylcholine | Improves performance, decreases fatigue and enhances fat metabolism | No supporting evidence |
| Chromium (chromium picolinate) | Micronutrient that potentiates insulin action | Promotes fat oxidation and muscle building | No supporting evidence |

*(Continued)*

**Table 4.4. Ergogenic aids: supplements used by athletes—Cont'd**

| Substance | Description | Claimed ergogenic effect | Supporting evidence |
|---|---|---|---|
| Coenzyme Q10 | Part of the electron transport chain in the mitochondria | Improves aerobic capacity and cardiovascular dynamics | No supporting evidence |
| Ginseng | Root of the Araliaceous plant | Improves strength, performance, stamina, and cognitive functioning; reduces fatigue | No supporting evidence |
| Inosine | Nucleoside found naturally in brewer's yeast and organ meats | Increases ATP stores, improve strength, training quality, and performance | No supporting evidence |
| Medium-chain triacylglycerols (MCT) | Triglycerides containing fatty acids with a carbon chain length of 6-10 | Improves energy supply, reduces rate of muscle glycogen breakdown, and improves performance | No supporting evidence |
| Pyruvate | End-product of aerobic glycolysis | Improves endurance capacity and recovery; increases glycogen storage | Limited supporting evidence |
| Polylactate | Polymer of lactate | Provides energy | No effects on performance |
| Wheat germ oil | Wheat embryo extract | Improves endurance | No supporting evidence |

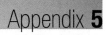

# Hormones

**Table 5.1. Hormones**

| Site of production | Name of hormone | Main targets | Involved in regulating: | Secretion controlled by: |
|---|---|---|---|---|
| Hypothalamus | Releasing and inhibiting hormones | Anterior pituitary (via local blood vessels) | Secretion of anterior pituitary hormones | Other brain regions; feedback re regulated hormones and their actions |
| | *Neurohormones released from posterior pituitary:* | | | |
| | Oxytocin | Uterus, breasts | Labour and lactation | Afferent information from target organs |
| | Antidiuretic hormone (ADH, vasopressin) | Kidneys | Water loss: ECF volume and osmolality | Hypothalamic osmoreceptors |
| Anterior pituitary | (Human) growth hormone (H)GH | Most cells | Growth and metabolism | Hypothalamic releasing and inhibiting hormones |
| | Prolactin | Breasts | Milk production | via local blood vessels |
| | *Trophic hormones:* Thyroid-stimulating (TSH) | Thyroid gland | Thyroid secretions | |
| | Gonadotrophins | Ovary or testis | Germ cell maturation and hormone secretions | |
| | Adrenocorticotrophic (ACTH) | Adrenal cortex | Cortisol secretion | |

| | | | |
|---|---|---|---|
| Pineal body | Melatonin | Widespread, including brain, thymus, etc. | Sleep/wake cycle Antioxidant Immune system | Hypothalamus; varying light input from retina |
| Thyroid | Thyroxine Triiodothyronine | Most cells | Cellular oxidative metabolism | TSH from anterior pituitary. Negative feedback from blood hormone concentration |
| | Calcitonin | Bone, kidneys, gut | Decreases ECF [Ca$^{2+}$] | ECF [Ca$^{2+}$] |
| Parathyroids | Parathormone | Bone, kidneys, gut | Calcium and phosphorus absorption, secretion and turnover in bone. Increases ECF [Ca$^{2+}$] | ECF [Ca$^{2+}$] |
| Adrenal: Cortex | Cortisol | Most cells | Metabolism Response to stress | ACTH from anterior pituitary |
| | Aldosterone | Kidneys | Na and K balance | ECF [Na$^+$] [K$^+$] Renin-angiotensin |
| | Androgens | Gonads & other tissues | Sex characteristics and reproductive function | ACTH |
| Medulla | Adrenaline Noradrenaline | Heart, smooth muscle, glands | Cardiovascular and metabolic adjustments to activity and stress | Sympathetic nervous system |
| Atrial wall | Atrial natriuretic hormone | Kidneys | Blood volume; increases sodium (therefore also water) loss in urine | Stretch of atrial wall by venous pressure |

*(Continued)*

461

## Table 5.1. Hormones—Cont'd

| Site of production | Name of hormone | Main targets | Involved in regulating: | Secretion controlled by: |
|---|---|---|---|---|
| **Gonads:** Testis | Androgens (mainly testosterone) | Genitalia and other tissues | Reproductive function and sex characteristics | Anterior pituitary gonadotrophins |
| Ovary | Oestrogens Progesterone | Uterus, breasts and other tissues | Menstrual cycle, pregnancy, lactation | |
| **Pancreas** | Insulin, glucagon | Most cells | Blood levels, storage and cellular uptake of nutrients, notably glucose, but also proteins and fats | Blood levels of nutrients; autonomic nervous system; other gastrointesinal hormones |
| | Somatostatin | Other secretory cells in the pancreas | | |
| **Alimentary tract** Stomach | Gastrin | Gastric acid-secreting cells | Gastrointestinal functions: motility, digestive juices and other secretions | Local chemical and mechanical factors in the alimentary tract |
| Small intestine | Secretin Cholecystokinin-pancreozymin (CCK-PZ) Somatostatin, motilin Other peptide hormones including vasoactive intestinal peptide (VIP) | Widespread on GI tract | Several GI functions including bile flow, pancreatic enzyme and exocrine secretions | Ingestion of food, distension of GI tract |

# Drugs: drugs and the law, use and abuse of drugs in sport and drugs in common use

## Drugs and the law

The main acts governing the use of medicines in the UK in relation to sport and exercise are the Medicines Act 1968, the Misuse of Drugs Act 1971 and the Medicinal Products: Prescription by Nurses Act 1992.

### The Medicines Act 1968

This act identifies doctors, dentists and veterinary surgeons as the only appropriate practitioners to prescribe medicines and deals with drugs in three groups.

- Prescription Only Medicines (POM): includes most of the potent drugs in common use, supplied or administered to a patient on the instructions of the appropriate practitioner.
- Pharmacy Only Medicines (P): licensed drugs supplied under the control and supervision of a registered pharmacist. Examples include ibuprofen, antihistamines and glyceryl trinitrate.
- General Sales List Medicines (GSL): commonly used drugs such as aspirin and paracetamol, available through many retail outlets such as supermarkets.

The Medicines Act 1968 also makes provision for various other substances such as potent herbal medicines (not available for unrestricted sale to the public) used in complementary therapies. However, many homeopathic preparations, food supplements, herbal and traditional medicines from non-European countries are not presently covered by the licensing process.

## The Misuse of Drugs Act 1971

This act imposes controls on those drugs liable to produce dependence or cause harm if misused. It prohibits certain activities in relation to controlled drugs (CD). Only doctors and dentists can prescribe CDs, which are divided into three classes (A, B and C) that reflect the level of harm caused by each drug if misused.

Further to the 1971 act, the Misuse of Drugs Regulations 1985 identify those who may supply and possess controlled drugs while acting in their professional capacity and ordain the conditions under which these activities may be carried out; they also further subdivide drugs into five schedules, each detailing the requirements for import, export, production, supply, possession, prescribing and record keeping.

## Further reading and information sources

British Medical Association and the Royal Pharmaceutical Society of Great Britain, London.
British National Formulary (revised twice yearly – March and September). www.bnf.org.uk

# Use and abuse of drugs in sport

Drug use in sport was first recorded around 300 BC. Prior to this sport was considered to be part of a balanced lifestyle but as mass spectator sport grew, it became 'professionalized', with greater rewards for success. A variety of substances were used, many of which contained alcohol. It has been suggested that the breakdown of the ancient Olympic Games was in part due to drug use and abuse to gain 'unfair' advantage. In the modern era, drug use in sport first arose as the Industrial Revolution led to a structure in sport, which became more commercial and professional.

The early 1900s saw some high-profile drug-related deaths in sport, including that of the runner Hicks during the 1904 London Olympic marathon as a result of a combination of brandy and strychnine. The 1930s brought the use of stimulant drugs (short-acting drugs such as amphetamines) to improve performance on the day, and the 1950s saw the introduction of anabolic steroids, used largely during training to allow the athlete to train 'harder, faster and for longer' (both now banned). The 1960s saw a more liberal approach to drug use in general in society, coinciding with a major expansion of drug development within the pharmaceutical industry and thus the opportunity to enhance performance beyond that achieved by hard work and training alone. Modern legislation concerning drug use in sport is based on the harmful effects on the athlete, potential performance-enhancing effects and legality.

Formal restriction and control of the use of drugs in sport were first introduced by the International Olympic Committee (IOC) in the 1960s and resulted in the production of their list of doping classes and methods. This covered not only certain drugs which were prohibited but also areas such as blood doping and pharmacological, chemical and physical manipulation. In recent years, increasing public concern about the use of drugs has led to the formation of the World Anti-Doping Agency (WADA). This body reflects a joint effort by governments, international federations and governing bodies to work together in the fight against drugs. WADA has produced its anti-doping code, which upholds sport's 'strict liability' policy whereby athletes are responsible for any banned substance found in their body, regardless of how it got there. The burden of proof is now placed on athletes to contest positive drug findings. A single list of banned substances, which is intermittently updated, has been created, with exemptions granted for therapeutic reasons only.

For further information see www.wada-ama.org.

# Drugs used (or *banned*) in sport and of general relevance to sportsmen and women

*See table facing.*

## Drugs used (or *banned*) in sport and of general relevance to sportsmen and women

| Drug groups and subgroups | Examples | Indications |
|---|---|---|
| **Anabolic steroids** | Nandrolone, stanozolol | *Banned in sport* |
| **Analgesics** | | |
| Non-opioids (see also NSAIDs) | Aspirin, paracetamol | Mild to moderate pain, e.g. simple headache; pyrexia |
| Opioids | Diamorphine, dihydrocodeine, fentanyl, morphine, etc. | *Banned in sport* |
| **Angiotensin-converting enzyme (ACE) inhibitor** | Captopril, ramipril, etc. | Heart failure and other clinical cardiovascular problems |
| **Antacids** | Aluminium hydroxide, magnesium trisilicate | Dyspepsia |
| **Antibiotics** (antibacterials) include: | | Infections, by many different bacteria, at various sites |
| Penicillins | e.g Ampicillin | |
| Sulphonamides | Co-trimoxazole | |
| Tetracyclines | Doxycycline | |
| **Antidiarrhoeals** | Codeine phosphate, loperamide (antimotility drugs) | Adjuncts to rehydration in acute diarrhoea |
| **Antiemetics** | | Nausea and vomiting in: |
| Dopamine ($D_2$)-receptor antagonists | Metoclopramide | gastrointestinal disorders |
| $H_1$-receptor antagonists | Cinnarizine | Motion sickness |
| Muscarinic antagonists | Hyoscine | Motion sickness |

*(Continued)*

## Drugs used (or *banned*) in sport and of general relevance to sportsmen and women—Cont'd

| Drug groups and subgroups | Examples | Indications |
|---|---|---|
| **Antiepileptic** (anticonvulsant) | Phenytoin | Epilepsy control |
| **Antihistamine** | Chlorphenamine (H₁-receptor antagonist) | Hay fever, emergency treatment of anaphylactic reactions |
| **Anti-inflammatory drugs** *See also* analgesics, NSAIDs | | *Banned in sport* |
| Corticosteroids | | *Banned in sport* |
| **Antipyretics** *See also* NSAIDs | Aspirin | Pyrexia |
| **Antithyroid** | Carbimazole | Hyperthyroidism |
| **Antivirals** | e.g. Aciclovir | Herpes simplex |
| **Anxiolytics** Benzodiazepines | Diazepam | Short term for anxiety and insomnia, acute alcohol withdrawal, etc. |
| **Beta-adrenceptor antagonists (beta blockers)** | Atenolol Propranolol | *Banned in sport* |
| **Bronchodilators** Beta₂-receptor agonist | Salbutamol | Asthma |
| Corticosteroids | Prednisolone | Asthma, rheumatic conditions *Banned in sport* |
| **Decongestant** | Pseudoephedrine (oral), ephedrine hydrochloride (nasal drops), etc. | Nasal congestion |
| **Diuretics** | e.g. Furosemide, bendroflumethiazide | *Banned in sport* |
| **5HT₁-agonists** | Sumatriptan | Migraine |

| | | |
|---|---|---|
| **Hypoglycaemics** (oral) | | Diabetes |
| Alpha ($\alpha$)-glucosidases inhibitor | Acarbose | |
| Biguanides | Metformin | |
| Sulphonylureas | Glipizide | |
| **Insulin** | Short-, intermediate- or long-acting preparations | Diabetes |
| **Laxatives (aperients)** | | Constipation |
| Bulk-forming laxatives | Ispaghula, methylcellulose | |
| Faecal softeners | Arachis oil (enema) | |
| Osmotic laxative | Lactulose | |
| Stimulant | Senna | |
| **Nitrates** | Glyceryl trinitrate (sublingual, transdermal) | Angina |
| **NSAIDs** | | Pain relief, antipyretic, reduction of inflammation and stiffness in arthritis, etc. |
| Fenamates | Mefenamic acid | |
| Oxicams | Piroxicam | |
| Propionic acids | Ibuprofen | |
| Pyrazolones | Azapropazone | |
| Salicylates and paracetamol | Aspirin, paracetamol | |

# Abbreviations and acronyms

| | |
|---|---|
| ABC | airway, breathing and circulation |
| ACE | angiotensin converting enzyme |
| ACh | acetylcholine |
| ACTH | adrenocorticotrophic hormone |
| ACSM | American College of Sports Medicine |
| ACPSM | Association of Chartered Physiotherapists in Sports Medicine |
| ADH | antidiuretic hormone |
| ADP | adenosine diphosphate |
| AIDS | acquired immune deficiency syndrome |
| Ala | alanine |
| ALA | alpha linolenic acid |
| AMI | acute myocardial infarction |
| AMP | adenosine monophosphate |
| ANOVA | analysis of variance |
| ANS | autonomic nervous system |
| AP | action potential |
| AT | anaerobic threshold |
| ATP | adenosine triphosphate |
| ATPS | ambient temperature and pressure saturated |
| AV | atrioventricular |
| A-V | arteriovenous |
| BAS | behavioural activation system |
| BASES | British Association for Sport and Exercise Science |

| | |
|---|---|
| BCAA | branched-chain amino acid |
| BIS | behavioural inhibition system |
| BMA | British Medical Association |
| BMD | bone mineral density |
| BMI | body mass index |
| BMR | basal metabolic rate |
| cal | calorie |
| cAMP | cyclic adenosine monophosphate |
| CBT | cognitive behaviour therapy |
| CCK | cholecystokinase |
| CHO | carbohydrate |
| CFS | chronic fatigue syndrome |
| CK | creatine kinase |
| CNS | central nervous system |
| CO | cardiac output |
| CoG | centre of gravity |
| CoM | centre of mass |
| CPAP | continuous positive airway pressure |
| CPR | cardiopulmonary resuscitation |
| CPK | creatine phosphokinase |
| Cr | creatine |
| CrP | creatine phosphate |
| CSF | cerebrospinal fluid |
| CT | computed tomography |
| CVP | central venous pressure |
| CVS | cardiovascular system |
| DBP | diastolic blood pressure |
| DEXA | dual emission X-ray absorptiometry |
| DHA | docosahexaenoic acid |

| | |
|---|---|
| DNA | deoxyribonucleic acid |
| 2,3-DPG | 2,3-diphosphoglycerate |
| DOMS | delayed-onset muscle soreness |
| DRV | dietary reference values |
| DVT | deep vein thrombosis |
| EAMC | exercise-associated muscle cramp |
| EAR | estimated average requirement |
| ECG | electrocardiogram |
| ECF | extracellular fluid |
| EEG | electroencephalogram |
| EFA | essential fatty acids |
| EMG | electromyogram |
| ENT | ear, nose and throat |
| EPA | eicosapentaenoic acid |
| EPOC | elevated postexercise oxygen consumption |
| ESR | erythrocyte sedimentation rate |
| ETT | exercise tolerance test |
| ERV | expiratory reserve volume |
| f | frequency of breathing |
| FAD | flavine adenine dinucleotide |
| FEV | forced expiratory volume |
| FFA | free fatty aids |
| FFM | fat-free body mass |
| FRC | functional residual capacity |
| FSH | follicle-stimulating hormone |
| FVC | forced vital capacity |
| g | gram |
| GABA | gamma aminobutyric acid |

| | |
|---|---|
| GAS | general adaptation syndrome |
| GCS | Glasgow Coma Scale |
| GDA | guideline daily amount |
| GFR | glomerular filtration rate |
| GH | growth hormone |
| GI | gastrointestinal/glycaemic index |
| $G_6PD$ | glucose-6-phosphate dehydrogenase |
| HDL | high-density lipoprotein |
| HGH | human growth hormone |
| HIV | human immunodefiiency virus |
| HK | hexokinase |
| HMB | beta-hydroxy-beta-methylbutyrate |
| HMM | heavy meromyosin |
| HOCM | hypertrophic obstructive cardiomyopathy |
| HR | heart rate |
| HRR | heart rate reserve |
| HRT | hormone replacement therapy |
| 5-HT | 5-hydroxytryptamine |
| ICF | intracellular fluid |
| ICP | intracranial pressure |
| IOC | International Olympic Committee |
| IRV | inspiratory reserve volume |
| IV | intravenous |
| IVC | inferior vena cava |
| IMTG | intramuscular triacylglycerol |
| IZOF | individual zone of optimal functioning |
| J | joule |
| jnd | just noticeable difference |

| | |
|---|---|
| kcal | kilocalorie |
| kg | kilogram |
| kJ | kilojoule |
| KP | knowledge of performance |
| KR | knowledge of results |
| L (l) | litre |
| LBM | lean body mass |
| LDH | lactic dehydrogenase |
| LDL | low-density lipoproteins |
| LH | luteinizing hormone |
| LRNI | lower reference nutrient intake |
| LT | lactate threshold |
| m | metre |
| MAOI | monoamine oxidase inhibitor |
| MBC | maximum breathing capacity |
| MCT | medium chain triglycerides |
| ME | myalgic encephalitis |
| MET | metabolic equivalent |
| mg | milligram |
| MHC | myosin heavy chain |
| mL (ml) | millilitre |
| MLC | myosin light chain |
| MLSS | maximum lactate steady state |
| mm | millimetre |
| mmHg | millimetres of mercury |
| mmol | millimole |
| mol | mole |
| MRI | magnetic resonance imaging |
| mRNA | messenger ribonucleic acid |

| MVC | maximal velocity of contraction |
| MVV | maximum voluntary ventilation |
| MSH | melanocyte stimulating hormone |
| N | newton |
| NAD | nicotinamide adenine dinucleotide |
| NADP | nicotinamide adenine dinucleotide phosphate |
| NEFA | non-esterified fatty acids |
| nm | nanometre |
| NSAID | non-steroidal anti-inflammatory drug |
| NSP | non-starch polysaccharides |
| OA | osteoarthritis |
| OBLA | onset of blood lactate accumulation |
| Pa | pascal |
| $P_i$ | inorganic phosphate |
| PAL | physical activity level |
| $P\mathrm{CO_2}$ | partial pressure of carbon dioxide |
| PCr | phosphocreatine |
| PCV | packed cell volume |
| PDH | pyruvate dehydrogenase |
| PEFR | peak expiratory flow rate |
| PFK | phosphofructokinase |
| PMS | premenstrual syndrome |
| PNF | proprioceptive neuromuscular facilitation |
| PNS | peripheral nervous system |
| PRL | prolactin |
| $P\mathrm{O_2}$ | partial pressure of oxygen |
| PTH | parathyroid |

| PUFA | polyunsaturated fatty acids |
| RBC | red blood cell |
| RDA | recommended daily allowance |
| RER | respiratory exchange ratio |
| Rh | Rhesus |
| RICE | rest, ice, compression, elevation |
| RMR | resting metabolic rate |
| RNA | ribonucleic acid |
| RNI | reference nutrient intake |
| ROM | range of movement |
| ROS | reactive oxygen species |
| rRNA | ribosomal ribonucleic acid |
| RQ | respiratory quotient |
| RSI | repetitive strain injury |
| RV | residual volume |
| SA | sinoatrial |
| SAD | seasonal affective disorder |
| $S_aO_2$ | arterial oxygen saturation |
| SBP | systolic blood pressure |
| SDH | succinate dehydrogenase |
| SI | Système International; sacroiliac |
| SR | sarcoplasmic reticulum |
| SSRI | selective serotonin reuptake inhibitor |
| STD | sexually transmitted disease |
| STPD | standard temperature and pressure dry |
| SV | stroke volume |
| $T_3$ | triiodothyronine |
| $T_4$ | thyroxine |

| | |
|---|---|
| TCA | tricyclic antidepressants |
| TEA | thermic effect of activity |
| TEF | thermic effect of food |
| TENS | transcutaneous electrical nerve stimulation |
| TG | triacylglycerol (triglyceride) |
| TLC | total lung capacity |
| tRNA | transfer ribonucleic acid |
| TT | tetanus toxoid |
| TUE | therapeutic use exemption |
| TV | ($V_T$) tidal volume |
| URT | upper respiratory tract |
| USS | ultrasound scan |
| v | volt |
| V | volume (of gas) |
| $\dot{V}$ | volume (of gas) per unit time |
| VC | vital capacity |
| VLDL | very low-density lipoprotein |
| VT | ventilatory threshold |
| $V_T$ (TV) | tidal volume |
| W | watt |
| WADA | World Anti-Doping Agency |
| WBC | white blood cell |
| WHO | World Health Organization |
| WHR | waist–hip ratio |
| WPW | Wolff–Parkinson–White syndrome |
| XB | cross-bridge |
| ZOF | zone of optimal functioning |

# Useful addresses and websites

**American College of Sports Medicine**

PO Box 1440, Indianapolis, IN 46206–1440, USA

www.acsm.org

Official journal: *Medicine and Science in Sports and Exercise*:
www.acsm-msse.org

**Biomechanics classes on the web:**

http://darkwing.uoregon.edu/~karduna/biomechanics/

**British Association of Sport & Exercise Medicine (BASEM)**

BASEM Central Office,
15 Hawthorne Avenue, Norton, Doncaster DN6 9HR

Tel/fax: 01302 709342

Email: basemcentral@basem.co.uk

www.basem.co.uk

**British Association of Sport and Exercise Sciences (BASES)**

(Executive officer: Dr Claire Palmer)

Leeds Metropolitan University, Carnegie Faculty of Sport and Education, Headingly Campus,
Beckett Park, Leeds LS6 3QS

Tel: 0113 283 6162

Email: cpalmer@bases.org.uk

www.bases.org.uk

**British Psychological Society**

St Andrews House, 48 Princess Road East,
Leicester LE1 7DR

Tel: 0116 252 9555

www.bps.org.uk

Division of Sport and Exercise Psychology:
www.bps.org.uk/spex/

**European College of Sport Science (ECSS)**

(Managing Director: Thomas Delaveaux)

German Sport University Cologne, Carl-Diem Weg 6, 50933 Köln, Germany

Tel: + 49(0)221 4982 7640

Email: info@ECSS.de

www.ecss.de

**International Olympic Committee:**
www.olympic.org

**International Society of Biomechanics:**
www.isbweb.org

**International Society of Biomechanics in Sports:**
www.isbs.org

**Nutrition Society**

10 Cambridge Court, 210 Shepherds Bush Road, London W6 7NJ

www.nutritionsociety.org

**Sports medicine – how to find out:**
www.sprig.org.uk/htfo/htfosportsmed.html

**UK Sport**

40 Bernard Street, London WC1N 1ST

www.uksport.gov.uk

Drug information line: 0800 528 0004

Email: drug-free@uksport.gov.uk

**World Anti-Doping Agency (WADA)**

Email: info@wada-ama.org

www.wada-ama.org

# References and further reading

## Books

### Physiology and biochemistry of sport and exercise

American College of Sports Medicine 2005 ACSM's guidelines for exercise testing and prescription, 7th edn. Williams and Wilkins, Baltimore, MD

Armstrong N 2006 Paediatric exercise physiology. Elsevier, Edinburgh

Astrand PO, Rodahl K, Dahl HA, Stromme SB 2003 Textbook of work physiology: physiological bases of exercise, 4th edn. Human Kinetics, Champaign, IL

Davis B, Roscoe J, Roscoe D, Bull R 2005 Physical education and the study of sport, 5th edn. Mosby, St Louis, MO

Gleeson M, Maughan RJ 2004 The biochemical basis of sports performance. Oxford University Press, Oxford

Houston ME 2006 Biochemistry primer for exercise science, 3rd edn. Human Kinetics, Champaign, IL

Maughan RJ, Gleeson M, Greenhaff PL 1997 Biochemistry of exercise and training. Oxford University Press, Oxford

McArdle WD, Katch FI, Katch VL 2005 Essentials of exercise physiology, 3rd edn. Lea and Febiger, Philadelphia

Powers SK, Howley ET 2003 Exercise physiology: theory and application to fitness and performance, 5th edn. McGraw-Hill, Boston

Whyte G (ed) 2006 The physiology of training.
Elsevier, Edinburgh

Wilmore JH, Costill DL 2004 Physiology of sport and
exercise, 3rd edn. Human Kinetics, Champaign, IL

Winter EM, Jones AM, Davison RCR, Bromley PD, Mercer
TH (eds) 2007 Sport and exercise physiology testing
guidelines: the British Association of Sport and
Exercise Sciences guide, vol 1 sport testing, vol 2
exercise and clinical testing. Routledge, London

Wirhed R 2006 Athletic ability and the anatomy of
motion, 3rd edn. Mosby, St Louis, MO

Woolf-May K 2006 Exercise prescription: physiological
foundations. Churchill Livingstone, Edinburgh

## Skeletal muscle

Delavier F 2006 Strength training anatomy, 2nd edn.
Human Kinetics, Champaign, IL

Jones D, Round J, de Haan A 2004 Skeletal muscle from
molecules to movement.
Churchill Livingstone, Edinburgh

MacIntosh BR, Gardiner P, McComas AJ 2006 Skeletal
muscle form and function, 2nd edn. Human Kinetics,
Champaign, IL

Spurway NC, Wackerhage H 2006 Genetics and
molecular biology of muscle adaptation.
Elsevier, Edinburgh

## Biomechanics

Bartlett RM 1997 Introduction to sports biomechanics.
E&FN Spon, London

Bartlett RM 1999 Sports biomechanics: reducing injury and improving performance. E&FN Spon, London

Hamill J, Knutzen KM 2003 Biomechanical basis of human movement.
Lippincott, Williams and Wilkins, Philadelphia

Hay JG 1993 Biomechanics of sports techniques.
Prentice-Hall, Englewood Cliffs, NJ

McGinnis PM 1999 Biomechanics of sport and exercise.
Human Kinetics, Champaign, IL

## Sports medicine

Brukner P, Khan K (eds) 2006 Clinical sports medicine, 3rd edn. McGraw-Hill, New York

Gleeson M (ed) 2006 Immune function in sport and exercise. Elsevier, Edinburgh

MacAuley D (ed) 2006 Oxford handbook of sport and exercise medicine. Oxford University Press, Oxford

Maffulli N, Chan KM, Macdonald R, Malina RM, Parker AW 2001 Sports medicine for specific ages and abilities. Churchill Livingstone, Edinburgh

Maughan RJ (ed) 1999 Basic and applied sciences for sports medicine. Butterworth-Heinemann, Oxford

McClatchie G, Harries M, Williams C, King J (eds) 2000 ABC of sports medicine, 2nd edn.
BMJ Books, London

Scuderi GR, McCann PD, Bruno PJ (eds) 1997 Sports medicine: principles of primary care. Mosby, St Louis

## Nutrition in sport and exercise

Burke L, Deakin V 2006 Clinical sports nutrition, 3rd edn. McGraw-Hill, New York

Jeukendrup A, Gleeson M 2004 Sport nutrition. Human Kinetics, Champaign, IL

MacLaren D (ed) 2007 Nutrition and sport. Elsevier, Edinburgh

Maughan RJ (ed) 2000 Nutrition in sport: the encyclopaedia of sports medicine VII. IOC Medical Commission. Blackwell Science, Oxford

McArdle WD, Katch FI, Katch VL 2005 Sports and exercise nutrition, 2nd edn. Williams & Wilkins, Baltimore, MD

Williams C, Devlin JT 1992 Foods, nutrition and sports performance. E & FN Spon, London

## Philosophy

McNamee M (ed) 2005 Philosophy and the sciences of exercise, health and sport: critical perspectives on research methods. Routledge, London

## Physiotherapy

Kolt GS, Snyder-Mackler (eds) 2003 Physical therapies in sport and exercise. Churchill Livingstone, Edinburgh

Zuluaga M, Briggs C, Carlisle J et al (eds) 1995 Sports Physiotherapy: applied science and practice. Churchill Livingstone, Edinburgh

## Sport and exercise psychology

Acevedo EO, Ekkekakis P 2006 Psychobiology of physical activity. Human Kinetics, Champaign, IL

Hagger M, Chatzisarantis N 2005 The social psychology of exercise and sport. Open University Press, Buckingham

Roberts GC 2001 Advances in motivation in sport and exercise, 4th edn. Human Kinetics, Champaign, IL

Schmidt RA, Lee TD 2006 Motor control and learning: a behavioural emphasis. Human Kinetics, Champaign, IL

Weinberg RS, Gould D 2007 Foundations of sport and exercise psychology, 4th edn. Human Kinetics, Champaign, IL

## Journals

British Journal of Sports Medicine: www.bjsm.bmj.com

Clinical Journal of Sport Medicine: www.cjsportmed.com

Exercise and Sport Sciences Reviews: www.acsm.org

International Journal of Behavioral Nutrition and Physical Activity: www.ijbnpa.org

International Journal of Sport Nutrition and Exercise Metabolism: www.humankinetics.com/IJSNEM

International Journal of Sport Psychology: www.ijsp-online.com

International Journal of Sports Medicine: www.thieme-connect.com/ejournals/toc/sportsmed

Journal of Applied Biomechanics: www.humankinetics.com/JAB

Journal of Biomechanics: www.elsevier.com/locate/jbiomech

Sports Biomechanics: www.twu.edu/biom/isbs/sb.htm

Journal of Sports Sciences: www.tandf.co.uk/journals/rjsp

Journal of Motor Behavior: www.heldref.org/jmb.php

Journal of Physical Activity and Health: www.humankinetics.com/JPAH

Journal of Sport and Exercise Psychology:
    www.humankinetics.com/JSEP

Journal of Sport Behavior (no website)

Journal of Strength and Conditioning Research:
    http://nsca.allenpress.com/nscaonline/
    ?request=index.html

Medicine and Science in Sports and Exercise:
    www.acsm-msse.org

Motor Control: www.humankinetics.com/MC

Physician and Sports Medicine:
    www.blackwellpublishing.com/medicine/sports.asp

Psychology of Sport and Exercise:
    www.elsevier.com/locate/psychsport

Research Quarterly for Exercise and Sport:
    www.highbeam.com/browse/Health-Fitness-
    Research + Quarterly + for + Exercise + and + Sport

Sportscience Journal: www.sportsci.org

The Sport Psychologist: www.humankinetics.com/TSP